CLINICAL BIOCHEMISTRY

for Medical Students

CLINICAL BIOCHEMISTRY
for Medical Students

M.F. Laker MD, DipBiochem, FRCPath
Reader in Clinical Biochemistry and Metabolic Medicine
Department of Clinical Biochemistry and Metabolic Medicine
The Medical School, University of Newcastle upon Tyne

Consultant in Clinical Biochemistry
Royal Victoria Infirmary and Associated Hospitals NHS Trust
Newcastle upon Tyne

W.B. Saunders Company Limited

London Philadelphia Toronto
Sydney Tokyo

W.B. Saunders Company Ltd   24–28 Oval Road
London NW1 7DX, UK

The Curtis Center
Independence Square West
Philadelphia, PA 19106-3399, USA

Harcourt Brace & Company
55 Horner Avenue
Toronto, Ontario M8Z 4X6, Canada

Harcourt Brace & Company, Australia
30–52 Smidmore Street
Marrickville, NSW 2204, Australia

Harcourt Brace & Company, Japan
Ichibancho Central Building
22-1 Ichibancho
Chiyoda-ku, Tokyo 102, Japan

British Library Cataloguing in Publication Data is available

ISBN 0-7020-1690-X

This book is printed on acid-free paper

Typeset by P&R Typesetters Ltd, Salisbury, Wilts
Printed and bound in Great Britain by Butler and Tanner, Frome, Somerset

CONTENTS

PREFACE

The main functions of clinical biochemistry departments are to provide laboratory services for the investigation and management of biochemical disorders, to interpret these investigations and, increasingly, to provide clinical services for patients with metabolic diseases. Although the timing of clinical biochemistry courses varies somewhat between medical schools, these generally follow the basic medical sciences and develop themes first introduced in subjects such as biochemistry and cell biology, integrating these with clinical teaching.

Each chapter in the present book includes a brief review to reinforce the relevant basic science before considering the pathophysiology of important biochemical disorders. Laboratory tests are described in the context of clinical features together with other investigations and, where relevant, the principles of management are outlined. Learning is reinforced in two ways. First, key points are highlighted throughout the text, and second, case histories are included at the end of each chapter as an aid to revision. Analytical methods have not been considered, except where these are relevant to the use or interpretation of particular investigations.

This book is intended primarily for undergraduate medical students and the order of chapters reflects this, building on earlier teaching. The clinical relevance of subjects such as intermediary metabolism is often not apparent and experience suggests' that this is clarified by early consideration of disorders of carbohydrate and lipid metabolism. Leaving a chapter which reviews factors that affect the interpretation of biochemical tests in clinical practice until the end of the book is not intended to underrate its importance. The alternative was to place it first, as some other authors have done, but it was felt that introducing the subject at that point would not relate to other teaching. Thus, the relevance of this very important topic would not be obvious but should be more so when the basis of biochemical investigation was understood.

Despite the focus on medical students it is hoped that the clinical orientation of the book will prove helpful to those preparing for postgraduate examinations in clinical biochemistry, medicine and other specialties. It should also prove useful for scientists preparing for professional examinations or degrees in clinical biochemistry.

Finally, it is a pleasure to acknowledge the very helpful advice and support received from the publishers, particularly Steven Handley, Tracy Breakell and Rachael Miller.

Mike Laker

CARBOHYDRATE METABOLISM

INTRODUCTION

Carbohydrates are distributed widely in the body, and have both metabolic and structural functions. Man can synthesize some carbohydrate from substrates such as glycerol and amino acids but most is derived from plant sources. Glucose is the principal form in which dietary carbohydrate is absorbed and is the major fuel for cellular metabolism. It is also the precursor of other sugars, such as ribose which is found in nucleic acids, and of the carbohydrate moieties of glycoproteins and glycosaminoglycans.

Disorders of carbohydrate metabolism include diabetes mellitus, hypoglycaemia and inherited metabolic diseases.

BLOOD GLUCOSE HOMEOSTASIS

Sources

Blood glucose is maintained from several sources, including the diet and by glycogenolysis and gluconeogenesis (**Figure 1.1**).

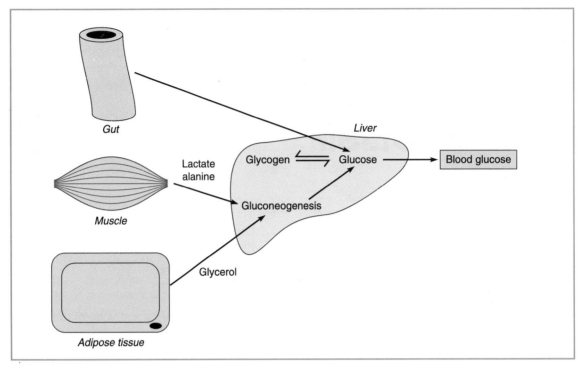

Figure 1.1 Origins of blood glucose. Some glucose arising from digestion contributes directly to blood levels which are also maintained by glycogen breakdown and synthesis from lactate, alanine and glycerol (gluconeogenesis).

Diet

Ingested carbohydrate includes both digestible and nondigestible forms, the latter being dietary fibre. Most digestible dietary carbohydrate is starch or disaccharides which, after digestion, are absorbed as glucose, galactose or fructose. These are transported by the portal vein to the liver, where galactose and fructose are converted to glucose.

The Liver

The liver is an important organ in blood glucose homeostasis as it stores some excess glucose as glycogen after feeding and, through glycogenolysis and gluconeogenesis, maintains blood levels in the fasted state. The hepatic uptake and output of glucose is controlled by the concentration of key intermediates and the activity of enzymes. In contrast to most extrahepatic tissues glucose enters liver cells relatively freely. In hepatocytes, glucose phosphorylation is promoted by glucokinase which has a lower affinity (higher K_m) than hexokinase, the equivalent enzyme in extrahepatic tissues; little glucose is therefore taken up by the liver at normal blood glucose concentrations but it is extracted more effectively by other tissues, such as the brain. The activity of glucokinase increases with high blood glucose levels and the liver thus removes glucose from the portal blood after a meal. After uptake and phosphorylation, excess glucose is stored in the liver as glycogen.

Glycogenolysis In well-fed individuals hepatic glycogen stores can account for up to 10% of organ weight. It forms a buffer which maintains blood glucose levels between meals. The process by which glucose is released from the liver is glycogenolysis, the key regulating enzyme being phosphorylase a, the activity of which is affected by several hormones.

Gluconeogenesis Other compounds are also converted to glucose in the liver; lactate, glycerol and amino acids, particularly alanine, are gluconeogenic substrates. Lactate is continually produced by partial oxidation of glucose in muscle and erythrocytes and is reconverted to glucose in the liver by the Cori cycle. Alanine is formed in muscle by transamination of pyruvate, which is derived from glucose by partial glycolysis. The liver has a high capacity to extract alanine from the blood.

Hormonal regulation

Blood glucose concentrations are normally maintained within fairly narrow limits, typical fasting values being 3.0–4.5 mmol l^{-1} in whole blood with postprandial values being 6.5–7.8 mmol l^{-1}. In addition to directly enhancing cellular uptake of glucose by the liver, a carbohydrate-rich meal also affects the release of several hormones. Insulin is the major hypoglycaemic hormone while other hormones, including glucagon, growth hormone, cortisol and adrenaline, are counter-regulatory; these antagonize the effects of insulin and have gluconeogenic effects.

Insulin Insulin is a peptide hormone that contains 51 amino acids and consists of two chains linked by three disulphide bridges. It is synthesized by the B (or β) cells in the islets of Langerhans of the pancreas, initially as a pre-prohormone which is rapidly converted to proinsulin by the removal of a peptide. Proinsulin consists of two chains of insulin which are linked by a peptide and most is further cleaved in the cell to equimolar amounts of active insulin and C-peptide. These are stored in granules, which are secreted by exocytosis. Glucose stimulates insulin release, although secretion is greater in response to oral compared with intravenous glucose. This is because gastrointestinal hormones which are secreted in response to a meal, particularly gastric

inhibitory polypeptide (GIP, synonym glucose-dependent insulinotrophic peptide), potentiate the effect of glucose. Glucagon and amino acids, particularly arginine and leucine, also stimulate insulin secretion. Vagal stimulation promotes insulin release, while sympathetic stimulation is inhibitory. Secretion is also inhibited by somatostatin. Insulin is an anabolic hormone which stimulates glucose uptake by muscle and adipose tissue, and increases protein synthesis, glycogen synthesis and lipogenesis (**Figure 1.2**).

Glucagon Glucagon is synthesized in the A (or α) cells of the pancreas. Secretion is stimulated by hypoglycaemia and gluconeogenic amino acids, and inhibited by glucose, insulin and somatostatin. Glucagon stimulates glycogenolysis and gluconeogenesis, thus raising blood glucose concentrations.

Growth Hormone Growth hormone secretion is stimulated by hypoglycaemia and its actions include increased hepatic glucose production and reduced glucose uptake by some tissues. It is possible that this latter effect is the result of increased lipolysis, raising plasma NEFA (nonesterified fatty acid) levels. NEFAs are utilized by some tissues as an energy source in preference to glucose.

Adrenaline Hypoglycaemia is a potent stimulus for adrenaline secretion. Catecholamines cause glycogenolysis and adrenaline inhibits insulin secretion, thus raising blood glucose concentrations. In addition, adrenaline stimulates adipose tissue lipolysis, increasing NEFA production.

Cortisol Cortisol inhibits hepatic glycogenolysis and stimulates gluconeogenesis. It promotes adipose tissue lipolysis and NEFA release.

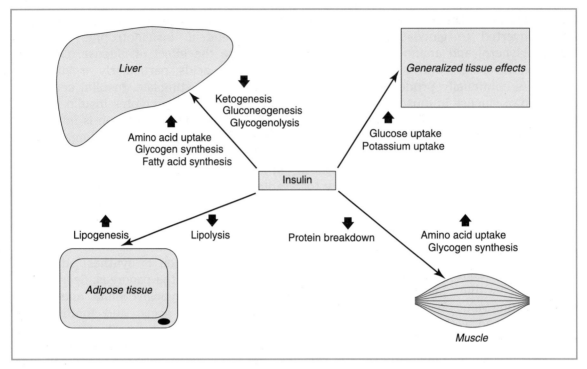

Figure 1.2 Principle actions of insulin. Insulin is an anabolic hormone, increasing cellular uptake of glucose and amino acids and promoting fat, protein and glycogen synthesis. Ketogenesis, gluconeogenesis and glycogenolysis are inhibited.

INTERRELATION OF GLUCOSE, NONESTERIFED FATTY ACID AND KETONE BODY METABOLISM

Muscle has a higher rate of fuel utilization than other organs during exercise, while the brain, kidney and intestine utilize a higher percentage of available glucose at rest. Alternative fuels are required during prolonged fasting or starvation since, if gluconeogenesis were the only process supplying tissue requirements, body protein would be consumed very rapidly. Muscle can utilize fatty acids directly but the brain is unable to do so. The ketone bodies acetoacetate and 3-hydroxybutyrate, derived from fatty acid metabolism in the liver, are an alternative fuel for the brain and are also utilized by other organs. Under conditions of starvation the muscle, brain and other tissues oxidize alternative fuels as blood concentrations of these rise, thus reducing glucose utilization.

The supply of fatty acids to organs where they are utilized is largely determined by the rate of release of NEFA from adipose tissue, this being controlled by the activity of hormone-sensitive lipase. Insulin inhibits this enzyme and is thus antilipolytic while adrenaline, growth hormone, glucagon and cortisol are lipolytic. Small amounts of NEFA are released from adipose tissue if carbohydrate supplies are adequate while, because of associated hormone changes, greater fluxes of NEFAs occur if carbohydrate availability is limited. NEFAs are transported in blood bound to albumin; about 30% is extracted by the liver. In the liver, NEFAs are either re-esterified to form triglycerides or metabolized by β-oxidation in mitochondria to form acetyl CoA. This can enter the citric acid cycle or, when large amounts of NEFA are available, form ketone bodies (**Figure 1.3**). Insulin and glucagon affect the proportion of fatty acid being re-esterifed or undergoing β-oxidation because

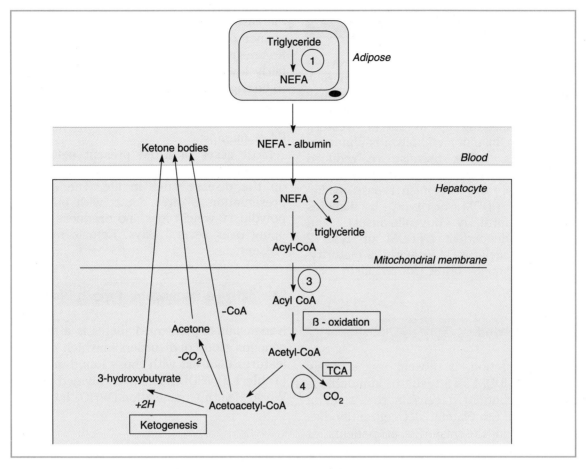

Figure 1.3 Control of ketogenesis. Key stages in regulation are numbered. (1) Lipolysis is stimulated if insulin is deficient but counter-regulatory hormone activity is high. (2) The rate of re-esterification of fatty acids to triglycerides (and phospholipids) depends on the availability of substrates and (3), the activity of mitochondrial carnitine palmitoyl-transferase I activity. This is increased by a decrease in the [insulin]/[glucagon] ratio. (4) Excess acetyl coenzyme A (CoA) cannot be metabolized by the tricarboxylic acid cycle as the capacity to store chemical energy as adenosine triphosphate (ATP) is limited; hence ketogenesis occurs. NEFA, nonesterified fatty acid; TCA, tricarboxylic acid cycle.

insulin inhibits and glucagon stimulates mitochondrial carnitine palmitoyl transferase I activity. This enzyme enhances the transfer of fatty acids into mitochondria and thus, if the ratio of glucagon to insulin is increased, more fatty acids are metabolized by β-oxidation. The concentrations of NEFA are also important, as with increased fluxes, proportionally greater amounts are converted to ketone bodies and less is oxidized by the citric acid cycle.

KEY POINTS

KETONE BODIES

- Ketone bodies are produced from NEFA in the liver

- Ketone bodies are an alternative fuel for brain metabolism

- In starvation many organs utilize ketones, sparing glucose

DIABETES MELLITUS

Diabetes mellitus is a heterogeneous group of disorders characterized by hyperglycaemia, glycosuria and associated abnormalities of lipid and protein metabolism. It is common, affecting up to 2% of Western populations. Insulin metabolism is abnormal in diabetes, either because of reduced secretion or owing to insensitivity to its effects. There are two main types, insulin-dependent (IDDM or type 1 diabetes mellitus, formerly juvenile-onset) and non-insulin-dependent (NIDDM or type 2 diabetes mellitus, formerly maturity-onset), although other forms also exist (**Table 1.1**).

Insulin-Dependent (Type 1) Diabetes

Insulin secretion is absent or severely reduced in IDDM as a result of immunological destruction of β cells in the islets of Langerhans. Circulating islet cell antibodies are found in the majority of patients at presentation and infiltration of the islets by T lymphocytes also occurs. Genetic factors are important in the development of IDDM: individuals with human leukocyte antigen (HLA) system antigens DR3 and DR4 have

Table 1.1 Clinical classification of diabetes mellitus

Insulin-dependent diabetes mellitus
Non-insulin-dependent diabetes mellitus
◆ Obese
◆ Non-obese
Malnutrition-related diabetes mellitus
Diabetes associated with other disorders
◆ Pancreatic disease
◆ Endocrine diseases
◆ Congenital disorders
Gestational diabetes mellitus
Impaired glucose tolerance

increased susceptibility, although the chance of a child developing IDDM when a first-degree relative has the condition is fairly low (5–10%). The disease is thought to be triggered by an environmental event in susceptible individuals. This is usually a viral infection, particularly with Coxsackie B4 or mumps.

Most cases of IDDM present before 30 years of age, although some patients develop the disease later in life. The clinical presentation is often acute, with polyuria, polydipsia, weight loss and tiredness developing over several days. Ketosis may be present.

Non-Insulin-Dependent (Type 2) Diabetes

Non-insulin-dependent diabetes is a heterogeneous group of disorders in which several features contrast with those found in IDDM (**Table 1.2**). NIDDM has been divided by the World Health Organisation (WHO) into two

Table 1.2 Typical features of insulin-dependent and non-insulin-dependent diabetes mellitus (IDDM and NIDDM, respectively)

Feature	IDDM (Type 1)	NIDDM (Type 2)
Age of onset	<30 years (peak 5)	>40 years
Rate of onset	Rapid	Slow
Weight	Lean	Obese or normal
Ketosis	Prone	Rare
Serum insulin	Low or absent	Normal or slightly reduced
Pancreatic β cell mass	Much reduced	Slightly reduced
Family history of diabetes	Rare	Common
HLA associations	Present	Absent
Islet cell antibodies	Common	Absent

HLA, human leukocyte antigen.

main groups, obese and non-obese. Insulin secretion is retained, although it is inadequate to control blood glucose levels. In addition, there is resistance to the effects of insulin in target organs, due to reduced insulin receptors and a postreceptor defect in insulin action within cells.

Genetic factors are a more important aetiological factor in NIDDM than IDDM. Identical twins have a near 100% concordance rate and the risk of developing NIDDM is higher than IDDM if a parent has the disease. There are no HLA associations and no islet cell antibodies are found. Although not all patients with NIDDM are overweight, there is a clear association with obesity. Obesity is associated with hyperinsulinism in the absence of NIDDM, and it is possible that obese patients who develop NIDDM either have diminished pancreatic reserve or a secretory defect in the pancreatic β cells, resulting in a failure to respond normally to glucose.

Clinical onset is usually in middle age and the prevalence increases with age. Occasionally, younger patients may be affected (non-insulin-dependent diabetes in the young; NIDDY). NIDDM is often detected by urine testing during a routine medical examination, or during the course of another illness. Patients may complain of polyuria and polydipsia. Ketosis is rare, although it can be precipitated if an acute illness occurs in a subject with NIDDM. Type 2 diabetic patients may present in hyperosmolar nonketotic coma (see below).

Malnutrition-Related Diabetes Mellitus

There are two types of malnutrition-related diabetes which are found mainly in developing countries, fibrocalculous and protein-deficient diabetes. The aetiology of these is not clear, although the extensive pancreatic duct calculi which are found in fibrocalculous diabetes are thought to be associated with cassava root consumption.

Diabetes Associated with Other Disorders (Secondary Diabetes)

Diabetes may occur in association with other conditions, particularly pancreatic disease and endocrinopathies. Pancreatic disorders such as chronic pancreatitis and haemochromatosis may cause destruction of β cells, while endocrine disorders which result in increased secretion of counter-regulatory hormones can induce insulin resistance. Congenital abnormalities of insulin receptors and antibodies to these are rare causes of diabetes. Diabetes occurs in association with several genetic disorders, including Turner's syndrome and Down's syndrome.

Gestational Diabetes Mellitus

Gestational diabetes occurs for the first time in pregnancy. Glycosuria without diabetes is common because the renal threshold for glucose is reduced. As complications can occur which are related to blood glucose concentrations in both the mother and fetus, diagnosis and appropriate treatment of diabetes are important. Glucose tolerance reverts to normal after delivery in most cases, although many later develop frank diabetes.

Impaired Glucose Tolerance

Impaired glucose tolerance (IGT) is an asymptomatic condition which is diagnosed on the basis of the response of blood glucose to the ingestion of a standard oral glucose solution (oral glucose tolerance test, OGTT), the values being intermediate between normal and diabetic (see below). Impaired glucose tolerance was previously known as chemical, latent or subclinical diabetes but these terms are misleading as IGT is associated with health risks. These risks include atherosclerosis and progression to diabetes mellitus.

Diagnosis of Diabetes and Impaired Glucose Tolerance

Diabetes may be suggested by the clinical features, particularly in IDDM, and a random venous whole-blood glucose value ≥ 10.0 mmol l^{-1} or a fasting value ≥ 6.7 mmol l^{-1} will confirm the diagnosis in symptomatic patients. Results from two blood tests are required to confirm the diagnosis in asymptomatic patients. Diabetes is unlikely if a result <4.4 mmol l^{-1} is obtained.

When the diagnosis is uncertain an oral glucose tolerance test should be performed (**Table 1.3**). Diagnostic criteria for diabetes mellitus and IGT have been defined by the WHO on the basis of blood glucose results following the administration of a glucose load containing the equivalent of 75 g anhydrous sugar (**Table 1.4**).

KEY POINTS

DIABETES MELLITUS

- Type 1 diabetes mellitus is characterized by insulin deficiency

- Type 2 diabetes mellitus is characterized by insulin resistance

- Diabetes mellitus is diagnosed by clinical features and blood glucose measurement or an oral glucose tolerance test

Table 1.3 Indications, protocol and factors influencing the oral glucose tolerance test (OGTT)

Indications	Protocol	Factors influencing results
Equivocal fasting or random blood glucose concentrations	Patient fasts overnight	*Previous diet*
	Patient rests during test	Glucose tolerance may be abnormal if the patient has been on a weight reducing diet. Diet should be normal for 3–4 days before oral glucose tolerance test (OGTT)
Unexplained glycosuria in pregnancy	Smoking is not permitted	
Clinical features of diabetes with normal blood glucose levels	Fasting blood sample taken	
	Oral glucose solution given (75 g in 300 ml water)	*Time of day*
	Blood and urine samples taken at 2 h	Diagnostic values are for morning tests. Glucose values are higher in the afternoon.
		Drugs
		Medication, e.g. steroids and diuretics may cause impaired glucose tolerance

Table 1.4 Diagnostic criteria for diabetes mellitus and impaired glucose tolerance

	Glucose concentration (mmol l^{-1})			
	Venous sampling		Capillary sampling	
	Whole blood	Plasma	Whole blood	Plasma
Diabetes mellitus				
Fasting sample	≥ 6.7	≥ 7.8	≥ 6.7	≥ 7.8
2 h after glucose load	≥ 10.0	≥ 11.1	≥ 11.1	≥ 12.2
Impaired glucose tolerance				
Fasting sample	<6.7	<7.8	<6.7	<7.8
2 h after glucose load	6.7–10.0	7.8–11.1	7.8–11.1	8.9–12.2

Glucose Estimation

Glucose may be estimated in either plasma or whole blood. Whole-blood values are lower because the volume of distribution of glucose is lower, as erythrocytes contain less free water than plasma. Samples for glucose can be obtained either by venepuncture or by a fingerprick technique, such samples being collected in capillary tubes. Capillary plasma values are significantly greater than concentrations in venous plasma samples at higher blood glucose levels. Blood cells continue to metabolize glucose after venepuncture and thus samples must either be separated rapidly to obtain valid results, or a preservative that inhibits glycolysis should be used. Sodium fluoride, together with potassium oxalate as an anticoagulant, is used for this purpose. Test strips which measure blood glucose can be useful in obtaining an indication of blood glucose concentrations, but diagnosis should be based on laboratory measurements. Glycated haemoglobin is useful for assessing diabetic control but is not reliable for diagnosis (see below).

Urine Testing

Urine testing is used to screen for diabetes although it has limitations, even if test strips which contain an enzyme specific for glucose are used (see chapter 23).

Management

The management of diabetes is directed at alleviating symptoms and preventing acute metabolic disturbances and long-term complications. Self-management by patients is an important part of treatment and education is therefore central, since changes in lifestyle are necessary and skills for monitoring and managing the condition must be acquired. Dietary treatment is important in both types of diabetes and may be the only form of therapy used in NIDDM, where weight reduction is a key objective. Refined sugar and fat intake is limited and the ingestion of complex carbohydrates, starch and fibre is increased.

Oral hypoglycaemic drugs are used in NIDDM patients who continue to have poor control after dietary therapy. Two main classes are used, sulphonylureas (e.g. tolbutamide), which increase insulin release and receptor binding, and biguanides (e.g. metformin), the mechanisms of action of which are unclear. Insulin injection is required in IDDM and is also needed in some type 2 diabetic patients.

Biochemical Monitoring of Management

Good control of blood glucose concentrations is important, particularly in younger patients, as this helps to prevent the development of long-term complications. The control of symptoms does not ensure normoglycaemia and therefore monitoring, which includes clinical assessment, weighing and biochemical measurements is essential.

Urine Analysis

Urinary glucose excretion may be determined using quantitative reagent strips and is useful in NIDDM, provided the renal threshold for glucose is normal. Urinary glucose gives an indication of the integrated blood glucose concentration above the renal threshold since the bladder was last emptied, although there is considerable individual variation in the renal threshold for glucose. Self-monitoring in IDDM is more usually undertaken by blood glucose monitoring. Most patients prefer blood to urine monitoring, as it is perceived to be more hygienic. In addition, it is the only method of monitoring that can be used to confirm hypoglycaemia.

Blood Glucose Analysis

Monitoring blood glucose at the diabetic clinic is less informative than home monitoring owing to the infrequency of visits. Measurement at home may be undertaken using blood obtained by fingerprick and reagent strips. Colour charts are available for reading the result, or a small meter can be used. Careful instruction is needed if reliable results are to be obtained. The frequency of monitoring depends on the clinical state of the patient – more frequent readings are taken during stabilization than in well-controlled subjects. Profiles throughout the day, which include preprandial and bedtime values, are preferable to random readings. Values are used to calculate insulin doses and must also be recorded and discussed with medical or nursing staff.

Glycated Proteins

Haemoglobin (Hb) in most normal adults consists of one major component, HbA_0, and several minor fractions, including glycated haemoglobin. This is formed after reticulocytes have been released from the bone marrow by the action of glucose on haemoglobin. Several different HbA_1s are found, the major fraction being HbA_{1c} in which glucose binds to the terminal valine of the β chain. Normally, about 5% of circulating haemoglobin is glycated, the amount depending on the average blood glucose concentrations over the previous 2 months. The measurement of glycated haemoglobin therefore gives an indication of the overall degree of blood glycaemic control, in contrast to glucose measurements which give information for a single time-point.

Other proteins are also glycated at a rate which depends on blood glucose concentrations. The period of glycaemic control they represent also depends on the half-life of the proteins. Fructosamine is a measure of glycated serum proteins, mainly albumin which has a half-life of 20 days. Its measurement therefore represents glycaemic control over a shorter period than glycated haemoglobin.

Metabolic Complications

Metabolic complications, particularly diabetic ketoacidosis and hypoglycaemia, are life-threatening and can cause permanent

Table 1.5 Causes of impaired consciousness in diabetic patients

Specific for diabetes
◆ Diabetic ketoacidosis
◆ Hyperosmolar nonketotic coma
Higher incidence in diabetes
◆ Metabolic
Hypoglycaemia
Lactic acidosis
◆ Nonmetabolic
Vascular
Infective
Causes with same incidence in nondiabetic populations
e.g. alcohol-induced, head injury

neurological damage. They must be considered if diabetic patients present with impaired consciousness, although this may be caused by other conditions (**Table 1.5**).

Diabetic Ketoacidosis

Diabetic ketoacidosis (DKA) was responsible for 70% of diabetic deaths before the advent of insulin therapy and mortality rates are still up to 7%. Although it is mainly a recognized complication of IDDM, DKA can also occur in NIDDM, particularly if severe infection or other major illness occurs. This is because insulin requirements increase in acute stress. The clinical features of DKA result from insulin deficiency and increases in counter-regulatory hormones, which produce major changes in fuel, water and electrolyte metabolism (**Figures 1.4** and **1.5**). If there is a deficiency of insulin, glycogenolysis and gluconeogenesis occur, leading to increased hepatic glucose output. Increased secretion of counter-regulatory hormones, either as a result of the initiating stress or due to the metabolic disturbance, also increases hepatic glucose output. Tissue uptake of glucose is reduced, contributing to the hyperglycaemia. As glucose does not enter cells, the extracellular osmotic pressure tends to rise, causing water to transfer from the intracellular to extracellular compartment. The renal

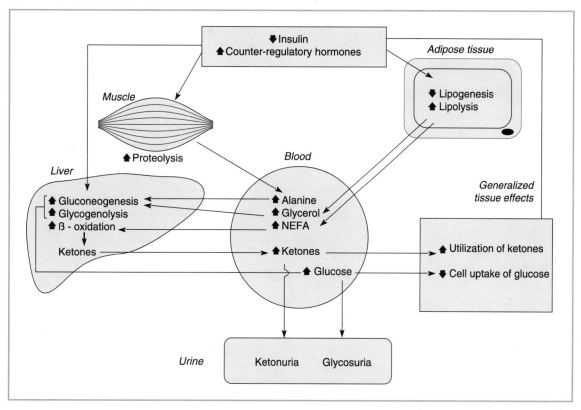

Figure 1.4 Major changes in fuel metabolism in diabetic ketoacidosis. Decreased insulin and increased counter-regulatory hormone levels inhibit anabolic processes, leading to increased proteolysis and lipolysis. These lead to increased gluconeogenesis and ketone body formation which, together with decreased cellular uptake of glucose, causes hyperglycaemia and ketonaemia. These lead to glycosuria and ketonuria. NEFA, nonesterified fatty acid.

threshold for glucose is exceeded and glycosuria occurs. The presence of excess nonabsorbed solute in the glomerular filtrate causes an osmotic diuresis which interferes with tubular reabsorptive function, leading to water, sodium and potassium depletion (see chapters 5 and 6).

Lipolysis results from insulin deficiency, this process being enhanced by increased cortisol and catecholamine action. NEFAs are released and transported to the liver where reduced insulin and increased glucagon concentrations lead to greater amounts of fatty acids being metabolized by β-oxidation. The capacity of the citric acid cycle to metabolize acetyl CoA is exceeded and increased amounts of ketone bodies are formed. Acetoacetate and 3-hydroxybutyrate are weak acids and increase the H$^+$ concentration in blood, exceeding the buffering capacity and causing acidosis. The H$^+$ ions exchange with potassium across cell membranes, causing hyperkalaemia in some patients. However, total body potassium is reduced because increased losses occur through the kidney due to the osmotic diuresis interfering with normal tubular reabsorptive function. A further effect of acidosis is direct stimulation of the respiratory centre by H$^+$, causing deep sighing hyperventilation (Kussmaul breathing).

Reduced consciousness is more common than frank unconsciousness. A recent history of polyuria, polydipsia, fatigue and vomiting is often obtained and there may be indications of a recent infection, these often precipitating DKA. Physical signs include dehydration, tachycardia, warm

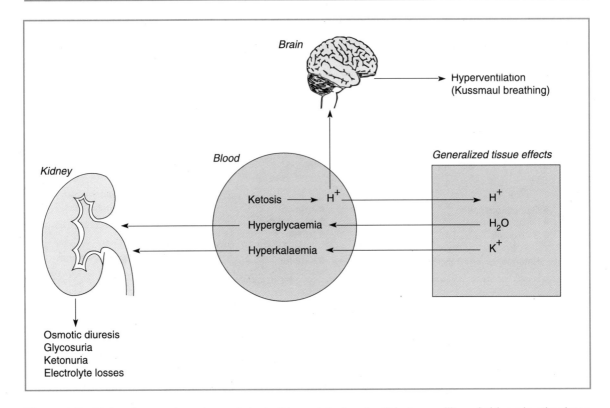

Figure 1.5 Major changes in water and electrolyte metabolism in diabetes mellitus. Acidaemia stimulates the respiratory centre and, by exchanging with cellular potassium, causes hyperkalaemia. Hyperglycaemia attracts water from cellular compartments by osmosis and causes an osmotic diuresis, leading to dehydration and electrolyte loss.

skin (vasodilatation being induced by ketones), Kussmaul respiration and the odour of acetone on the breath. Biochemical findings include hyperglycaemia which may be established initially using reagent strips, although confirmation by laboratory investigation is required. The presence of ketosis may also be established by testing plasma with reagent strips. Other laboratory investigations are required to assess electrolyte imbalance and to allow the response to treatment to be monitored. These include plasma electrolytes, urea, and blood gases.

Management Diabetic ketoacidosis is a medical emergency. The aim of treatment is to replace fluids and electrolytes, and to restore metabolic control. In addition to insulin replacement, patients typically require several litres of isotonic saline to be infused. However, hypernatraemia can occur during treatment and if this develops, half-normal saline should be given. Most patients are treated with intravenous insulin infusion, initially 6 units h^{-1}; this amount is increased if the blood glucose concentration does not respond after 2 h. Plasma potassium levels, which are normal or high at presentation, fall rapidly with effective treatment. This is caused by insulin increasing potassium uptake by cells, extracellular volume expansion and correction of the acidaemia. Intravenous potassium supplements may therefore be required, the rates depending on the plasma potassium values. Monitoring patients by ECG gives a useful guide to changes in potassium status (see chapter 6). Bicarbonate is sometimes infused to correct the metabolic acidosis in severely affected patients (pH<7.0),

DIABETIC KETOACIDOSIS

- Diabetic ketoacidosis (DKA) is a medical emergency

- Patients with DKA are dehydrated, sodium depleted and acidotic

- Plasma potassium levels should be monitored during treatment

although this may accentuate hypokalaemia. Precipitating causes, such as an infection or myocardial infarction, should be sought. General medical measures are also important and the possibility of pooling of fluid in the stomach should be considered and aspirated if necessary, particularly in unconscious or semiconscious patients.

Monitoring   After initial blood samples have been taken and treatment initiated, blood glucose levels should be monitored hourly using test strips. Laboratory analysis of glucose and electrolytes should be done after 2 h and then four-hourly until the patient is stable. Blood gases should also be monitored periodically.

Hyperosmolar Nonketotic Coma

Hyperosmolar nonketotic coma (HONK) occurs mainly in elderly patients with NIDDM. The pathogenesis of the condition is unclear, although it is thought that it occurs when there is sufficient insulin to limit increased hepatic β-oxidation of NEFA but not enough to prevent hyperglycaemia. Some degree of ketosis may be detected although ketone body concentrations are much lower than those seen in DKA, and are similar to values found in ketosis accompanying starvation. Hyperglycaemia is more severe than in DKA, with values of glucose commonly above 50 mmol l^{-1}. This is accompanied by dehydration and many patients have hypernatraemia. Fluid replacement is needed – the average deficit is 10 l. Isotonic saline is given initially, followed with half-normal saline if the plasma sodium

concentration is raised. Insulin is used to correct the metabolic abnormality and potassium replacement is often necessary. The condition has a high mortality, over 50%, and thromboembolic events are common.

Lactic Acidosis

There are two main types of lactic acidosis, type A which is associated with anoxia, and type B which has various causes (see chapter 7). Type B lactic acidosis may occur in diabetes mellitus associated with biguanide therapy. This was associated particularly with phenformin therapy, although this agent has now been replaced with metformin. Lactic acidosis is rare with metformin use and is usually associated with renal failure. It is thought to be due, in part, to increased peripheral anaerobic glycolysis, and also to inhibition of gluconeogenesis from lactate.

Long-term Complications

Tissue damage occurs in many organs in diabetes which is probably caused by poor metabolic control. Long-term complications may result from microvascular changes, macrovascular disease, or other causes (**Table 1.6**). Microvascular disease is relatively specific to diabetes. The pathological processes underlying macrovascular disease are similar to atherosclerotic vascular disease which occurs in nondiabetic subjects (see chapter 2), although the prevalence is greater.

The exact mechanisms of complications are unclear although several have been proposed.

1. Changes in the glycoproteins of basement membranes of capillaries, leading to thickening and increased permeability.
2. Accumulation of sugar alcohols which are formed from glucose. These cause tissue damage, either directly, or by osmotic attraction of water. The latter

Table 1.6 Long-term complications in diabetes mellitus

Pathophysiology	Organ	Lesion
Microangiopathy	Eye	Retinopathy
		Maculopathy
	Kidney	Nephropathy
	Nerves	Neuropathy
Macroangiopathy	Heart	Coronary heart disease
	Vessels	Cerebrovascular disease
		Peripheral vascular disease
		Hypertension
Other	Skin	Skin thickening
	Lens	Cataracts

is a possible mechanism for cataract formation.

3. Glycation of structural proteins. Such changes alter the properties of collagen and could be responsible for damage to skin and connective tissue.
4. Several factors contribute to atherosclerosis including hypertension and dyslipidaemia and, in NIDDM, insulin resistance.

Proteinuria in Diabetes

Many fit people excrete small quantities of protein in urine, typically around 10 mg day^{-1} of mainly low molecular weight proteins such as albumin. These amounts are too small to be detected by screening for proteinuria with dipsticks, since these react positively to >100 mg l^{-1} albumin (see chapter 8). Frank proteinuria occurs in diabetic patients who develop overt nephropathy. Some diabetic patients develop albumin excretion rates >30 μg min^{-1} but these are less than amounts detected by albustix. Very sensitive assays are required to measure such amounts and excretion in this range is classed as microalbuminuria.

Microalbuminuric patients are at risk of developing frank proteinuria, renal failure and accelerated vascular disease. Improved control in such patients may prevent or delay the progression of complications.

HYPOGLYCAEMIA

Hypoglycaemia is dangerous because glucose is a vital primary fuel for the brain. Deficiency produces disordered function and, if prolonged or severe, can cause tissue damage or death. In fasting, the brain still has an energy requirement equivalent to 80 g glucose 24 h^{-1}, which cannot be provided by NEFA, the immediately available alternative fuel. The brain can utilize ketone bodies but these are not produced rapidly enough to protect against acute hypoglycaemia.

Hypoglycaemia is defined as a fasting venous whole-blood glucose level of less than 2.2 mmol l^{-1} (plasma glucose <2.5 mmol l^{-1}), when measured by a glucose-specific (enzymatic) method. However, such a definition is somewhat arbitrary, as it gives only an approximate indication of the levels at which symptoms occur. Some, mainly elderly, patients develop symptoms at higher concentrations, while infants appear to tolerate lower levels.

Clinical Features

Symptoms fall into two main categories, those produced by excessive secretion of adrenaline, and those caused by dysfunction of the central nervous system. Symptoms caused by adrenaline release usually occur earlier in acute hypoglycaemia and include nervousness, weakness, headache, sweating, dizziness, tremor, tachycardia, palpitations, anxiety and hunger. Features resulting from disordered central nervous system function (neuroglycopaenia) include visual symptoms, headache, blunted mental acuity, loss of motor function, confusion, abnormal behaviour, fits and loss of consciousness.

Causes

It has been traditional to classify hypoglycaemia as conditions that produce low blood glucose levels during fasting, or those that are reactive to particular stimuli. There is some overlap however, as reactive hypoglycaemia can occur together with fasting hypoglycaemia. An alternative approach is to base classification on the pathophysiology of hypoglycaemia, particularly reduced gluconeogenesis and increased utilization of glucose (**Table 1.7**).

Decreased Output of Glucose

Hypoglycaemia may result from impaired glycogenolysis or reduced gluconeogenesis. Although the kidney makes a small contribution, under fasting conditions gluconeogenesis occurs mainly in the liver. Gluconeogenesis may be impaired because of reduced formation from amino acids and glycerol or decreased recycling from lactate. Quantitatively, the latter is the most important.

Liver Disease Hypoglycaemia might be expected to be a complication of liver disease because of the role of this organ in gluconeogenesis. It is, however, an unusual cause because of the great hepatic functional reserve, although hypoglycaemia may be seen with massive hepatocellular destruction in paracetamol poisoning.

Alcohol Abuse Alcohol inhibits gluconeogenesis and symptoms of hypoglycaemia following alcohol ingestion are particularly likely if hepatic glycogen stores are depleted, as occurs in malnourished subjects. This condition is probably underdiagnosed, as the symptoms of neuroglycopaenia and alcohol intoxication can be similar.

Table 1.7   Causes of hypoglycaemia

Decreased glucose output
Liver disease
Alcohol abuse
Inherited metabolic disorders
◆ Glycogen synthase deficiency
◆ Glycogen storage diseases
◆ Galactosaemia
◆ Hereditary fructose intolerance
◆ Impaired recycling of glycolytic intermediates
Endocrine disease
◆ Growth hormone deficiency
◆ Cortisol deficiency

Increased glucose utilization
Reduced fat stores
◆ Prematurity
◆ Malnutrition
Impaired fatty acid oxidation
◆ Defective transport into mitochondria
◆ Oxidative defects
◆ Impaired production or utilization of ketone bodies

Decreased output and increased utilization of glucose
Hyperinsulinism
◆ Exogenous administration
◆ Endogenous production
    Insulinoma
    Nesidioblastosis
    Islet cell hyperplasia
Sulphonyiureas
Nonpancreatic tumours
Postgastrectomy

Inherited Metabolic Disorders Reduced hepatic glucose output can occur in several inherited metabolic disorders (see below). Liver glycogen is severely reduced in glycogen synthase deficiency, predisposing to fasting hypoglycaemia. The release of glucose from glucose-6-phosphate is defective in type I glycogen storage disease (glucose-6-phosphatase deficiency). Glucose release during fasting is impaired type III glycogen storage disease because the debranching enzyme (amylo-1,6-glucosidase) is deficient: only the outermost 1,4-linked glucose molecules in glycogen polymers can be released.

In hereditary fructose intolerance and galactosaemia, ingestion of the relevant sugar causes hypoglycaemia, possibly caused by the effects of intermediates which accumulate, such as sugar phosphates. Several other enzyme deficiencies are rare causes of hypoglycaemia, including defects of recycling of glycolytic intermediates to glucose.

Endocrine Disease Deficiency of counter-regulatory hormones is an uncommon cause of hypoglycaemia. It occurs in cortisol deficiency, due either to primary adrenal failure or secondary to adrenocorticotrophic hormone (ACTH) deficiency, and in growth hormone deficiency. Impaired gluconeogenesis is the most likely reason.

Decreased Ketone Body Production

Continued utilization of glucose by the brain can cause hypoglycaemia when the production of ketone bodies is defective.

Reduced Fat Stores Low fat stores allow only limited ketogenesis and this may contribute to hypoglycaemia in premature infants, in malnutrition, and in starvation.

Impaired Fatty Acid Oxidation Activated long-chain fatty acids are transported by carnitine into mitochondria for oxidation, this being facilitated by two carnitine acyltransferases (**Figure 1.3**). Deficiency of carnitine or inactivity of one of these enzymes may cause impaired oxidation of long-chain fatty acids. Intramitochondrial fatty acids are oxidized by a group of acyl dehydrogenases (long-chain (LCAD), medium-chain (MCAD) and short-chain (SCAD) acyl dehydrogenases), each of which preferentially metabolizes fatty acids of a particular chain length. Single and multiple deficiencies of these enzymes occur causing hypoglycaemia on fasting or during a stress such as infection. Both carnitine and acyl dehydrogenase abnormalities cause elevated NEFA levels in plasma.

Decreased Output and Increased Utilization of Glucose

Insulin Insulin reduces blood glucose acutely, mainly by increasing cellular uptake and utilization; therefore, excess administration causes hypoglycaemia. Lipolysis, and thus ketogenesis, is also suppressed, but this occurs at much lower concentrations.

Hyperinsulinaemia may also result from inappropriate endogenous production. Insulinomas, which are common causes of hypoglycaemia in adults, are tumours of pancreatic β cells. Nesiodioblastosis is a diffuse increase in pancreatic endocrine cells and is an important cause of hypoglycaemia in infancy. This condition must be differentiated from hyperinsulinism in infants born to mothers with poorly controlled diabetes which occurs as a result of sustained intrauterine hyperglycaemia leading to hyperplasia of the islets.

Sulphonylureas Sulphonylureas increase glucose-stimulated insulin release and hypoglycaemia is the most commonly observed side-effect. It is frequent in patients who are losing weight or have impaired renal function.

Nonpancreatic Tumours Some nonpancreatic tumours, particularly large mesenchymal neoplasms or primary liver carcinomas, occasionally cause hypoglycaemia. This is thought to result from increased glucose utilization by the tumour and production of humoral factors with insulin-like actions, such as growth factors and somatomedins.

Postgastrectomy Hypoglycaemia approximately 2 h after a meal rich in carbohydrate is common in patients with a partial gastrectomy. It occurs because of rapid passage of sugar into the small intestine and enhanced release of enteric hormones which augment glucose-stimulated insulin release. This excessive release of insulin causes hypoglycaemia.

Other Causes

Idiopathic hypoglycaemia was, by definition, of unknown cause. Since the introduction of insulin assays many patients formerly diagnosed as having idiopathic hypoglycaemia have been shown to have nesidioblastosis. Previously, leucine sensitivity has been described as a specific cause of hypoglycaemia, although it now appears unlikely that this is a distinct entity. Leucine stimulates insulin secretion and many patients diagnosed as having this condition probably had hyperinsulinism – either nesidioblastosis or an insulinoma. Ketotic hypoglycaemia occurs in starvation or in an illness in which liver glycogen stores are depleted. It appears to be an extreme response to food deprivation. Hypoglycaemia following the ingestion of a large carbohydrate meal is a normal physiological response which may be exaggerated following gastric surgery. Symptoms such as fatigue, poor concentration and confusion have been ascribed to such reactive hypoglycaemia although it is unclear whether this is a genuine disease state. Some patients who show reactive hypoglycaemia with a glucose tolerance test later develop diabetes mellitus. The response is thought to be due to a delay in insulin secretion, followed by exaggerated release of the hormone.

Investigation of Hypoglycaemia in Adults

The causes of hypoglycaemia differ according to the age of the patient, insulinoma being common in adults while inherited metabolic diseases are extremely rare.

Some causes of hypoglycaemia, particularly those following a stimulus (reactive hypoglycaemia) may be suggested by the history. These include drugs, particularly insulin, alcohol ingestion and postgastrectomy. Hypoglycaemic episodes in insulin-treated diabetic patients and with sulphonylurea treatment do not usually cause diagnostic problems. However, both diabetic and nondiabetic patients sometimes deliberately induce hypoglycaemia by insulin injection (factitious hypoglycaemia) and this must be differentiated from insulinoma.

Patients with insulinomas sometimes present with bizarre psychiatric symptoms, resulting from chronic neuroglycopaenia, and hypoglycaemia may not at first be considered. In patients with unexplained psychiatric symptoms a relationship between these and fasting or exertion should be sought. Once the diagnosis is considered blood glucose and insulin should be measured after an overnight fast on three consecutive occasions: hypoglycaemia with inappropriately high insulin levels is being demonstrated by such a protocol in over 90% of cases of insulinoma. For some patients an extended fast of up to 72 h is needed, and glucose and insulin concentrations should be determined every 4–6 h, or when the patient has symptoms.

In nondiabetic patients, symptoms of factitious hypoglycaemia may mimic those of insulinoma. The conditions may be differentiated by measuring C-peptide and insulin in blood. These are secreted in equimolar amounts, with C-peptide being the more stable of the two. C-peptide is an index of endogenous insulin secretion as little is present in therapeutic preparations of insulin. Levels are suppressed by exogenous insulin administration but are inappropriately high when excess endogenous insulin secretion occurs e.g. insulinoma.

Hypoglycaemia due to non-islet cell tumours is usually very severe and tumours may often be detected by physical examination or imaging techniques. Plasma insulin, C-peptide and proinsulin levels are very low.

Hypoglycaemia in Infancy and Childhood

Hypoglycaemia is a common metabolic abnormality in infancy and early recognition is important to prevent brain damage. Hypoglycaemia often occurs transiently at birth, as normal blood glucose control is established after a few days. Adaptation to enteral feeding is required with the development of the ability to mobilize glucose and ketone bodies. This adaptation is often delayed in premature infants, or when there has been intrauterine growth retardation. Prolonged and severe hypoglycaemia suggests a pathological cause. Most neonates with persistent hypoglycaemia have hyperinsulinism, deficiency of a counter-regulatory hormone, or an enzyme deficiency affecting gluconeogensis or glycogenolysis. In older children hyperinsulinism, growth hormone or cortisol deficiency, or accelerated starvation are important causes. The last of these conditions is not fully understood but occurs in small children, usually between the ages of 1 and 5 years, who are small, with low glycogen stores. Under conditions of increased glucose utilization, such as intense exercise or intercurrent infection, glucose production is limited and hypoglycaemia develops.

Investigation Careful planning of investigations is required owing to the constraints imposed by the size of the patients and their blood volumes. The minimum investigations are blood glucose, serum insulin and blood or urinary ketone bodies (the first urine specimen passed after hypoglycaemia is identified is collected). In addition, it may be necessary to estimate growth hormone, cortisol, lactate, NEFA, and other intermediary metabolites, together with urinary reducing sugars.

Ketosis is a physiological response to hypoglycaemia, and the lack of ketosis suggests hyperinsulinism or impaired oxidation of fatty acids. Elevated levels of both NEFA and ketones occur when insulin secretion is inhibited and fat stores are being mobilized. Causes include accelerated starvation, cortisol deficiency, growth hormone deficiency or impaired glucose production due to an inherited metabolic disorder. Increased blood lactate concentrations suggest disorders such as type I glycogen storage disease or defects in

recycling glycolytic intermediates. Reducing sugars in urine occur in galactosaemia and fructose intolerance, while the pattern of urinary metabolite excretion is often characteristic in inherited metabolic diseases.

INHERITED METABOLIC DISORDERS OF CARBOHYDRATE METABOLISM
Glycogen Storage Diseases (Glycogenoses)

Glycogen storage diseases are a group of inherited conditions characterized by tissue deposits of glycogen that are abnormal in amount or structure. Glycogen is found principally in liver and muscle, and is synthesized from glucose by different enzymes from those which mediate glycogenolysis (**Figure 1.6**). During synthesis, glycogen synthase promotes the addition of glucose-1-phosphate in $(1 \rightarrow 4)$ linkages,

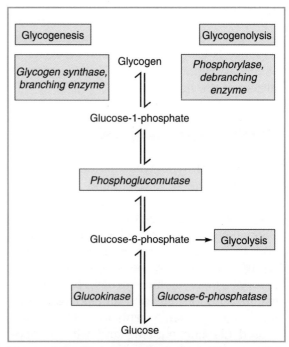

Figure 1.6 Glycogen metabolism. The enzymes promoting glycogen synthesis are different from those involved in glycogenolysis.

Table 1.8   Features of glycogen storage diseases

Type	Principle tissues involved	Enzyme deficiency	Features
I (von Gierke)	Liver	Glucose-6-phosphatase	Hypoglycaemia, lactic acidosis, hepatomegaly, hyperuricaemia
II (Pompe)	Heart, liver, muscle	Lysosomal (1-4) glucosidase	Muscle weakness, cardiac hypertrophy, normoglycaemia
III (Cori)	Liver, muscle	Debranching enzyme	Hypoglycaemia, hepatomegaly
IV	Liver	Branching enzyme	Cirrhosis
V (McArdle)	Muscle	Phosphorylase	Muscle fatigue after exercise, myoglobinuria
VI (Hers)	Liver, muscle	Phosphorylase	Hepatomegaly
VII	Muscle	Phosphofructokinase	Muscle fatigue after exercise, myoglobinuria
IX	Liver, muscle	Phosphorylase kinase	Hepatomegaly

forming straight chains. Glycogen also contains branch points, these being introduced as (1 → 6) linkages by branching enzyme. Degradation is mediated by the combined actions of the phosphorylase complex, which cleaves the (1 → 4) linkages, and debranching enzyme, which removes the (1 → 6) linkages. Type I glycogenosis (von Gierke's disease) is caused by a deficiency in glucose-6-phosphatase, which results in impaired glucose release from glycogen and thus hypoglycaemia. Glycogen accumulates in the liver, leading to hepatomegaly. Lactate metabolism is also impaired as it is converted to glucose via glucose-6-phosphate in the Cori cycle. Thus metabolic acidosis is a clinical feature. Hyperuricaemia is also seen, partly due to increased metabolism of glucose-6-phosphate via the pentose phosphate pathway, forming ribose-5-phosphate and hence purines. Lactate also interferes with the renal excretion of urate, causing hyperuricaemia.

Features of the other glycogen storage diseases are outlined in **Table 1.8**. Type II

glycogenosis differs from the others in that it is a defect in a lysosomal rather than a cytoplasmic enzyme. In glycogen synthase deficiency, which is extremely rare, very little glucose is converted to glycogen, although conversion to lactate does occur, with hyperglycaemia and hyperlactataemia being features of this deficiency.

Galactosaemia

Impaired metabolism of galactose may result from three enzyme defects (**Figure 1.7**). The most common is galactose-1-phosphate uridyl transferase deficiency in which feeding difficulties, vomiting and hypoglycaemia occur soon after birth. Later, hepatomegaly, jaundice, ascites, cataracts, mental retardation and disordered renal tubular function, particularly glycosuria and aminoaciduria, develop. Cataracts are caused by the conversion of galactose to galactitol by aldose reductase in the lens, resulting in osmotic swelling. The other features appear to be caused by excess

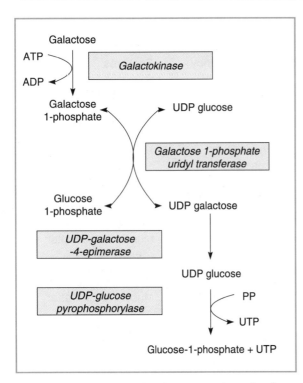

Figure 1.7 Pathway for the conversion of galactose to glucose. A deficiency of any of the three enzymes causes galactosaemia although the severity of the condition varies. ADP, adenosine diphosphate; ATP, adenosine triphosphate; PP, pyrophosphate; UDP, uridyl diphosphate; UTP, uridyl triphosphate.

galactose-1-phosphate, since hepatic, renal and brain changes do not occur in galactokinase deficiency, a mild condition in which galactitol but not galactose-1-phosphate accumulates. The clinical features of epimerase deficiency resemble those of transferase deficiency.

Disorders of Fructose Metabolism

Hereditary Fructose Intolerance

Hereditary fructose intolerance is due to a deficiency of fructose-1-phosphate aldolase B which converts fructose into two 3-carbon units, mainly in the liver. Symptoms do not develop until sucrose is introduced into the diet, when hypoglycaemia, vomiting and lethargy occur, probably as a result of intracellular accumulation of fructose-1-phosphate. Fructose is excreted in the urine, giving a positive reaction for reducing substances although not for glucose (see chapter 23).

Essential Fructosuria

This condition is caused by a deficiency of fructokinase which phosphorylates fructose. The condition is benign, fructose being excreted in urine. It is usually found after testing urine for reducing substances.

FURTHER READING

Dungar DB, Holton JB. Disorders of carbohydrate metabolism. Chapter 2. In Holton JB (ed.). *The Inherited Metabolic Diseases* (2nd edn). Edinburgh: Churchill Livingstone, 1994, pp. 21–65

Gregory JW, Aynsley-Green A. Hypoglycaemia in the infant and child. *Baillière's Clinical Endocrinology and Metabolism* 1993; **7**: 683-704

Hall R, Besser M. Chapters 14, 15 & 16. *Fundamentals of Clinical Endocrinology*. Edinburgh: Churchill Livingstone, 1989

Marks V, Teale JD. Hypoglycaemia in the adult. *Baillière's Clinical Endocrinology and Metabolism* 1993; **7**: 705–30

Nathan DM. Long-term complications of diabetes mellitus. *New England Journal of Medicine* 1993; **328**: 1676–85

Senior B, Sadeghi-Nejad A. Hypoglycaemia: a pathophysiological approach. *Acta Paediatrica Scandinavia* 1989; Suppl. 352: 1–27

The Diabetes Control and Complications Trial Research Group. The effect of intensive treatment of diabetes on the development and progression of long-term complications in insulin-dependent diabetes mellitus. *New England Journal of Medicine* 1993; **329**: 977–86

Wiener K. The diagnosis of diabetes mellitus, including gestational diabetes. *Annals of Clinical Biochemistry* 1992; **29**: 481–93

CASE 1.1

A 26-year-old patient expecting her second child was found to have glycosuria on routine testing of her urine in the antenatal clinic. An oral glucose tolerance test was carried out with the following results:

fasting blood glucose	4.9 mmol l^{-1}
1-h blood glucose	6.4 mmol l^{-1}
2-h blood glucose	5.2 mmol l^{-1}

Why was the OGTT performed and what do the results indicate?

CASE 1.2

A 27-year-old patient with IDDM was admitted in a drowsy and confused state. The breath smelled of acetone and a history of a chest infection was obtained from a relative. Initial investigations showed the following:

sodium	137 mmol l^{-1}
potassium	5.7 mmol l^{-1}
total CO_2	11 mmol l^{-1}
urea	11.4 mmol l^{-1}
blood glucose	23 mmol l^{-1}

What is the explanation for the low total CO_2 result and why were the plasma potassium and urea levels increased?

CASE 1.3

A 21-year-old nurse was found to have recurrent hypoglycaemic episodes. On investigation the following results were obtained:

Specimen	Blood glucose (mmol l^{-1})	*C*-peptide (pmol l^{-1})
1	<1.0	0.00
2	<1.0	0.01
3	<1.0	0.00
4	<1.0	0.00

What is the most likely diagnosis?

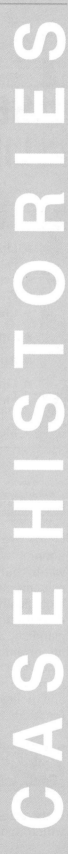

SERUM LIPIDS AND LIPOPROTEINS

INTRODUCTION

Lipids are a heterogeneous group of compounds which are relatively insoluble in water but dissolve in nonpolar organic solvents such as chloroform. They include biologically active substances, such as steroid hormones, bile acids and prostaglandins, and compound lipids which have important structural functions, e.g. sphingosine. The major lipids found in blood are cholesterol, triglycerides, phospholipids and nonesterifed fatty acids (NEFAs). The functions of these are outlined in **Table 2.1**.

LIPID AND LIPOPROTEIN STRUCTURE

Fatty Acids

Fatty acids are carboxylic acids, most of which have straight hydrocarbon chains.

The majority of those which occur naturally have an even number of carbon atoms: C2–6 are short-chain, C8–12 medium-chain and C14–24 long-chain acids. The nomenclature of fatty acids is cumbersome, chain positions being designated by both numeric and Greek characters (**Figure 2.1**). Carbon atoms are numbered from the carboxylic group (C1), the highest number being the terminal methyl carbon. The second carbon atom is designated α, the third β and the terminal methyl group ω or n. The site of double bonds is related to the ω-end of the molecule, oleic acid is monounsaturated at the ω-9 position, and the polyunsaturated eicosapentaenoic acid has five double bonds sited between every third carbon atom from the ω end (ω-3 or n-3 polyunsaturated fatty acid).

The fat content of diets varies in different geographical areas. Northern European

Table 2.1   Major serum lipids

Lipid	Function
Cholesterol	Component of cell membranes, precursor of steroid hormones, vitamin D and bile acids
Triglycerides	Storage and transport of energy, thermal insulation
Phospholipids	Component of cell membranes and lipoproteins
Fatty acids	Energy metabolism, precursors of prostanoids, component of triglycerides and phospholipids

diets contain a high proportion of animal fat rich in saturated acids, such as stearic acid, while Mediterranean diets include a high content of olive oil, rich in oleic acid. The mainstay of the traditional Eskimo is fish, together with seal and whale meat, which contain a high proportion of ω-3 polyunsa-turated fatty acids (PUFAs). The fatty acid content of diets contributes to the prevalence of coronary heart disease in a community, saturated acids are proatherogenic while oleic acid and PUFAs are antiatherogenic. Unsaturated fatty acids possibly exert their effects by actions on lipoprotein metabolism and clotting factors. Polyunsaturated fatty acids are precursors of the eicosanoids (prostaglandins, prostacyclins and leukotrienes). PUFAs are essential dietary components in man as endogenous synthesis is inadequate for eicosanoid synthesis.

Fatty acids are components of triglycerides and phospholipids and are also transported in blood from adipose tissue to sites of metabolism, mainly liver and muscle. They are complexed with but not esterified to albumin and in this form are designated nonesterified (or, less accurately, free) fatty acids (NEFAs). This transport mechanism is

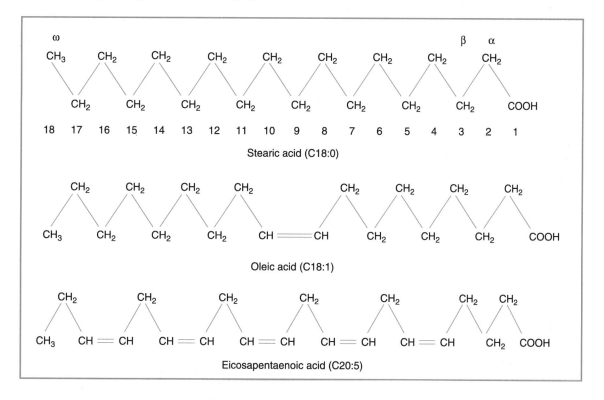

Figure 2.1   Structure of fatty acids. Stearic acid is a saturated fatty acid with 18 carbon atoms. The position of carbon atoms is designated by either Greek letters or numbers, the position of unsaturated bonds being numbered from the methyl terminal end of the molecule. Oleic acid is an ω-9 monounsaturated fatty acid and eicosapentaenoic acid an ω-3 polyunsaturated fatty acid.

necessary because fatty acids have limited solubility in water.

Triglycerides (Triacylglycerols)

Triglycerides are fatty acid esters of glycerol which usually contain a mixture of fatty acids (**Figure 2.2**). A typical Western diet contains 70–150 g triglyceride per day, this component being important for the palatability of food. Storage of energy as triglyceride in adipose tissue is very efficient because of its high calorific value and low water content. If energy reserves were all stored as glycogen rather than triglyceride a 70 kg man would weigh 210 kg!

Triglycerides are apolar lipids with no free ionizable groups. In common with phospholipids and cholesterol, which also have limited solubility in water, they are transported through lymph and blood from sites of synthesis to sites of catabolism in lipoprotein particles.

Phospholipids

Phospholipids are similar in structure to triglycerides except that phosphate and an additional polar group, such as an alcohol, are substituted on the third carbon atom of glycerol (**Figure 2.2**). This structure results in a polar and an apolar section of the molecule and thus phospholipids have detergent-like properties. Because of this, phospholipids play a key role in stabilizing hydrophobic lipids in blood, and are the main lipid constituent of cell membranes.

Cholesterol

Cholesterol is a sterol which occurs either in a free or esterified form (**Figure 2.3**). Free cholesterol is a component of cell membranes, while cholesterol ester predominates in serum, and is also the form in which cholesterol occurs in atheromatous plaques. Free cholesterol has a single polar group (-OH), the steroid ring being apolar. Esterified cholesterol is apolar.

LIPOPROTEINS

Because of their limited solubility in the aqueous environment of plasma, lipids must be stabilized for transport. Lipoproteins are

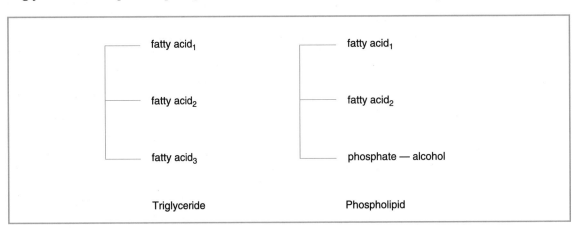

Figure 2.2 Structure of triglycerides and phospholipids. The 'skeleton' of each molecule is glycerol, this being esterified with three fatty acid molecules in triglycerides. Most naturally occurring triglycerides contain mixtures of fatty acids. Triglycerides are stored without associated water and are the most efficient form of energy store. The substitution of a polar grouping for the third fatty acid in phospholipids confers mixed physicochemical properties, part of the molecule being lipid soluble, the other part water soluble. This enables phospholipids to act as biological detergents, solubilizing triglycerides and cholesterol esters in the aqueous medium of plasma.

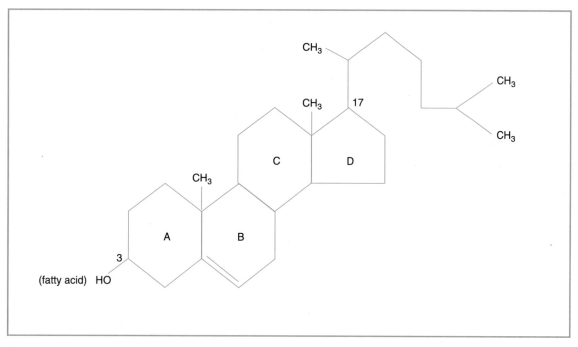

Figure 2.3 The structure of cholesterol. Cholesterol has a steroid nucleus, a hydroxyl group being attached to the third carbon atom in the A ring. There is also a hydrocarbon side-chain on C-17 in the D ring. In free cholesterol the hydroxyl group is unsubstituted while a fatty acid is esterified in this position in cholesterol ester.

particulate complexes which transport lipids in blood (**Figure 2.4**). Each lipoprotein class consists of similar components which are present in different amounts. There is an inner core of apolar lipids (cholesterol ester and triglycerides) and an outer shell containing lipids with polar groups (phospholipids and free cholesterol) and proteins (apolipoproteins), which have important structural and metabolic functions.

Lipoproteins are usually classified on the basis of their physicochemical characteristics, particularly density differences (**Table 2.2**). Thus, five lipoprotein classes are defined using ultracentrifugation, chylomicrons, very-low-density lipoprotein (VLDL), low-density lipoprotein (LDL), intermediate-density lipoprotein (IDL), and high-density lipoprotein (HDL). Chylomicrons and VLDL are the largest lipoproteins and have the highest triglyceride and lowest protein contents, expressed as a percentage of composition. Because of the high triglyceride and low protein content they are the

least dense particles. Cholesterol is mainly found in LDL, while HDL has the lowest triglyceride and highest protein contents. Lipoprotein classes may be separated on the basis of charge differences (electrophoresis) in addition to density; lipoproteins defined by these techniques are similar although not identical (**Table 2.2**).

The main lipoproteins found in the plasma of healthy fasting subjects are VLDL, LDL and HDL. Chylomicrons, the lipoproteins which transport dietary lipids, are found in the circulation postprandially. Intermediate-density lipoproteins are particles formed during the conversion of VLDL to LDL and are rapidly cleared from the circulation in normal subjects. Thus, only trace amounts are found unless IDL metabolism is disturbed.

It is important to recognize that lipoproteins defined by physicochemical characteristics are heterogeneous, subclasses of which have different metabolic origins and fates.

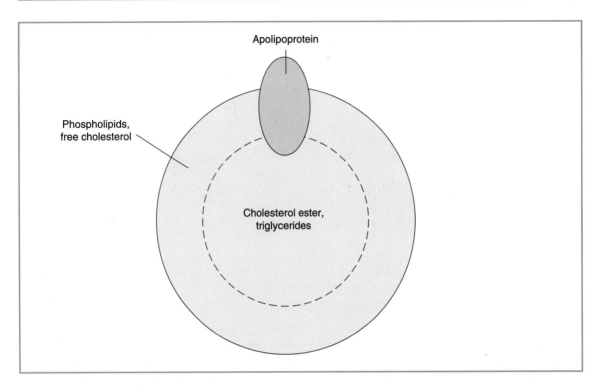

Figure 2.4 Schematic representation of the structure of a lipoprotein particle. All lipoproteins have a similar structure, an inner core of apolar lipids and an outer shell of polar lipids and apolipoproteins. The proportions of these vary in different lipoprotein species.

Table 2.2   Characteristics of lipoproteins

Lipoprotein	Diameter (Å)	Density (g ml^{-1})	Electrophoretic mobility	Composition	Major apolipoproteins	Origin
Chylomicrons	800–>1000	<0.95	origin		B-48, C, E	Intestine
Very-low-density (VLDL)	300–800	0.95–1.006	pre β		B-100, C, E	Liver, intestine
Intermediate-density (IDL)	250–300	1.006–1.019	broad β		B-100, E	VLDL
Low-density (LDL)	190–250	1.019–1.063	β		B-100	IDL
High-density (HDL)	45–190	1.063–1.21	α		A, C, E	Liver, intestine, VLDL, chylomicrons

☐ Protein, ☐ Phospholipid, ■ Cholesterol, ☐ Triglycerides

APOLIPOPROTEINS

Apolipoproteins (apos) are protein components of lipoproteins. They have three main functions:

1. As structural components apolipoproteins help stabilize apolar lipids in plasma.
2. Apolipoproteins bind to cell surface receptors, thus determining the sites of cellular uptake and degradation of lipoproteins.
3. Apolipoproteins regulate the activity of enzymes which are involved in lipoprotein metabolism (**Table 2.3**).

The main apoproteins are apos A, B, C and E, each with subclasses which have different metabolic functions. Subclasses of apos A and C are designated by Roman numerals. ApoB occurs in two forms, the larger apoB-100 and apoB-48, which has 48% of the molecular weight of the larger protein. ApoB-100 is the main apoprotein of LDL, while apoB-48 occurs only in chylomicrons. Interestingly, they are coded for by the same gene. ApoB mRNA in the gut is smaller, possibly because an enzyme changes a base in gut mRNA, producing a stop codon. Three

codominant isoforms of apoE occur, E2, E3 and E4, each coded for by a single gene. Thus, six phenotypes occur, E2/E2, E2/E3, E2/E4, E3/E3, E3/E4 and E4/E4.

LIPID AND LIPOPROTEIN METABOLISM

The metabolism of serum lipids is considered best by following the fate of lipoproteins from their synthesis to catabolism.

Metabolism of Exogenous (Dietary) Lipids

Chylomicrons

Dietary lipids are absorbed as monoglycerides, NEFAs and free cholesterol. They are re-esterified in the smooth endoplasmic reticulum within enterocytes and combine with an apoprotein, apoB-48, which is synthesized in the rough endoplasmic reticulum. After further intracellular processing chylomicrons, which also contain apoA, are secreted into the lymphatic system. Here, transfer of apoproteins between lipoproteins occurs: chylomicrons acquire apoC-II and apoE, mainly from HDL, to which apoA is transferred from chylomicrons. Chylomicrons drain into the subclavian vein with other contents of the thoracic duct.

Chylomicrons are metabolized mainly in adipose tissue and skeletal muscle (**Figure 2.5**). ApoC-II in chylomicrons activates lipoprotein lipase, which is located on the capillary endothelium in tissues, particularly adipose tissue and skeletal muscle, but also cardiac muscle and the lactating breast. Lipoprotein lipase hydrolyses triglycerides in chylomicrons, releasing fatty acids to the tissues, where they are used for synthesizing triglycerides or as a source of energy. Glycerol is also released and is transported in the blood to the liver, where it is converted to glucose. Chylomicrons shrink

Table 2.3 Properties of apolipoproteins

Property	Apolipoprotein	Particle/enzyme
Lipoprotein	B	LDL
structure	A-I	HDL
Lipoprotein	B	LDL
receptor	E	IDL, chylomicron
binding		remnants
Regulation	C-II	Lipoprotein
of enzyme		lipase
activity	A-I	Cofactor for
		LCAT

LDL, low-density lipoprotein; HDL, high-density lipoprotein; IDL, intermediate-density lipoprotein; LCAT, lecithin: cholesterol acyl transferase

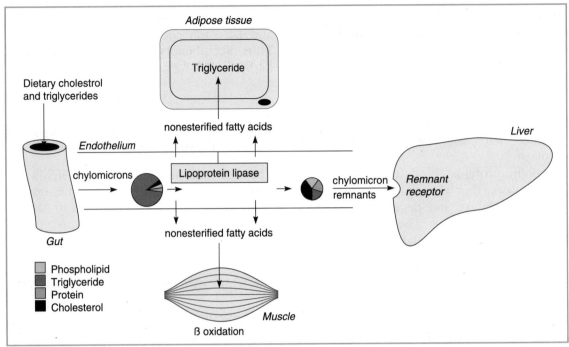

Figure 2.5 Metabolism of exogenous lipids. Dietary fats are, after digestion and absorption, resynthesized in enterocytes and secreted as chylomicrons. Triglycerides are removed and metabolized in peripheral tissues, particularly adipose tissue and muscle, while dietary cholesterol remains in the chylomicron remnant until its uptake by the liver.

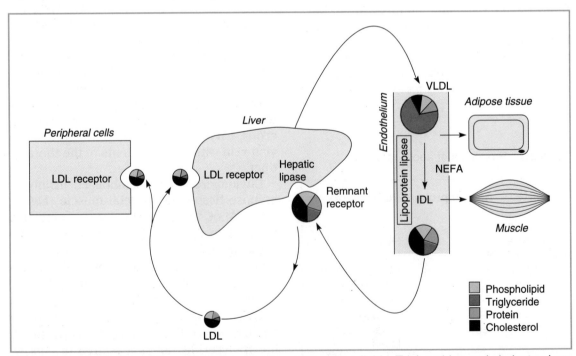

Figure 2.6 Metabolism of lipoproteins transporting endogenous lipids. Triglycerides and cholesterol are incorporated into very-low-density lipoprotein (VLDL) in the liver. VLDL is converted to intermediate-density lipoprotein (IDL) after removal of triglyceride; IDL is converted to low-density lipoprotein (LDL) by hepatic lipase. LDL is taken up and removed by specific receptors on cell surfaces, the highest density of these being in the liver. NEFA, nonesterified fatty acid.

in size as triglycerides are removed and part of the outer shell, containing phospholipids, free cholesterol and apoproteins, is split off and incorporated into HDL particles. As cholesterol ester is not removed, this component forms an increased proportion of the core lipid in chylomicron remnants. These remnants are cleared from ﺝ the circulation by the liver, after particles bind to receptors (remnant receptors) on the surface of hepatic cells. ApoE is the ligand in remnants which binds to the receptors, the particles being internalized after binding and their contents are released by enzymatic breakdown. Thus, dietary cholesterol and the remaining triglyceride in chylomicrons enter hepatic lipid pools.

Metabolism of Endogenous Lipids

Endogenous lipids are those synthesized within the body, rather than originating from the diet. Lipids synthesized in the liver are transported to peripheral tissues for metabolism, during which process three lipoprotein classes are formed: VLDL, IDL and LDL (**Figure 2.6**). The fourth lipoprotein class, HDL, is also involved in endogenous lipid metabolism.

VLDL

Triglycerides are synthesized in many tissues of the body but, with the exception of the intestine, only the liver secretes significant amounts into the blood. Triglycerides are synthesized from fatty acids which arise from three sources, *de novo* synthesis from acetyl-CoA, uptake of NEFAs from the blood, and hydrolysis of triglyceride in chylomicron remnants. The liver has a limited capacity to store triglyceride and excess is secreted into the blood in VLDL, which also contain phospholipid, cholesterol and apo B-100. Cholesterol in VLDL is derived from the diet (via chylomicron remnants) and is also synthesized in the liver. VLDL supplies peripheral tissues with triglyceride, and thus fatty acids, in the fasting state.

After secretion, VLDL acquire apoproteins, particularly apoC and apoE, from HDL. Initial metabolism is similar to that of chylomicrons – removal of triglycerides from the core of the particle by lipoprotein lipase in peripheral tissues, with uptake and metabolism of the NEFAs which are released. As VLDL shrink in size, transfer of surface components to HDL occurs and the remaining lipoprotein particles become IDL.

IDL

Intermediate density lipoproteins are sometimes referred to as VLDL remnants and are mostly converted to LDL. This involves binding of apoE in IDL to hepatic remnant receptors and removal of triglyceride from the particle, probably by hepatic lipase. This enzyme, which is also involved in HDL metabolism, differs from lipoprotein lipase. ApoE is also lost from IDL and LDL is formed.

LDL

Cholesterol is the major lipid of LDL and apoB-100 the major apoprotein. LDL is removed from the circulation by cellular uptake, mostly as a result of binding of LDL to cell-surface receptors. There are two types of receptor: one provides high-affinity binding while the other provides low-affinity binding. Uptake via the high-affinity receptor pathway occurs following binding of apoB-100 to the LDL receptors which are found in pits which occur on the surfaces of most cells. The highest density of LDL receptors is in organs that require cholesterol as a precursor for the synthesis of other steroids – the liver, adrenals and gonads. The low-affinity receptor takes up little LDL under normal conditions. However, uptake by this receptor is increased, particularly by macrophages, if the lipids and protein in LDL are altered by oxidation. This process is thought to be important in atherogenesis.

Intracellular Cholesterol Metabolism

All cells need a supply of free cholesterol since, in addition to being a precursor of

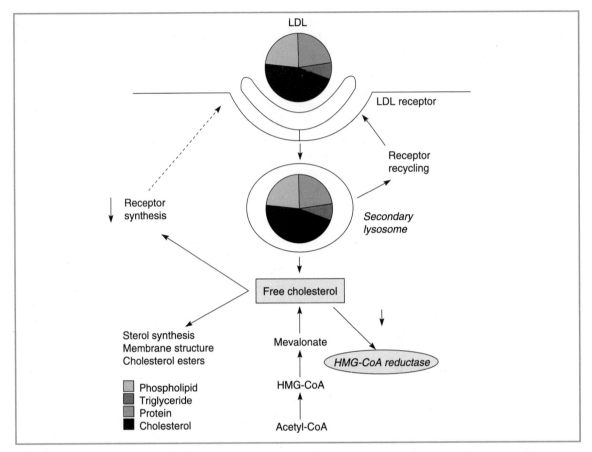

Figure 2.7 Intracellular cholesterol metabolism. (a) Intracellular cholesterol is derived from two sources, circulating low-density lipoprotein (LDL) and synthesis from acetyl coenzyme A (CoA). High intracellular free cholesterol levels limit further accumulation by inhibiting hydroxymethyl glutaryl (HMG)-CoA reductase activity and LDL receptor synthesis. Free cholesterol is continually utilized for sterol synthesis, maintaining membrane structure and for cholesterol ester synthesis.

other steroids, it is an essential component of cell membranes. Most cells are able to synthesize cholesterol from acetyl coenzyme A (CoA) by a complex biochemical pathway. Three molecules of acetyl CoA combine to form hydroxymethylglutaryl CoA (HMG CoA), which in turn can be converted into either ketone bodies or mevalonate, a precursor of cholesterol. Because mevalonate is the first intermediate committed to cholesterol formation the enzyme controlling this reaction, HMG-CoA reductase, is rate-limiting for the synthesis of cholesterol. The activity of HMG-CoA reductase is regulated by negative feedback from the end-product of the metabolic

pathway, free cholesterol. Cellular free cholesterol also regulates LDL receptor synthesis by negative feedback (**Figure 2.7**). Free cholesterol is metabolized continually, as it is required for membrane repair, in specialized cells for bile acid or steroid hormone synthesis, and is also converted to cholesterol esters.

After internalization of LDL the particles are degraded enzymatically in secondary lysosomes and the proteins, which are lysed to form amino acids, and free cholesterol are released. Free cholesterol from LDL has the same metabolic activity as cellular cholesterol, including regulation of HMG-CoA reductase activity. Under normal cir-

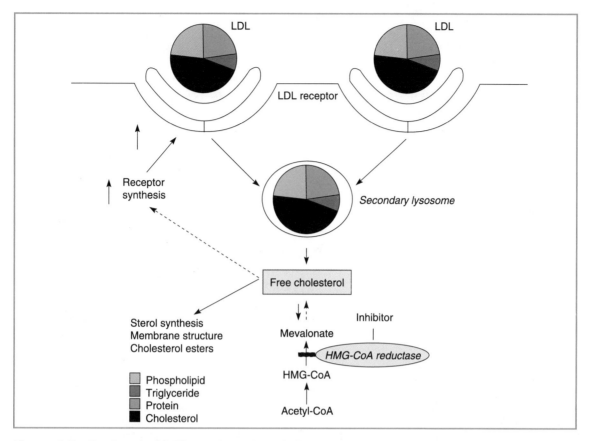

Figure 2.7 Continued. (b) The action of HMG-CoA reductase inhibitors is to reduce intracellular cholesterol synthesis by reducing mevalonate synthesis: therefore the continual losses of cholesterol must be replaced largely from LDL. LDL receptor synthesis is increased, more LDL is bound to the cell surface and internalized, thus reducing circulating LDL levels.

cumstances cholesterol synthesis is largely inhibited in peripheral tissues, requirements being met by hepatic synthesis and lipoprotein delivery, rather than being produced *de novo* in the cells.

HDL

There are several types of HDL particles which have distinct metabolic properties. Precursor or nascent particles arise from the liver, intestine and from surface components of chylomicrons and VLDL which are released as they are catabolized (**Figure 2.8**). The precursor nascent discs contain apoE, apoC, phospholipid and free cholesterol. The enzyme LCAT (lecithin:cholesterol acyl transferase) is associated with HDL and esterifies the free cholesterol; the esterified

cholesterol moves to the centre of the particle and forms a small spherical subclass of HDL, HDL_3.

An important function of HDL is transfer of cholesterol from peripheral cells to the liver – this is reverse cholesterol transport. The liver is the only organ capable of excreting significant amounts of cholesterol; this occurs in the form of bile acids, which are produced from cholesterol, and neutral sterols in the bile. Reverse cholesterol transport is thought to be antiatherogenic. Free cholesterol diffuses into HDL_3 from cells and is esterified by LCAT to form cholesterol ester. HDL increases in size as it acquires more lipid (**Figure 2.9**). This larger form of HDL, HDL_2, transfers cholesterol to the liver by at least two routes. The more

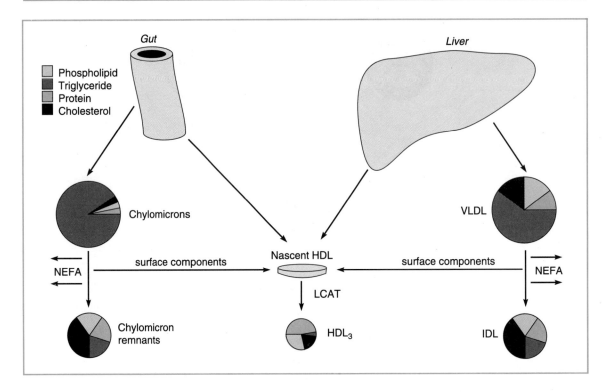

Figure 2.8 Origins of high-density lipoprotein. Nascent or precursor high-density lipoprotein (HDL) is secreted by the liver and intestine, and is also derived from the surface components of chylomicrons and very-low-density lipoprotein (VLDL). Nascent HDL is converted to HDL₃ by lecithin:cholesterol acyl transferase (LCAT) which also promotes further incorporation of free cholesterol from tissues which, after esterification, causes larger HDL₂ particles to be formed. NEFA, nonesterified fatty acids.

significant, quantitatively, is the exchange of HDL cholesterol ester with triglyceride in VLDL, a process facilitated by a protein which is found in serum, cholesterol ester transfer protein. As a result, VLDL is enriched with cholesterol ester, which remains with the particle during its conversion to LDL. As the liver has a higher density of LDL receptors than other organs a large proportion of this cholesterol is transferred to the liver.

The second route of transfer of cellular cholesterol to the liver is by HDL itself. During transfer of cholesterol ester to VLDL, HDL acquires triglyceride. Some HDL₂ is taken up by the liver by a receptor-mediated process which probably involves binding by apoE in HDL. Not all HDL₂ is removed from the circulation in this manner; some reappears in the circulation as HDL₃, which is regenerated by the removal of triglyceride from HDL₂ by hepatic lipase.

KEY POINTS

LIPOPROTEINS

- Lipoproteins consist of cholesterol, triglycerides, phospholipids and proteins (apolipoproteins)

- Apolipoproteins play key regulatory roles in lipoprotein metabolism

- Chylomicrons transport dietary lipids

- VLDL, IDL and LDL transport endogenous lipids from sites of synthesis to sites of metabolism

- HDL is involved in reverse cholesterol metabolism

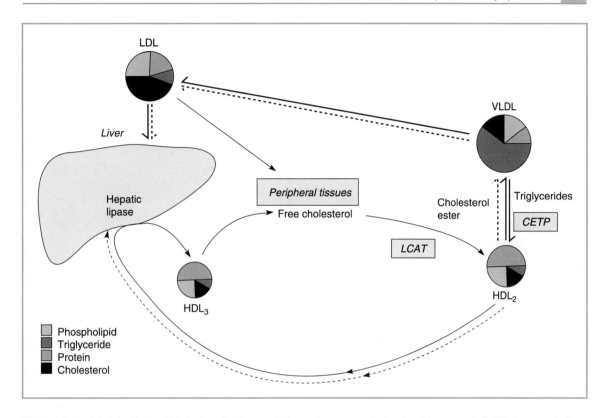

Figure 2.9 Metabolism of high density lipoprotein and reverse cholesterol transport. (HDL$_3$) accepts free cholesterol from cell membranes of peripheral tissues which is esterified to cholesterol ester by lecithin:cholesterol acyl transferase (LCAT), thus converting HDL$_3$ to HDL$_2$. Cholesterol ester is transferred to the liver directly by HDL and indirectly by transfer to very-low-density lipoprotein (VLDL) and thus low-density lipoprotein (LDL), this transfer being facilitated by cholesterol ester transfer protein (CETP). The dashed lines represent the routes of transfer of tissue cholesterol to the liver. HDL$_2$ is reconverted to HDL$_3$ by the action of hepatic lipase.

SERUM LIPIDS, LIPOPROTEINS AND DISEASE

Serum lipids and lipoproteins are important clinically because hyperlipidaemia is a risk factor for disease, hypercholesterolaemia for coronary heart disease (CHD) and hypertriglyceridaemia for pancreatitis.

There are several risk factors for CHD, some of which are modifiable while others cannot be changed (**Table 2.4**). The term risk factor implies a statistical association between the factor and CHD without necessarily indicating a causal relationship. Serum cholesterol concentrations rise with age and CHD is more prevalent in the elderly. Thus, the association between cholesterol levels

and CHD could be due to both occurring as an ageing phenomenon. However, elevated cholesterol levels do cause heart disease, this relationship being demonstrated by five lines of evidence.

1. Histopathology. Atherosclerotic lesions, which cause CHD, contain LDL cholesterol.
2. Animal Studies. Man has higher cholesterol levels than other members of the animal kingdom. If high levels are induced in animals they develop atherosclerosis.
3. Epidemiological Investigations. A clear relationship between serum cholesterol and CHD has been demonstrated when

Table 2.4 Risk factors for coronary heart disease

Nonmodifiable	Modifiable
Age	Cigarette smoking
Male sex	Hyperlipidaemia
Family history	Hypertension
Previous heart attack	Diabetes mellitus
	Diet
	Exercise patterns
	Obesity
	High fibrinogen levels

concentrations have been measured in large groups of subjects and the occurrence of subsequent diseases recorded (**Figure 2.10**).

4. Genetic Conditions. Familial hypercholesterolaemia is a genetic condition in which there is a deficiency of LDL receptors. This leads to very high cholesterol levels, which cause premature CHD.

5. Reducing Serum Cholesterol Levels. Reducing serum cholesterol levels by dietary or drug treatment reduces the incidence of CHD, the reduction being proportional to the degree of cholesterol lowering.

Total serum cholesterol is related to CHD because most cholesterol is found in LDL and LDL is atherogenic. When LDL levels are high, particles are taken up by macrophages in subendothelial spaces of arteries, forming foam cells. These aggregate to form fatty streaks, the precursors of atherosclerotic lesions. Macrophages do not contain receptors which bind normal LDL and uptake occurs either as a result of nonspecific binding or via a receptor which binds LDL which has been modified in some way. The uptake of LDL particles by macrophages is increased if the particles are modified by oxidation.

There is an inverse relationship between HDL cholesterol and CHD; thus, HDL is antiatherogenic and although this may be related to its role in reverse cholesterol transport, the precise reason for this association is not known.

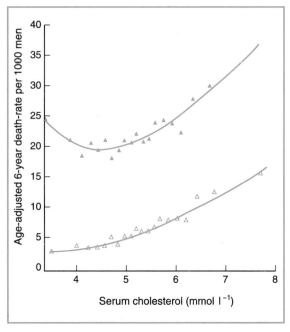

Figure 2.10 Relationship of increasing serum cholesterol concentrations to coronary heart disease and total mortality. In the MRFIT study (multiple risk factor intervention trial) cholesterol was measured in 360 000 men who were then followed up for 6 years. For concentrations above 5.2 mmol l^{-1} both total (▲) and coronary heart disease (CHD) mortality (△) increased with rising blood cholesterol. (Reproduced with permission from Martin MJ *et al. Lancet*, 1986; ii: 933–936.)

High serum triglyceride levels are associated with CHD in many studies although it is still not clear how strong this relationship is when allowance is made for high LDL cholesterol and low HDL cholesterol concentrations. These tend to occur together with high serum triglyceride concentrations. Serum triglyceride concentrations greater than 10 mmol l^{-1} are a risk factor for pancreatitis, one possible explanation being that large triglyceride-rich lipoproteins interfere with the pancreatic microcirculation.

DISORDERS OF LIPOPROTEIN METABOLISM

Disorders of lipoprotein metabolism include hyperlipidaemias, hypolipidaemias and lipid storage disorders. Hyperlipidaemias are very common and only these will be considered in detail.

HYPERLIPIDAEMIA

Definitions of Hyperlipidaemia

Reference ranges for biochemical investigations are usually determined by estimating values in a large number of disease-free men and women, ensuring that the possibility of age-related changes is considered (see chapter 24). When such measurements are made for cholesterol in the UK, 60% have values >5 mmol l^{-1}, 25% have levels >6.5 mmol l^{-1} and 10% have concentrations >7.3 mmol l^{-1}. Thus, many people without obvious heart disease have cholesterol values that are high enough to be associated with the later development of CHD (**Figure 2.10**). For this reason hypercholesterolaemia is usually defined in risk bands, levels <5.2 mmol l^{-1} indicating low risk of CHD, 5.2–6.4 mmol l^{-1} moderate risk and ≥6.5 mmol l^{-1} high risk. However, the chance of developing CHD is also affected by other risk factors (**Table 2.4**) and all of these must be considered in individual patients.

Total cholesterol concentrations are low at birth, usually <3.0 mmol l^{-1}. These rise with age, the pattern being different in men and women. In men, cholesterol levels rise through early and middle years, falling in the elderly. The concentrations increase more slowly in women until the menopause, although they then rise to overtake those in men (**Figure 2.11**). This is due to sex hormones: oestrogens lower LDL cholesterol in postmenopausal women and androgens raise total cholesterol.

Triglyceride values depend on the prandial state, fasting values being <2.0 mmol l^{-1}. Higher levels occur after a meal, owing to intestinal secretion of chylomicrons. Blood for triglycerides should be taken after a 14-h fast to ensure that there is no

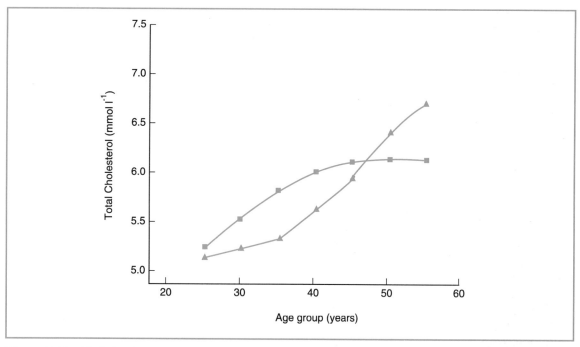

Figure 2.11   Variation in mean blood total cholesterol concentrations with age in adults. Total cholesterol levels increase in adult men (■) until middle age. Levels increase more slowly in women (▲) until the menopause, when they overtake those in men.

effect from a meal. HDL cholesterol reference values are 1.0–1.5 mmol l^{-1} in men and 1.3–1.8 mmol l^{-1} in women.

Classification of Hyperlipidaemias

The terms hyperlipidaemia and hyperlipoproteinaemia are sometimes used interchangeably although the former would be more appropriate when considering total lipid levels and the latter when lipoproteins have been fractionated. Dyslipidaemia or dyslipoproteinaemia refer to disordered lipid or lipoprotein metabolism and include conditions when lipoproteins are raised or abnormal in some other way, e.g. altered composition.

Hyperlipidaemias may occur as primary conditions or secondary to other disorders. Primary hyperlipidaemias are caused either by a genetic abnormality or are due to the interaction of diet with genetic factors. Secondary hyperlipidaemias are due to an abnormality of lipoprotein metabolism resulting from another condition (**Table 2.5**).

Primary hyperlipidaemias may be classified in more than one way (**Table 2.6**). The simplest method is to categorize the type of lipid abnormality, hypercholesterolaemia, hypertriglyceridaemia or, if both are raised, combined hyperlipidaemia. The choice of therapeutic agent is based largely on this classification if drug treatment is undertaken and it is therefore particularly useful in primary care. It does not, however, identify specific syndromes which have different modes of inheritance and varying risks of associated diseases. The second classification is based on the appearance of lipoproteins when serum proteins are separated by electrophoresis and stained for lipid content. The bands detected in this way are roughly equivalent to lipoprotein fractions obtained by ultracentrifugation (**Table 2.2**). Five patterns, designated by Roman numerals, were originally described by Fredrickson and coworkers (1967), type II hyperlipoproteinaemia subsequently being subdivided in the later WHO classification. This is still not a diagnostic but rather a phenotypic classification and conditions with different metabolic causes may have the same electrophoretic pattern. A further difficulty with the Fredrickson classification is that the phenotype may change in an

Table 2.5 Common causes of secondary dyslipoproteinaemia

Condition	Major lipid abnormality		
	Cholesterol	Triglycerides	HDL cholesterol
Diabetes mellitus	(↑)	↑	↓
Obesity	(↑)	↑	↓
Alcohol abuse		↑	↑
Hypothyroidism	↑		
Chronic renal failure		↑	
Nephrotic syndrome	↑		
Biliary obstruction	↑		
Drug induced			
β-Blockers		↑	↓
Thiazide diuretics		↑	↓
Retinoids		↑	

HDL, high-density lipoprotein.
( ), Slight changes.
↑ increased.
↓ decreased.

Table 2.6 Classification of primary hyperlipoproteinaemias

Type of lipid
◆ Hypercholesterolaemia
◆ Hypertriglyceridaemia
◆ Mixed (combined) hyperlipidaemia

Phenotypic classification
◆ Fredrickson (WHO) types I–V

Genetic (metabolic) classification
◆ Familial hypercholesterolaemia
  (Familial defective apoB-100
◆ Polygenic hypercholesterolaemia
◆ Familial combined hyperlipidaemia
◆ Familial dysbetalipoproteinaemia
◆ Familial hypertriglyceridaemia
◆ Chylomicronaemia syndrome
◆ Hyperalphalipoproteinaemia

individual with treatment and different patterns may be seen in relatives with the same condition.

With increased knowledge of the pathophysiology of hyperlipoproteinaemia the metabolic and genetic basis of these disorders is becoming clearer. Even though the precise nature of the metabolic defect is not understood in all conditions, this is the most satisfactory classification as it is more discriminatory with regard to associated disease risk (**Table 2.7**).

Familial Hypercholesterolaemia (and Familial Defective Apolipoprotein B-100)

Familial hypercholesterolaemia (FH) is an autosomal dominant condition, the heterozygous state affecting 1 in 500 of the population. It is thus one of the most common genetic disorders. There are a

Table 2.7 Genetic classification of primary hyperlipoproteinaemias

Condition	Metabolic defect	Phenotype	Serum lipids (lipoproteins)	Associated diseases
Familial hypercholesterolaemia	LDL receptor defect (apoB mutation)	IIa or IIb	↑ chol (LDL) (↑) trig	CHD+++
Polygenic hypercholesterolaemia	Interaction of genetic and dietary factors	IIa or IIb	↑ chol (LDL) (↑) trig	CHD+
Familial combined hyperlipidaemia	Increased production of apoB	IIa, IIb or IV	↑ trig (VLDL) ↑ chol (LDL)	CHD+
Familial dysbetalipoproteinaemia	Nonfunctioning apoE + overproduction of IDL	III	↑ chol (β-VLDL) ↑ trig	CHD++ Peripheral vascular disease
Familial hypertriglyceridaemia	Increased triglyceride production	IV or V	↑ trig (VLDL ± chylomicrons)	Pancreatitis +
Chylomicronaemia syndrome	Deficiency of lipoprotein lipase or apoC-II	I or V	↑↑ trig (chylomicrons + VLDL)	Pancreatitis +++
Hyperalphalipoprotein-aemia	Heterogeneous		↑ chol (HDL)	None

(↑) slight increase.
↑ increased.
+ slight increase in disease risk.
+++ marked increase in disease risk.

large number of different mutations which lead to FH, the effect of all of these being to reduce the number of high-affinity receptors for clearing LDL from blood by about 50% in heterozygotes. Structural defects in apoB can produce a similar effect as high-affinity uptake of LDL is reduced if apoB is defective (familial defective apoB-100). High serum cholesterol levels occur in heterozygous FH, typically 8–15 mmol l^{-1}. As high-affinity uptake is reduced increased amounts are bound nonspecifically by cells and if these are taken up by macrophages in arterial walls, atherogenesis occurs. The risk of premature CHD is increased greatly, patients aged 25–39 years having a 100-fold greater risk than unaffected subjects of the same age. Deposits of cholesterol often cause palpable swellings (xanthomas) in extensor tendons, particularly on the dorsum of the hand, the elbow or in the Achilles tendon. Xanthelasmas (cutaneous cholesterol deposits around the eye) and premature white rings in the cornea (corneal arcus) are less specific physical signs because these occur due to other causes of hypercholesterolaemia and also in subjects with normal lipid levels (**Plates 1–3**).

Homozygous FH, in which there is a total absence of functioning LDL receptors, occurs in 1 in 10^6 births. Cholesterol levels in blood are 15–30 mmol l^{-1} and severe atheroma can occur in childhood. Patients rarely live beyond their 20s without aggressive treatment.

KEY POINTS

FAMILIAL HYPERCHOLESTEROLAEMIA (FH)

- Heterozygous FH is common, affecting 1 in 500 of the population

- The risk of developing coronary heart disease is increased 100-fold

- Physical signs of FH include deposits of cholesterol (xanthomas) on extensor tendons

Polygenic Hypercholesterolaemia

Serum cholesterol concentrations are under the control of many genes and, if particular variants of these cluster within an individual, polygenic hypercholesterolaemia may result, particularly if dietary fat intake is high. Such genes include those coding for the LDL receptor, apoB and apoE. Polygenic hypercholesterolaemia is commoner than FH, the incidence being determined largely by the definition of the upper limit of the cholesterol reference range. The risk of coronary disease is lower than in FH and tendon xanthomas are not a feature.

Familial Combined Hyperlipidaemia

Familial combined hyperlipidaemia is characterized by variable patterns of hyperlipidaemia, hypercholesterolaemia, hypertriglyceridaemia and combined hyperlipidaemia. There is no characteristic biochemical marker although high production rates of apoB-100 occur. Diagnosis is made through detecting variable types of hyperlipidaemia in first-degree relatives. Premature coronary heart disease, xanthelasmas and premature corneal arcus are clinical features, although xanthomas do not occur and LDL receptor activity is normal.

Familial Dysbetalipoproteinaemia

This condition is also called broad beta disease or type III hyperlipoproteinaemia because of the characteristic electrophoretic pattern which occurs in most cases. It occurs in subjects who are homozygous for apoE2. This variant has a lower affinity for the remnant receptor than other apoE isoforms, thus the conversion of IDL to LDL is reduced. This leads to hyperlipidaemia when the E2/E2 phenotype is combined with overproduction of VLDL, which occurs in approximately 10% of individuals who are homozygous for this apolipoprotein. Overproduction of VLDL occurs in diabetes mellitus, obesity or hypothyroidism and these conditions are associated with familial dysbetalipoproteinaemia. Cutaneous

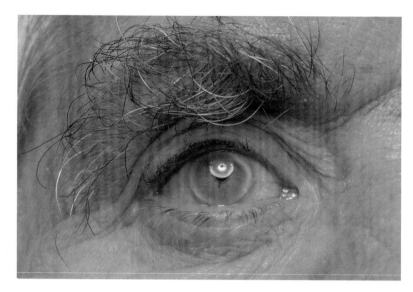

Plate 1 Corneal arcus in a patient with familial hypercholesterolaemia.

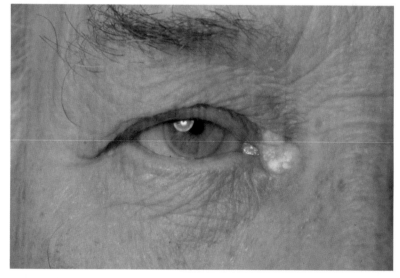

Plate 2 Xanthelasma in a patient with polygenic hypercholesterolaemia.

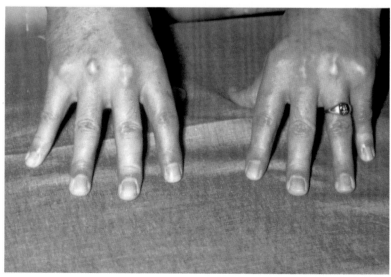

Plate 3 Tendon xanthomas in a patient with familial hypercholesterolaemia.

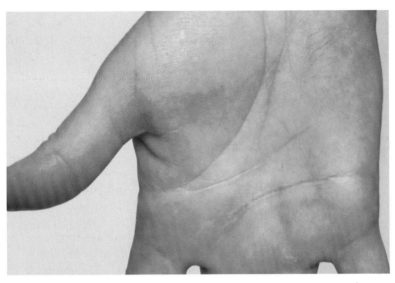

Plate 4 Xanthomas in the palmar creases of a patient with familial dysbetalipoproteinaemia.

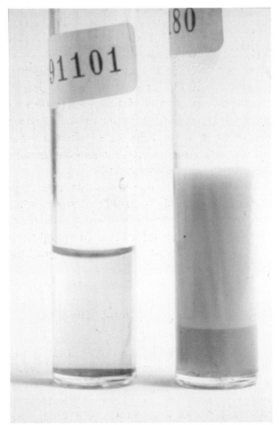

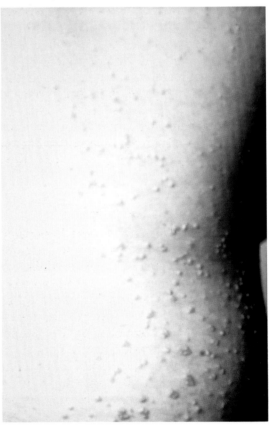

Plate 5 The plasma of a patient with chylomicronaemia syndrome (right) compared with normal plasma. The plasma stood at 4°C overnight. The top creamy layer is chylomicrons while the opalescent lower layer is due to the presence of very-low-density lipoprotein (VLDL).

Plate 6 Eruptive xanthomas on the back of a patient with chylomicronaemia syndrome.

xanthomas occur and one characteristic clinical sign is yellow streaks on the palms (palmar xanthomas; **Plate 4**). Combined hyperlipidaemia is found due to the accumulation of an abnormal cholesterol-enriched form of VLDL (β-VLDL). Familial dysbetalipoproteinaemia predisposes to both CHD and peripheral vascular disease.

Familial Hypertriglyceridaemia

Familial hypertriglyceridaemia results in high serum triglycerides, due to increased VLDL or VLDL plus chylomicrons, the latter being accompanied by more severe hypertriglyceridaemia. The pathophysiological defect is overproduction of triglyceride; in severe cases this is also accompanied by delayed removal of triglyceride-rich lipoproteins. Low HDL cholesterol levels are also found owing to a reduction in the release of the surface components of triglyeride-rich lipoproteins. Hyperlipidaemia is more severe in patients who are obese or abuse alcohol. There is an associated risk of acute pancreatitis in severe hypertriglyceridaemia.

Chylomicronaemia Syndrome

This is characterized by severe hypertriglyceridaemia which results from the accumulation of chylomicrons. The defect is impaired chylomicron clearance from blood caused by an absence of functioning lipoprotein lipase or an abnormality of apoC-II, the apolipoprotein which activates lipoprotein lipase. Triglyceride levels may be as high as 100 mmol l^{-1}, although values in the range 20–70 mmol l^{-1} are more usual. Chylomicronaemia causes a creamy appearance in plasma which becomes apparent as erythrocytes sediment (**Plate 5**). The main clinical features are recurrent acute pancreatitis, eruptive xanthomas (cutaneous punctate lesions; **Plate 6**), lipaemia retinalis (pale retina) and hepatosplenomegaly, which results from clearance and accumulation of chylomicrons in the reticuloendothelial system. Severe chylomicronaemia may also occur secondary to alcohol abuse or, rarely, uncontrolled type I diabetes mellitus.

Hyperalphalipoproteinaemia

Mild hypercholesterolaemia may sometimes be due to high HDL cholesterol levels. There appear to be several patterns of inheritance of this condition, the importance of which being that it does not result in an increased incidence of coronary heart disease.

Investigation of Hyperlipidaemia

Dyslipoproteinaemias are characterized by measuring total cholesterol, triglycerides and HDL cholesterol in blood. Clotted blood specimens are often used for total cholesterol and triglycerides although EDTA is used as an anticoagulant in blood collection tubes for HDL cholesterol, as values change after a short period if no preservative is used. Fasting blood is required for triglyceride analysis since values rise after a meal, although nonfasting blood is satisfactory for measuring cholesterol alone.

Although some physical signs are characteristic diagnosis of primary hyperlipidaemias usually involves eliminating secondary causes. Therefore additional investigations should be undertaken for the conditions listed in **Table 2.5**.

Management of Lipoprotein Disorders

The cornerstone of treatment is diet and lifestyle management; other forms of treatment being available for patients who do not respond to this initial therapy (**Table 2.8**). The decision to treat hyperlipidaemia with drugs should not be undertaken lightly as drug therapy is expensive, potentially life-long and the benefits should outweigh any risks. There is controversy concerning the long-term benefits of drug treatment to lower cholesterol levels. The objective of such treatment is to prevent the occurrence of serious disease, particularly CHD but

Table 2.8   Treatment of hyperlipidaemia

Diet

Drugs
◆ Predominantly cholesterol lowering
  Bile acid sequestering resins e.g.
  cholestyramine
  Hydroxymethyl glutaryl coenzyme A
  (HMG-CoA) reductase inhibitors e.g.
  simvastatin
◆ Predominantly triglyceride lowering
  ω-3 polyunsaturated fatty acids
◆ Lowering both triglycerides and cholesterol
  Fibric acid analogues, e.g. bezafibrate
  Nicotinic acid and analogues

Extracorporeal lipid removal
◆ Apheresis
◆ Plasmapheresis

Surgery
◆ Partial ileal bypass
◆ Liver transplantation

also, in appropriate cases, pancreatitis. Drug treatment reduces the number of heart attacks but has been shown to prolong life only in patients who are at very high risk. Patients at greatly increased risk include those with existing coronary disease and hyperlipidaemia, those in whom multiple risk factors are present or who have a genetic disorder of lipid metabolism, particularly FH or familial dysbetalipoproteinaemia. The benefit of increased life expectancy has not been demonstrated for treating isolated modest hypercholesterolaemia with lipid-lowering drugs, if no other risk factors are present.

It is important to investigate patients to establish whether secondary hyperlipidaemia is present, as treatment of these conditions is directed initially at the primary disorder. Lipid-lowering treatment is not usually needed unless patients also have a coexistent primary hyperlipidaemia.

Diet and Lifestyle Management

Most patients with hyperlipidaemia will respond to appropriate dietary measures, particularly if they are obese or have polygenic hypercholesterolaemia. The average UK diet includes 2400 calories of which 42% is fat (mainly saturated fat). Dietary measures should reduce intake to around 2000 calories per day (less for obese patients) with less fat, and increased fibre. Fat should contribute less than 35% of calories with approximately 30% as saturated, 30% as monounsaturated and 30% as polyunsaturated fat (see chapter 4). In practice this may be achieved by limiting intake of dairy produce and red meat, choosing lean cuts of meat, eating reasonable amounts of fish and chicken and increasing the intake of fresh fruit and vegetables. Fried food should be limited and olive oil and polyunsaturated oils used for cooking in place of lard. Alcohol is a rich source of calories and intake should be limited.

Other lifestyle measures which are important include counselling to give up smoking and encouraging regular exercise. Additional risk factors, such as hypertension and diabetes mellitus, should be detected and treated appropriately.

Drugs

The main cholesterol-lowering drugs are bile acid sequestrants and HMG-CoA reductase inhibitors. Bile acid sequestrants bind bile acids in the gut, limiting their absorption in the terminal ileum and leading to increased faecal loss. As a result, the liver synthesizes more bile acids from cholesterol to replace those lost, lowering serum cholesterol levels. Bile acid sequestrants have an unpleasant texture and often cause gastrointesinal side-effects. The HMG-CoA reductase inhibitors reduce cellular cholesterol synthesis, thus leading to increased uptake of LDL via the LDL receptors, particularly in the liver (**Figure 2.7b**).

The ω-3 fatty acid preparations are derived from fish oils and reduce hepatic triglyceride synthesis but do not reduce serum cholesterol. Fibric acid analogues decrease VLDL, increase lipoprotein lipase activity and increase biliary cholesterol excretion. They lower both cholesterol and triglycerides and raise HDL cholesterol levels. Nicotinic acid reduces VLDL synthesis by decreasing lipolysis in adipose tissue, thus reducing NEFA fluxes to the liver. Triglycerides and cholesterol are lowered and HDL cholesterol levels are increased. Nicotinic acid is a B vitamin but much larger doses (gram) quantities are needed for its lipid-lowering effect. Cutaneous flushing is a troublesome side-effect.

Extracorporeal Lipid Removal

Apheresis is a technique in which blood is passed from the patient to a machine that separates plasma from blood cells. LDL is then removed selectively, following which the plasma and cells are remixed and returned to the patient. The procedure is used to treat homozygous FH.

Surgery

Surgery is usually restricted to patients with severe hyperlipidaemia. The terminal ileum can be bypassed, interrupting the normal enterohepatic circulation of bile acids; these are normally reabsorbed in the distal part of the small intestine (see chapter 11). This reduces serum cholesterol levels by a mechanism similar to that described for bile acid sequestrants. Liver transplantation has been used to treat homozygous FH – the transplanted liver containing LDL receptors which are absent in this condition.

> ## KEY POINTS
>
> ## MANAGEMENT OF HYPERLIPIDAEMIA
>
> - Management should be decided on the basis of overall risk of developing disease
>
> - Initial treatment is based on dietary and lifestyle management
>
> - Lipid-lowering drugs should be prescribed only when the overall risk of disease is high

FURTHER READING

Betteridge DJ, Dodson PM, Durrington PN, *et al*. Management of hyperlipidaemia: guidelines of the British Hyperlipidaemia Association. *Postgraduate Medical Journal* 1993; **69**: 359–69

Durrington PN. *Hyperlipidaemia: Diagnosis and Management*. London: Wright, 1989

Fredrickson DS, Levy RI, Lees RS. Fat transport in lipoproteins – an integrated approach to mechanisms and disorders. *New England Journal of Medicine* 1967; **276**: 34–44, 94–103, 215–25, 273–81

Laker MF. Laboratory testing and biochemical analysis of hyperlipidaemias. *Postgraduate Medical Journal* 1993; **69** (Suppl. 1): S12–17

Law MR, Wald NJ, Thompson SG. By how much and how quickly does reduction in serum cholesterol concentration lower risk of ischaemic heart disease? *British Medical Journal* 1994; **308**: 367–73

O'Connor P, Feely J, Shepherd J. Lipid lowering drugs. *British Medical Journal* 1990; **300**: 667–72

Pownall HJ, Gotto AM Jr. Human plasma apolipoproteins in biology and medicine. Chapter 1. In: Rosseneu M (ed.), *Structure and Functions of Apolipoproteins*. Boca Raton: CRC Press, 1992, pp. 1–32

Shepherd J, Packard CJ. Lipid transport through the plasma: the metabolic basis of hyperlipidaemia. *Baillière's Clinical Endocrinology and Metabolism* 1987; **1**: 495–514

CASE HISTORIES *(vertical text in left margin)*

CASE 2.1

A 37-year-old man consulted his general practitioner because of concerns regarding a family history of coronary disease. His father had died at the age of 48 from myocardial infarction and a brother had suffered a nonfatal myocardial infarction at the age of 42. On examination he was found to have nodules in the extensor tendons on the dorsum of the hands and in the Achilles tendons. Blood lipids were measured:

total cholesterol	10.6 mmol l^{-1}
triglycerides	2.1 mmol l^{-1}
HDL cholesterol	1.1 mmol l^{-1}
LDL cholesterol	8.6 mmol l^{-1}

What action should be taken?

CASE 2.2

A 45-year-old man was found to be hypertensive and blood was taken to check his renal function. The laboratory reported that the blood was grossly lipaemic and therefore a further sample was taken for blood lipids. This showed:

total cholesterol	15.7 mmol l^{-1}
triglycerides	79 mmol l^{-1}

What are the possibilities?

CASE 2.3

A 39-year-old woman was seen in a 'well woman' clinic and blood cholesterol was measured, as her father had died of coronary disease at the age of 52. The result was:

total cholesterol	7.7 mmol l^{-1}

What action would you take?

CASE 2.4

A 53-year-old woman who was obese consulted her general practitioner because of nodules approximately 2 cm diameter which had appeared recently on the extensor surfaces of her elbows. On examination she was noted to have yellow streaks in the palm creases. Investigation showed:

total cholesterol	11.4 mmol l^{-1}
triglycerides	8.6 mmol l^{-1}
electrophoresis	Broad β-pattern

What type of hyperlipidaemia is present and how should it be treated?

PROTEINS IN PLASMA AND OTHER BODY FLUIDS

INTRODUCTION

The human body contains a vast number of different proteins – as many as 5000 occurring in a single cell. Proteins have diverse functions, many being important structural components of cells, while enzymes control cellular metabolism. Other proteins are secreted into body fluids, particularly plasma, and the concentrations of many of these are affected by pathological processes; they are therefore measured widely in the investigation of disease. Over 300 proteins have been detected in plasma but relatively few are estimated routinely. Most plasma proteins are glycoproteins, the amount of carbohydrate varying from <1% (albumin) to approximately 40% (α_1-acid glycoprotein). They contain disulphide bonds but few free thiol (–SH) groups: it is thought that this characteristic is important in preventing denaturation of proteins in plasma, which could occur due to the relatively high oxygen tension. Functions of plasma proteins include transport (**Table 3.1**), maintaining plasma oncotic pressure, buffering pH changes, humoral immunity, enzyme activity, clotting and the acute inflammatory response.

METABOLISM OF PLASMA PROTEINS

The concentration of plasma proteins is determined by three main factors: rate of synthesis; rate of catabolism; the volume of fluid in which proteins are distributed.

Table 3.1 Transport functions of plasma proteins

Substance	Protein
Hormones	
Thyroxine	Albumin, pre-albumin, thyroxine binding globulin
Cortisol	Transcortin, albumin
Metals	
Calcium	Albumin
Iron	Transferrin
Drugs	
Phenytoin	Albumin
Salicylates	Albumin
Sulphonamides	Albumin
Warfarin	Albumin
Lipids	
Cholesterol, triglycerides	Lipoproteins
NEFA	Albumin
Vitamin A	Retinol-binding protein, prealbumin
Water-insoluble excretory products	
Bilirubin	Albumin

NEFA, nonesterified fatty acid.

Synthesis

Most plasma proteins are synthesized in the liver although some are produced at other sites, e.g. immunoglobulins by lymphocytes, apolipoproteins by enterocytes and β_2-microglobulin, which is a cell surface protein, widely in the body. Approximately 25 g of plasma proteins are synthesized and secreted each day, there being no intracellular storage.

Distribution

In health, the total concentration of proteins in plasma is around 70 g l^{-1} and approximately 250 g protein are found in the vascular compartment of a 70-kg man. The total pool size in which plasma proteins are distributed is larger than the vascular space, as proteins are also found in extravascular interstitial fluid; this amount is around 350 g at any one time. Water passes more freely through capillary walls than proteins and therefore the concentration of proteins in the vascular space is affected by fluid distribution: concentrations fall with recumbency and rise on assuming the upright posture. Application of a tourniquet for extended periods leads to fluid loss from the occluded veins, increasing apparent plasma protein concentrations.

Catabolism

Plasma proteins are degraded throughout the body. A small proportion of albumin is broken down after leakage into the lumen of the gastrointestinal tract but most proteins are degraded after being taken up by cells within the body. The amino acids released are then available for the synthesis of cellular proteins.

ASSESSMENT OF PLASMA PROTEINS

Some knowledge of the methods of assessment of plasma proteins is necessary to understand changes in disease and to interpret investigations undertaken in clinical laboratories. Two types of technique are used: quantitative measurement of individual proteins or groups of proteins, and semiquantitative assessment of the proportions of different proteins present in plasma or serum.

Quantitative Measurement

Total protein is quantified by chemical methods which depend on the reaction of peptide bonds with a chemical reagent. Individual proteins are usually determined by methods which use either chemical or immunological reactions.

Semiquantitative Assessment

Proteins are separated from each other on the basis of their electrical charge. In the technique of electrophoresis, serum is applied to a support medium, usually cellulose acetate or a gel, and an electrical current applied. After a suitable period the medium is stained with a dye that visualizes the proteins. In normal subjects five or six discrete bands of proteins are seen (**Figure 3.1**) and altered patterns of these occur in various diseases. The most important abnormalities detected by electrophoresis are densely staining bands in the $\alpha_2-\gamma$ region – these are paraproteins, which result from monoclonal proliferations of B lymphocytes. Electrophoresis is usually carried out using serum rather than plasma since fibrinogen, which appears as a discrete band between the β and γ region and may thus resemble a paraprotein band, is removed during clotting. Albumin is the fastest-moving protein and is normally the most intensely staining band. The α_1-band consists almost entirely of α_1-antitrypsin while several proteins are contained in each of the other bands (**Table 3.2**). Most immunoglobulins are found in the γ region.

SPECIFIC PLASMA PROTEINS
Albumin

Albumin is present in higher concentrations than other plasma proteins, (approximately 40 g l^{-1} in normal adults). Albumin has a molecular weight of approximately 66 000 daltons and an effective molecular diameter of 7 nm. Very small amounts cross the

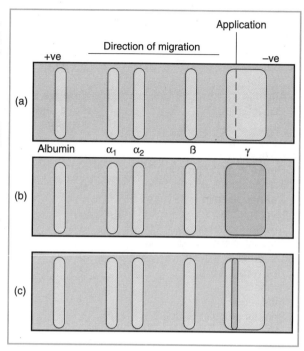

Figure 3.1 Diagrammatic representation of protein electrophoresis. (a) Normal pattern. Some subjects have two bands in the β region. (b) Diffuse hypergammaglobulinaemia. There is increased staining of proteins throughout the γ region. (c) Paraproteinaemia with decreases in other immunoglobulins (immune paresis). An intensely staining additional bands is seen in the γ region while there is less staining of the other immunoglobulins. Major contributors to each electrophoretic band are indicated in **Table 3.2.**

glomerular capillary wall, much less than would be expected from the diameter of the protein. This is because both albumin and the glomerular wall are negatively charged. Albumin is synthesized in the liver and has a half-life of approximately 20 days. Its synthesis is highly dependent on the supply of amino acids and therefore the production rate falls during periods of protein depletion. However, plasma albumin concentrations are relatively insensitive indicators of nutritional status, since the rate of catabolism also falls during starvation. The rate of catabolism of albumin increases as a result of injury, infection and surgery.

Table 3.2   Physical characteristics of plasma proteins

Protein	Electrophoretic mobility	Molecular mass (Da)	Concentration (g l^{-1})
Albumin	Discrete band	66 000	38–48
Prealbumin	Faint band before albumin	55 000	0.1–0.4
α_1-Antitrypsin	α_1	54 000	1.4–4.0
α_1-Acid glycoprotein	α_1	44 000	0.6–1.4
Retinol-binding protein	α_1	21 000	0.03–0.1
Transcortin	α_1	56 000	0.02–0.04
Caeruloplasmin	α_2	132 000	0.2–0.6
Haptoglobin	α_2	100 000	1.2–2.6
α_2-Macroglobulin	α_2	820 000	1.5–3.5
Thyroxine-binding globulin	α_2	61 000	0.01–0.04
C-Reactive protein	β	105 000	<0.003
β_2-Microglobulin	β	11 800	<0.002
Transferrin	β	77 000	1.8–2.7
Fibrinogen	β	341 000	2.0–4.5
Immunoglobulin G (IgG)	γ	150 000	8–16
IgA	γ	175 000–500 000	1–4
IgM	γ	900 000	0.6–2.6

Functions

The main functions of albumin are maintenance of plasma oncotic pressure, transport and buffering pH changes.

1. Oncotic pressure. Albumin is responsible for approximately 80% of the plasma oncotic pressure (the osmotic pressure due to proteins). This is a major determinant of the distribution of fluid between the intravascular and extravascular compartments and thus plasma volume.

2. Buffering. Plasma proteins, particularly albumin, have some buffering capacity although they do not make a major contribution to acid–base balance. However, increased H^+ binding to albumin does occur in acidotic states and, because of competition for binding sites, this may affect the transport of other substances.

3. Transport. Many substances are transported in blood bound to albumin, particularly lipid-soluble substances and certain ions. Substances transported include hormones, calcium, drugs, nonesterified fatty acid (NEFA) and bilirubin. Binding is by nonspecific mechanisms and some substances have a stronger affinity for the binding sites than others. Competition for binding may lead to displacement of drugs, altering their pharmacokinetic characteristics and increasing the concentrations of free drugs, and thus their therapeutic activity. In hyperbilirubinaemic neonates acidosis may weaken the binding of bilirubin, thus increasing the possibility that bilirubin may cross the blood–brain barrier, causing kernicterus (see chapter 12).

Reduced serum albumin levels are common, occurring in many conditions. Hyperalbuminaemia is rare and is usually caused by dehydration.

Causes of Hypoalbuminaemia

Hypoalbuminaemia may be due to artefactual, physiological or pathological factors (**Table 3.3**). As with any blood test the plasma concentration of albumin may appear low if the blood is diluted, as can occur

Table 3.3 Causes of hypoalbuminaemia

Artefactual
◆ Diluted specimen

Physiological
◆ Pregnancy
◆ Recumbency

Pathological
◆ Decreased production
  Reduced availability of amino acids
    Malnutrition
    Malabsorption
  Defective synthesis
    Analbuminaemia
    Chronic liver disease
◆ Increased volume of distribution
  Increased plasma water
    Overhydration
  Redistribution of albumin
    Liver disease
    Septicaemia
    Burns
◆ Increased loss
  From the kidney
    Nephrotic syndrome
  From the gastrointestinal tract
    Protein-losing enteropathy
  Increased catabolism
    Surgery
    Trauma
    Infection

if a sample is taken from an arm into which fluids are being infused, or if blood is taken from an indwelling cannula that has not been flushed adequately. Physiological causes include the later stages of pregnancy, in which the volume of distribution is increased, and levels are lower in recumbency than the erect posture for a similar reason.

Pathological hypoalbuminaemia may be due to decreased synthesis, increased volume of distribution, or increased losses.

Decreased Synthesis Analbuminaemia is a rare hereditary condition in which there is a failure of synthesis. Synthesis is sensitive to the supply of amino acids and thus malnutrition and, rarely, malabsorption may cause hypoalbuminaemia. Impaired hepatocyte function may result in impaired synthesis in chronic liver disease.

Increased Volume of Distribution Hypoalbuminaemia in liver disease may also result from an increased volume of distribution, particularly in cirrhosis when ascites is present, since secretion occurs into hepatic lymph and thus into ascitic fluid rather than into the hepatic vein. Increased capillary permeability leads to redistribution of albumin after trauma, operation and severe burns, and in septicaemia, although increased catabolism also occurs in these conditions.

Increased Losses Increased catabolism is common in many diseases, including infections. Protein-losing states include renal disease, particularly nephrotic syndrome, haemorrhage, severe burns and enteropathies. Loss from the gastrointestinal tract is common in many conditions and may be a relatively minor feature or the dominant abnormality. Losses are usually minor in inflammatory conditions such as Crohn's disease, whereas major losses occur where there is lymphatic obstruction, e.g. intestinal lymphangiectasia.

Consequences of Hypoalbuminaemia
These relate mainly to the osmotic and transport functions of albumin.

Oncotic Pressure Plasma concentrations less than 20 g l^{-1} are often associated with peripheral oedema although this is not inevitable, as oedema either does not occur or is mild in analbuminaemia owing to a compensatory increase in the concentration of serum globulins.

Transport The total plasma concentrations of substances transported by albumin, particularly thyroxine and calcium, will be reduced although the physiologically active fractions and thus the biological activities of these (free thyroxine and ionized calcium) are not affected. The possibility of reduced albumin should be considered when interpreting drug levels which are being measured to monitor the therapeutic effect. Phenytoin is 90% protein bound and in hypoalbuminaemia a greater proportion of the drug may be in the free form and thus pharmacologically active.

ALBUMIN

- Albumin is synthesized in the liver and has a half-life of approximately 20 days

- Calcium, unconjugated bilirubin, H^+ and drugs are transported by albumin

- Hypoalbuminaemia is caused by decreased synthesis, increased losses or an increased volume of distribution

---

Other Transport Proteins

Several other plasma proteins have important transport functions. Hormone-binding proteins are considered in the chapters on endocrine function and lipoproteins in the chapter on lipid metabolism. Retinol-binding protein and prealbumin transport vitamin A, the latter also transports some thyroxine. There are also transport proteins for vitamin B_{12} (transcobalamins) and vitamin D.

Transferrin

Transferrin is the major iron-transporting protein in plasma, binding up to two atoms of iron per molecule of protein. It is normally 30% saturated with iron. Its function is to transport iron from the intestine and between sites of synthesis and degradation of haemoglobin and other iron-containing proteins. It has a shorter half-life than albumin and its synthesis is more sensitive to the supply of amino acids. Thus, concentrations are reduced in malnutrition, liver disease, inflammatory conditions and malignancy. Iron deficiency results in increased hepatic synthesis. It is measured either as the specific protein or by determining the iron-binding capacity of serum.

Haptoglobins

The haptoglobins are a group of proteins that bind free haemoglobin to form complexes that are metabolized in the reticuloendothelial system: this has the effect of limiting iron losses which would otherwise occur because haemoglobin is small enough to be filtered by the glomerulus. Low plasma concentrations may be due to increased catabolism or decreased synthesis. Catabolism is increased in intravascular haemolysis, while decreased synthesis results from liver disease or genetic polymorphisms of the protein. Haptoglobin concentrations increase in acute inflammatory conditions – it is thus an acute-phase reactant (see below).

Retinol Binding Protein (RBP)

The function of this protein is to transport retinol (vitamin A). Although RBP is an α_1-globulin it normally circulates complexed with prealbumin. It has a shorter half-life than albumin and synthesis is more sensitive to the supply of amino acids. It is thus sometimes measured as an indicator of malnutrition. RBP has a molecular mass of 21 000 daltons (Da) and it is thus filtered by the glomeruli and reabsorbed by the renal tubules. Urinary RBP levels rise in the presence of tubular damage.

α_1-Antitrypsin and Other Protease Inhibitors

α_1-Antitrypsin (or α_1-protease inhibitor, API) is one of several plasma proteins (serpins) which inhibit proteases. These enzymes arise from several sources including endogenous production, leukocytes, and bacteria. Digestive enzymes such as trypsin and chymotrypsin are released into the circulation in small amounts and other endogenous proteases include elastase and thrombin. Infection leads to protease release from bacteria and from leukocytes, and bacterial proteases arise continually from the gut. In the absence of effective inhibitors these enzymes would cause considerable tissue damage. Deficiency of α_1-antitrypsin occurs as an inherited condition. It may be detected by noting the absence of an α_1 band on protein electrophoresis or by measuring the protein specifically. Other protease inhibitors include α_2-macroglobulin, which inactivates pepsin, and antithrombin III, which is effective against several clotting factors, in addition to trypsin.

Genetic Polymorphisms of α_1-Antitrypsin

Several genetically determined variants of α_1-antitrypsin occur, the phenotypes being designated by the prefix Pi (protease inhibitor) and over 30 alleles have been described, these being designated by a letter. The most common type is M and in the UK over 80% of the population are homozygous for this type (PiMM). Deficiency of circulating α_1-antitrypsin is most commonly found in the PiZZ phenotype with intermediate levels occurring in PiMZ. Synthesis of the defective α_1-antitrypsin occurs in the liver but there is a failure to secrete the protein; thus, it accumulates in hepatocytes and is deficient in plasma.

Clinical Consequences of α_1-Antitrypsin Deficiency

Neonatal hepatitis with evidence of cholestasis, childhood cirrhosis and emphysema in young adults result from α_1-antitrypsin deficiency. Emphysema is thought to occur because inhaled particles and infections stimulate phagocytic activity, leading to the local release of proteases. In the absence of inhibitors these damage lung tissue. Liver damage is caused by a different mechanism – granules containing immunoreactive α_1-antitrypsin accumulate in hepatic tissue and this increases susceptibility to damage from viruses or toxins. Tissue damage is most commonly found with the PiZZ and PiSZ phenotypes.

KEY POINTS

α_1-ANTITRYPSIN (α_1-PROTEASE INHIBITOR)

- α_1-Antitrypsin is an antiprotease

- Emphysema and childhood cirrhosis are associated with α_1-antitrypsin deficiency

- α_1-Antitrypsin is an acute-phase reactant

Acute-Phase Reactants

The plasma concentrations of several proteins increase in response to stresses such as myocardial infarction, inflammation, malignancy, trauma or major surgery. These proteins are termed acute-phase reactants and their synthesis is part of the body's response to injury. They include α_1-antitrypsin and some other protease inhibitors (C-reactive protein, haptoglobin, caeruloplasmin and fibrinogen). Plasma levels of acute-phase reactants increase within 24 h of injury in response to humoral mediators, particularly cytokines, which include interleukin-I (IL-1), IL-6, tumour necrosis factor α and β, the interferons, and platelet-activating factors. These are produced by tissue macrophages, monocytes and endothelial cells. They have diverse functions, including binding to polysaccharides in bacterial walls, activating complement and stimulating phagocytosis. Humoral effects of IL-1 and IL-6 include increased production of ACTH and thus cortisol, and inhibition of hepatic synthesis of proteins other than acute-phase reactants, including albumin, prealbumin and transferrin. The protease inhibitors probably inactivate enzymes released from lysosymes and minimize damage that these would otherwise cause.

The acute-phase response leads to increases in the α_1- and α_2-globulin bands on electrophoresis although this pattern, like the response, is nonspecific. Measurement of individual acute-phase proteins may be useful in detecting occult tissue damage or for assessing disease activity.

C-Reactive Protein

This protein is so-named because of its property of binding strongly to the C polysaccharide of pneumococcal cell walls. It is probably synthesized by macrophages. Very large increases in plasma C-reactive protein occur in many inflammatory conditions and it is measured to detect and monitor disease, e.g. rheumatoid arthritis.

α_1-Acid Glycoprotein

Plasma concentrations of α_1-acid glycoprotein, also called orosomucoid, rise in response to a variety of acute and chronic inflammatory stimuli. Its function is unknown but it is sometimes measured as an indicator of the acute-phase response.

Caeruloplasmin

The function of caeruloplasmin has not been clearly defined. It contains over 90% of serum copper, although the metal is tightly bound and does not exchange readily; thus it may not be a physiological transport protein. Caeruloplasmin is an oxidoreductase and it has been suggested that this property is important in the acute-phase response, as it is able to inactivate free radicals, which are highly reactive chemical species with unpaired electrons (e.g. OH$^{\bullet}$) derived from oxygen, capable of producing tissue damage. Free radicals are produced during bursts of oxidative metabolism such as occur during phagocytosis. Plasma levels of caeruloplasmin (and thus copper) are usually low in Wilson's disease, a genetic condition in which copper accumulation occurs in the liver, leading to cirrhosis, and in the basal ganglia of the brain causing choreoathetosis. Plasma caeruloplasmin concentrations are very sensitive to the effects of oestrogens, and rise during pregnancy and in response to oral oestrogens.

Immunoglobulins

The immunoglobulins (Igs), which are antibodies, are a heterogeneous group of plasma proteins produced by B lymphocytes. Most are found in the γ region on electrophoresis although some occur in the β and α_2 regions. Five classes of immunoglobulins are recognized (**Table 3.4**) which have a similar basic structure. Each immunoglobulin unit consists of four polypeptide chains, two heavy (mass 50 000–75 000 Da) and two light (mass 22 000 Da), which are linked by disulphide bridges. The heavy chains (γ, α, μ, δ, ϵ) are specific to a particular immunoglobulin class while there are two types of light chains (κ and λ) which occur in all immunoglobulin classes. When

Table 3.4 Characteristics of the major immunoglobulin (Ig) classes

I	IgG	IgA	IgM	IgD	IgE
Molecular weight	150 000	160 000 +dimer	900 000	185 000	200 000
Number of Ig units	1	1,2	5	1	1
Heavy chains	γ	α	μ	δ	ϵ
Light chains	κ,λ	κ,λ	κ,λ	κ,λ	κ,λ
Antigen-binding sites	2	2,4	5	2	2
Serum concentrations	7–16 g l^{-1}	0.7–4 g l^{-1}	0.4–2 g l^{-1}	<0.04 g l^{-1}	<0.5 mg l^{-1}

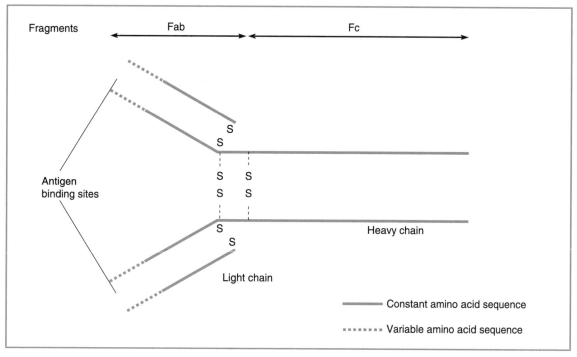

Fragments

Fab

Fc

Antigen binding sites

S
S

S　S
S　S

S
S

Heavy chain

Light chain

———— Constant amino acid sequence

········ Variable amino acid sequence

Figure 3.2　Diagrammatic representation of an immunoglobulin molecule. The molecule consists of two heavy chains which are one of five types (γ, α, μ, δ, or ϵ) which are specific for the immunoglobulin class and two light chains (κ or λ) which occur in each immunoglobulin class.

visualized, immunoglobulins have a Y-shaped structure, the arms of which (Fab fragments) consist of the light chains and part of the heavy chains, and contain the antibody-binding sites (**Figure 3.2**). The stem of the molecule (Fc fragment) consists of part of the heavy chains. The amino acid sequences of the *N*-terminal ends of both the light and heavy chains are highly variable while they are relatively constant in the remaining portions of the chains. Internal disulphide bonds in the peptide chains form loops or domains, several of which have specific functions. Thus, areas of the heavy chains which bind complement have been identified, while the *C*-terminal domain binds immunoglobulins to monocytes.

Immunoglobulin G

Approximately 75% of plasma immunoglobulins are IgG, these being the major antibodies produced during secondary immune responses. IgG diffuses more readily into extravascular spaces than other immunoglobulins and also crosses the placenta, conferring passive immunity on neonates for their first few weeks of life. They neutralize bacterial toxins and bind to microorganisms, enhancing phagocytosis.

Immunoglobulin A

IgA is the major class of antibodies in secretions, including tears, saliva and secretions of the respiratory, genitourinary and gastrointestinal tracts. They exist either as single immunoglobulin units or as dimers linked by a secretory unit (molecular weight 60 000) and an additional polypeptide chain (J chain, molecular weight 20 000). IgA coat microorganisms and inhibit their adherence to mucosal surfaces.

Immunoglobulin M

IgM is the major class of antibodies secreted in the early stages of a primary immune response. These immunoglobulins are polymers of five immunoglobulin units linked around a J chain. They are largely confined to the vascular space and are particularly effective agglutinating and cytolytic antibodies. After birth IgM is synthesized and levels rise progressively as the infant is exposed to antigenic stimuli. Measurement of neonatal IgM is a useful indicator of intrauterine infection.

Immunoglobulin D

IgD immunoglobulins are found on the surface of resting B lymphocytes where they probably function as receptors for antigens. Plasma concentrations are very low.

Immunoglobulin E

IgE antibodies are bound firmly to the surface of mast cells and present only in minute amounts in plasma. Binding of antigen results in degranulation of mast cells with release of active amines, including histamine, giving rise to hypersensitivity reactions, including hay fever.

Hypergammaglobulinaemia

Increased immunoglobulin levels may result from stimulation of many clones of B cells (polyclonal hypergammaglobulinaemia), relatively few clones (oligoclonal) or monoclonal proliferation (paraproteinaemia).

Polyclonal Hypergammaglobulinaemia

Stimulation of many B-cell clones produce a wide range of antibodies which appear as a diffuse increase in γ-globulin on electrophoresis (**Figure 3.1b**). Acute and chronic infections, autoimmune disease and chronic liver disease produce this type of response. These conditions may cause increases in one predominant immunoglobulin class although measurement of these is rarely helpful in diagnosis.

Oligoclonal Hypergammaglobulinaemia

A more restricted range of antibodies sometimes occurs in response to antigenic stimuli which can produce discrete bands in the γ-globulin region. Occasionally, these may resemble a paraproteinaemia although both types of light chains are found in oligoclonal hypergammaglobulinaemia.

Monoclonal Hypergammaglobulinaemia

Proliferation of a single B-cell clone produces a single immunoglobulin which appears as a discrete densely staining band (paraprotein or M band) on electrophoresis (**Figure 3.1c**). Although occasionally due to a benign cause paraproteins are characteristic of malignant B-cell proliferation (**Table 3.5**). Paraproteinaemia is rare in chronic lymphatic leukaemia and lymphomas.

Multiple Myeloma. Multiple myeloma, which is the commonest cause of paraproteinaemia, is a disseminated malignancy of plasma cells, although isolated lesions (plasmacytomas) occur occasionally. Multiple myeloma produces a wide range of pathological features (**Table 3.6**). Most secrete significant amounts of mature immunoglobulins, usually IgG or IgA which, because they are synthesized by a single clone, contain only one class of light chain. The amount of immunoglobulin produced, and thus the plasma concentration, is related to the tumour mass. Fragments of immunoglobulins may be produced, including dimers of free light chains (Bence–Jones protein); this is found in approximately 50% of cases and may be the only abnormal protein in 20% of cases of myeloma. These are found characteristically in urine, since they have a molecular weight of 44 000 and are thus cleared by the glomerulus.

Table 3.5 Causes of paraproteinaemia

Malignant
◆ Myeloma
◆ Plasmacytoma
◆ Waldenström's macroglobulinaemia
◆ Chronic lymphatic leukaemia
◆ Non-Hodgkin's lymphoma

Benign

Table 3.6 Features of Myeloma

Feature	Cause
Clinical	
Bone pain	Tumour proliferation, pathological fractures
Anaemia	Replacement of bone marrow
Recurrent infections	Reduced normal immunoglobulins
Renal failure	Proteinuria, hypercalcaemia, hyperuricaemia, amyloid
Hyperviscosity syndrome	Hyperproteinaemia
Biochemical	
High serum total protein	Paraprotein synthesis
Low serum immunoglobulins	Suppression of synthesis by tumour
Proteinuria	Bence–Jones protein
Fanconi syndrome	Renal tubular damage
Uraemia	Renal failure
Hypercalcaemia	Skeletal destruction
Hyponatraemia	Interference with measurement (see chapter 5)
Other	
Increased ESR	Rouleaux formation

ESR, erythrocyte sedimentation rate.

Occasionally, myelomas produce only heavy chains. Amyloidosis, a condition caused by tissue deposits of a fibrous protein, is a rare complication of myeloma. The protein deposits in amyloidosis may be of several different types but in myeloma they appear to be related to light chains.

KEY POINTS

MULTIPLE MYELOMA

- Multiple myeloma is caused by a malignant proliferation of B cells

- Bone pain and anaemia are common clinical features

- Abnormal proteins produced include monoclonal immunoglobulins (paraproteins) and Bence–Jones protein (light chain dimers)

Waldenström's Macroglobulinaemia This disease is a malignancy of plasma cells which produce IgM. In contrast to myeloma it does not cause bone pain or hypercalcaemia but is associated with lymphadenopathy and hepatosplenomegaly. The major clinical manifestations arise from hyperviscosity, which is due to hyperproteinaemia – IgM leads to higher plasma viscosity than the equivalent concentration of IgG. Hyperviscosity leads to impaired circulation of blood through capillaries causing headache, fatigue, visual disturbances, retinopathy and an increased tendency to thrombosis. Approximately 6% of IgM paraproteins are cryoglobulins (see below). Treatment includes, in addition to chemotherapy, plasmapheresis to remove the paraprotein and thus control the symptoms resulting from hyperviscosity. The prognosis is more favourable than in myeloma.

Benign Paraproteinaemia Some paraproteins are benign, although such a diagnosis is one of exclusion and conditions that appear benign initially may develop malignant features. Criteria supporting a benign paraproteinaemia include the absence of clinical features such as bone pain, which are suggestive of myeloma, a paraprotein concentration of less than 10 g l^{-1}, no Bence–Jones proteinuria, a normal bone-marrow biopsy, no lytic bone lesions and stable features on follow up.

Cryoglobulins

Cryoglobulins are immunoglobulins which precipitate when cooled to 4°C and which redissolve when warmed to 37°C. Approximately 50% of cryoglobulins are paraproteins while others are complexes of immunoglobulins and anti-immunoglobulins, these most often being produced by rheumatoid factor. Many cryoglobulins are simply curiosities although some which precipitate above 22°C can cause clinical symptoms. Such temperatures occur in the extremities in cold weather and cryoglobulinaemia is one of the causes of Raynaud's phenomenon (episodic ischaemic pain in the extremities precipitated by cold weather).

Investigation of Paraproteinaemia

Electrophoresis of serum is undertaken to establish whether a monoclonal band is present; these usually occur in the $\alpha_2–\gamma$ zone. Measurement of the paraprotein concentration is important, high or increasing levels increasing the probability of malignancy. Malignancy is also more likely if the concentrations of other immunoglobulins are reduced. Urine should be tested for Bence–Jones proteinuria, the presence of which is also strong indication of malignancy. Complications of myeloma include hypercalcaemia and impaired renal function, and it is therefore important to monitor these. Impaired renal function at presentation indicates a poor prognosis, as does anaemia. High serum β_2-microglobulin concentrations are also indicate a poor prognosis, as β_2-microglobulin reflects both tumour mass and impaired renal function.

Immunoglobulin Deficiency

Immunoglobin concentrations, except for IgG, are very low at birth but rise steadily during childhood years. Synthesis may be defective due either to congenital or acquired disorders. Congenital deficiencies are a heterogeneous group of syndromes which vary in severity from gross impairment of both humoral and cell-mediated immunity to partial defects of humoral immunity, affecting one or two immunoglobulin classes. Patients with defects in humoral immunity suffer from recurrent bacterial infections and also multiple bouts of viral infections in which an initial attack would be followed normally by permanent immunity, e.g. chickenpox. Diminished concentrations of one or more immunoglobulin classes are the most frequent abnormalities, although the wide range of values found in adults makes the lower limits of normal difficult to define. In addition to the measurement of immunoglobulin concentrations, evaluation of immune deficiency involves assessment of specific antibodies, complement components and cell studies, these being undertaken by specialized immunology units.

Secondary immunoglobulin deficiencies are more common than primary disorders. Neonates have a physiological deficiency which is more marked in premature infants, as transplacental transfer of IgG occurs in the last trimester of pregnancy. Decreased production of normal immunoglobulins is often found in lymphoid tumours, including multiple myeloma, Hodgkin's disease and chronic lymphatic leukaemia, while production is suppressed by steroid and cytotoxic drug therapy. Immunoglobulin losses occur in protein-losing states such as nephrotic syndrome or protein-losing enteropathy.

Complement

The complement system consists of a group of proteins that function together with immunoglobulins to eliminate foreign antigens from the body. They are activated by either the classical or alternative pathways. The classical pathway is initiated by antigen–antibody complexes while the alternative pathway is activated by products of the classical pathway or by stimuli such as bacterial lipopolysaccharides. Activated complement enhances lysis of bacteria and stimulates chemotaxis of phagocytes. The permeability of capillary walls is also increased allowing cells and other proteins, particularly immunoglobulins and acute-phase reactants, to reach affected areas. Complement components, particularly C3 and C4, are consumed during immune reactions and are sometimes measured in the investigation of immune complex disease, e.g. systemic lupus erythematosis (SLE) and mesangiocapillary glomerulonephritis.

Other Proteins

β_2-Microglobulin

This protein is synthesized by most tissues in the body and is part of the human leukocyte antigen (HLA) system which is found on cell surfaces. β_2-Microglobulin is a small protein (molecular weight 11 800 Da) that can be filtered by the glomerulus. It is normally reabsorbed almost completely by and degraded in the proximal tubule, although reabsorption is reduced if tubular function is impaired. β_2-Microglobulin is thus measured in urine as an indicator of tubular damage, although it is less stable than RBP. Serum levels of β_2-microglobulin increase in chronic renal failure owing to reduced glomerular clearance. Plasma levels are also useful in monitoring myeloma.

Proteins in Urine

The pathophysiology and investigation of proteinuria is discussed in chapter 8.

Proteins in Cerebrospinal Fluid

Cerebrospinal fluid (CSF) is an ultrafiltrate of plasma and normally contains low levels of protein (0.1–0.4 g l^{-1}) although higher levels (up to 0.6 g l^{-1}) occur in the elderly and also in neonates. Albumin is the main protein present in normal CSF. Contamination of the CSF with blood can occur during lumbar puncture and this will cause considerable elevations in protein concentrations, as values are 100-fold higher in plasma. Concentrations are raised in meningitis, mainly because of increased permeability caused by meningeal inflammation, although IgG synthesis and secretion into the CSF makes a small contribution. Higher values occur in pyogenic and tuberculous disease than in viral meningitis. Increased CSF protein concentrations also occur in cerebral tumours, with very high values (>5 g l^{-1}) being found if there is obstruction to the normal circulation of CSF (Froin's syndrome).

Local production of IgG in the subarachnoid space occurs in multiple sclerosis, neurosyphilis and various other conditions affecting the central nervous system, in addition to meningitis. This produces an increase in the IgG:albumin ratio. IgG synthesized in the central nervous system has limited heterogeneity, presumably because a small number of B cells are responsible. Thus, a small number of discrete bands are seen on electrophoresis (oligoclonal pattern).

FURTHER READING

Rees RC. Cytokines as biological response modifiers. *Journal of Clinical Pathology* 1992; **45**: 93–8

Roitt I. *Essential Immunology* (7th edn). Oxford: Blackwell, 1991

Whicher JT. Abnormalities of plasma proteins. Chapter 28. In Williams DL & Marks V, eds, *Biochemistry in Clinical Practice* (2nd edn). London: Heinemann, 1994

Whicher JT, Calvin J, Riches P, Warren C. The laboratory investigation of paraproteinaemia. *Annals of Clinical Biochemistry* 1987; **24**: 119–32.

Whicher JT, Spence CE. When is albumin worth measuring? *Annals of Clinical Biochemistry* 1987; **24**: 572–90

CASE HISTORIES

CASE 3.1

A 56-year-old man was referred for investigation of back pain which had been increasing for several weeks. On examination he appeared anaemic and the following results were obtained from blood tests:

total protein	98 g l^{-1}
albumin	32 g l^{-1}
total calcium	3.48 mmol l^{-1}
phosphate	1.10 mmol l^{-1}
alkaline phosphatase	94 U l^{-1}
haemoglobin	8.7 g dl^{-1}
erythrocyte sedimentation rate (ESR)	110 mm h^{-1}

Multiple myeloma was suspected. Are these results consistent with the diagnosis? What other investigations should be performed?

CASE 3.2

A 62-year-old woman was being investigated for bone pain and anaemia. Blood tests showed:

total protein	74 g l^{-1}
albumin	42 g l^{-1}
total calcium	2.34 mmol l^{-1}
phosphate	1.21 mmol l^{-1}
alkaline phosphatase	86 U l^{-1}
electrophoresis	densely staining band in γ region ? paraprotein

The investigations were repeated 2 days later, also testing for Bence–Jones protein in urine. The possible paraprotein band in serum had disappeared. What could be going on?

CASE 3.3

A patient with long-standing Crohn's disease was investigated for recurrent abdominal pain and weight loss. The following blood test results were obtained:

total protein	34 g l^{-1}
albumin	17 g l^{-1}
total calcium	1.90 mmol l^{-1}
phosphate	0.95 mmol l^{-1}
alkaline phosphatase	74 U l^{-1}

How may these results be explained?

NUTRITION

INTRODUCTION

Good nutrition is important for normal growth and development, and is also important in the prevention and treatment of disease. Disorders of nutrition may be due to dietary deficiencies or because excess nutrients are ingested. Nutritional factors contribute to three common disorders in developed societies: Type 2 diabetes mellitus and obesity, in which energy intake is in excess of requirements, and coronary heart disease (CHD), in which the fat content of the diet plays a role. Both generalized (e.g. protein–energy malnutrition) and specific (e.g. scurvy) deficiencies occur. Both are now rarer in affluent societies than previously, but they still occur all too commonly in third-world countries. In addition to primary deficiencies the nutritional state may be abnormal secondary to other conditions, particularly gastrointestinal and chronic debilitating diseases.

DIETARY CONSTITUENTS

Carbohydrates

Carbohydrates provide a major part of the energy intake in human diets, amounts varying from 40% of calories in affluent societies to 85% in poor countries. Neither of these extremes is desirable, since the fat intake is high in developed societies, while dietary protein is often deficient in poor countries. Current recommendations suggest 55–60% of energy intake should be in the form of carbohydrate. There are two forms of dietary carbohydrates: available, which are digested and absorbed in the small intestine, and nonavailable carbo-

Table 4.1 Available carbohydrates

Carbohydrate	Source	Constituent monosaccharides	Average daily intake (g)
Polysaccharides			
Starch	Cereals, root vegetables	Glucose	250
Glycogen	Meat	Glucose	Negligible
Disaccharides			
Sucrose	Cane sugar, beet	Glucose, fructose	100
Lactose	Milk	Glucose, lactose	15
Monosaccharides			
Glucose	Honey, fruits		5
Fructose	Fruits		5

hydrates (dietary fibre), which are metabolized by the bacterial flora in the large intestine (see chapter 10). Deficiencies of dietary carbohydrates are considered under malnutrition (see below). Available carbohydrates are outlined in **Table 4.1**.

Fats

Fats provide a concentrated source of energy, and are important for the palatability of food. Recommended daily intakes of the different types of fat and the role of dietary fat in the pathogenesis of CHD are considered in chapter 2.

Protein

Proteins contribute 10–15% of calories in a well-balanced diet, the intake being 70–100 g per day. The quality of dietary protein is important in addition to the amount, as man is unable to synthesize some amino acids and therefore these are essential dietary constituents. Protein intake should be varied because some animal and particularly vegetable proteins contain a relative lack of one of the essential amino acids. National and international agencies publish recommended daily dietary intakes which include special requirements for childhood, adolescence, pregnancy and lactation.

Vitamins

Vitamins are organic substances which are not synthesized in the body in sufficient quantities to meet requirements and are therefore needed in the diet, although in small amounts. The two main groups are fat-soluble and water-soluble vitamins. The major vitamins, together with their sources and daily requirements, are outlined in **Table 4.2**.

Water-Soluble Vitamins

Thiamin (Vitamin B$_1$) The most important dietary sources of thiamin are the seeds of plants. After absorption, thiamin is phosphorylated in the brain or liver and serves as a cofactor in oxidative decarboxylation of α-keto acids, including pyruvate, and in the transketolase reaction in the hexose monophosphate shunt. Thiamin is found in large amounts in tissues with very active carbohydrate metabolism, including skeletal and cardiac muscle, liver, kidney and brain. Deficiency occurs in chronic alcoholics, when poor nutrition, impaired absorption and storage, and increased losses of thiamin pyrophosphate are contributory factors. Increased losses also occur in dialysis. In developing countries, high intake of foods containing thiaminases, such as milled rice, may lead to deficiency.

Table 4.2 Vitamins

Vitamin	Sources	Recommended daily intakes for adults
Water-soluble vitamins		
Thiamin (B$_1$)	Cereals, nuts, pulses	0.4 mg (1000 kcal)$^{-1}$
Riboflavin (B$_2$)	Liver, dairy produce, green vegetables	0.55 mg (1000 kcal)$^{-1}$
Niacin	Meat, fish, cereals, pulses, endogenous synthesis	6.6 mg (1000 kcal)$^{-1}$
Pyridoxine	Cereals, vegetables, fruit, liver	2.2 mg
Biotin	Liver, pulses, eggs, enteric bacteria	300 μg
Folate	Liver, spinach, cabbage	400 μg, 500 μg in pregnancy
Vitamin B$_{12}$	Liver, egg yolks, milk	3 μg
Vitamin C	Fruit, green vegetables	30 mg
Fat-soluble vitamins		
Vitamin A	Dairy produce, liver, oily fish	750 μg
Vitamin D	Endogenous synthesis, liver, dairy produce	2.5 μg
Vitamin E	Vegetable oils	10 mg
Vitamin K	Leafy vegetables	40 μg

There are two major clinical manifestations of deficiency, wet beri-beri and neurological disease. Wet beri-beri predominantly affects the cardiovascular system, although neurological manifestations may also be present. Peripheral vasodilatation, myocardial failure and retention of sodium and water occur, leading to high output cardiac failure and peripheral oedema. Dietary deficiency is an important factor in its pathogenesis. The nervous system is often involved in thiamin deficiency affecting alcoholic patients. This may cause peripheral neuropathy, a psychosis (Korsakoff syndrome) or an encephalopathy (Wernicke's encephalopathy). A thiamin-responsive cardiomyopathy may also occur.

Urinary excretion of thiamin is a poor indicator of deficiency, as excretion falls to low levels before tissue depletion occurs. The most reliable method used to investigate possible thiamin deficiency is the measurement of the activity of an enzyme that is dependent on thiamin – erythrocyte transketolase is usually used.

Riboflavin (Vitamin B$_2$) Riboflavin is a component of flavin mononucleotide and flavin adenine dinucleotide coenzymes, these being essential for energy metabolism and cellular respiration. Riboflavin is widely available – meat, eggs, milk and cereals are rich sources. Deficiency is therefore rare, although it is seen occasionally in alcoholic patients, when the intake of other vitamins and nutrients may also be lacking. Clinical features of deficiency include glossitis, angular stomatitis, seborrhoeic dermatitis and anaemia. Deficiency is investigated by measuring the activity of glutathione reductase in erythrocytes, with and without added flavin adenine dinucleotide, an essential cofactor for the enzyme.

Nicotinic Acid Nicotinic acid (niacin) is an essential component of coenzymes which are required for many oxidation–reduction reactions, nicotinamide adenine dinucleotide (NAD) and nicotinamide adenine dinucleotide phosphate (NADP). Some nicotinic acid is produced endogenously from tryptophan, although the production of this is insufficient to meet all requirements. Deficiency causes pellagra which was endemic in countries in which there is a high intake of maize or millet, but is now rare as such diets are supplemented with other cereals. Pellagra is seen occasionally as a secondary condition in two disorders of tryptophan metabolism, carcinoid syndrome and Hartnup disease. In the carcinoid syndrome, large amounts of tryptophan are metabolized to 5-hydroxytryptamine, while the absorption of several amino acids, including tryptophan, is impaired in Hartnup disease. Clinical features of pellagra include weight loss, anaemia, photosensitive dermatitis, dementia and diarrhoea. Deficiency may be investigated by measuring the urinary excretion of nicotinic acid or its metabolite N'-methylnicotinamide. Plasma tryptophan levels are often low in Hartnup disease and carcinoid syndrome (chapter 17).

Pyridoxine (Vitamin B$_6$) Pyridoxine phosphate and its derivatives form coenzymes that are involved widely in amino acid metabolism, particularly transamination and decarboxylation reactions. It is also required for the synthesis of the haem precursor δ-aminolevulinic acid (see chapter 21). Isolated dietary deficiency is extremely rare in adults since many foods contain pyridoxine. Drugs affecting vitamin B$_6$ status include isoniazid, which is used in the treatment of tuberculosis. This combines with pyridoxine, causing deficiency which leads to peripheral neuropathy. Several inherited metabolic disorders respond to supplementation with large doses of vitamin B$_6$; these are due to defects in enzymes which require pyridoxine – large supplements overcome defective binding of the cofactor to the enzyme.

Deficiency may be investigated by determining the activity of a transaminase, usually aspartate aminotransferase, in haemolysates of erythrocytes with and without the addition of its cofactor, pyridoxal phosphate.

Biotin Biotin is the prosthetic group for carboxylase enzymes. These include pyruvate carboxylase, which is important in gluconeogenesis, and acetyl CoA carboxylase, a key enzyme in fatty acid synthesis. Biotin is synthesized by intestinal bacteria and is found in the whites of eggs, where it is bound by the protein avidin. Cooking releases the bound biotin but if raw eggs are ingested, avidin binds free biotin and deficiency may result. Deficiency may also occur during total parenteral feeding and causes dermatitis, anorexia, nausea and depression. Some inherited carboxylase deficiencies have been described which respond to administration of biotin.

Folic Acid Folic acid forms the functional group of a coenzyme which facilitates the transfer of single-carbon units from donors, such as methionine, to intermediates which require these for the synthesis of macromolecules, including nucleic acids. Folate is present in many fruits and vegetables, although prolonged heating and canning in food preparation can cause losses. Folate in the diet occurs mainly in a conjugated form. Free folate is released during digestion, and this form is absorbed from the upper small intestine.

Deficiency can occur for several reasons:

1. Inadequate intake e.g. alcohol abuse, the elderly.
2. Increased requirements. Folate requirements are greater in pregnancy and also increase in conditions in which increased cell turnover and nucleic acid synthesis occurs, such as occurs in leukaemias and haemolytic anaemia.
3. Malabsorption, particularly to conditions affecting the mucosa of the upper small intestine, such as coeliac disease and tropical sprue (see chapter 10).
4. Drugs affecting folate metabolism. These include anticonvulsant, drugs such as phenytoin and primidone, which interfere with folate absorption, and cytotoxic drugs which are folate antagonists (e.g. methotrexate).

The major consequence of folate deficiency is megaloblastic anaemia; in addition, folate supplements in pregnancy have been shown to reduce the incidence of neural tube defects. Megaloblastic anaemia, characterized by an increased mean corpuscular volume of erythrocytes, is also caused by vitamin B_{12} deficiency and drugs which inhibit deoxyribonucleic acid (DNA) synthesis, particularly cytotoxic drugs (e.g. azathiaprine) and antiviral drugs, particularly azidothymidine (AZT). Folate deficiency is diagnosed by measuring serum or erythrocyte folate levels. Serum folate levels are affected by short-term fluctuations in dietary intake; concentrations in erythrocytes reflect tissue stores more accurately.

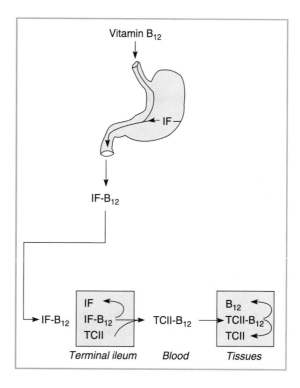

Figure 4.1   Absorption and metabolism of vitamin B_{12}. IF, intrinsic factor; TCII, transcobalamin II.

KEY POINTS

FOLIC ACID

- Folic acid is essential for the synthesis of DNA

- Folate deficiency causes megaloblastic anaemia

- Causes of folate deficiency include inadequate intake, malabsorption, increased requirements and drugs which interfere with folate metabolism

Cyanocobalamin (Vitamin B_{12})   Vitamin B_{12} is a complex molecule in which cobalt is bound within a porphyrin-like ring which is linked to a nucleotide and, in nature, a protein. It cannot be synthesized in the human body and the major dietary sources are animal products, particularly meats and dairy produce. Vitamin B_{12} is released during digestion and bound by intrinsic factor, a protein which is secreted by the parietal cells of the stomach (**Figure 4.1**). This complex is resistant to further digestion until it reaches the terminal ileum, where it is bound by receptors on the mucosal surface. The complex is internalized into ileal cells and intrinsic factor is destroyed, liberating vitamin B_{12} which is then transferred to a transport protein, transcobalamin II. This is released into the circulation and taken up by the liver and other tissues.

Vitamin B_{12} is an essential cofactor for the conversion of homocysteine to methionine and if this is defective, folate metabolism is impaired, interfering with the synthesis of DNA; vitamin B_{12} deficiency therefore causes megaloblastic anaemia. Methionine is also required for the production of phospholipids and a protein, both of which are necessary for myelin synthesis. Thus, vitamin B_{12} deficiency may cause neurological manifestations resulting from demyelination, this being unrelated to folate metabolism. The spinal cord, particularly the posterior and lateral columns, is characteristically affected (subacute combined degeneration of the cord), but peripheral nerves and the brain may also be involved. Vitamin B_{12} is also required for the conversion of methylmalonyl coenzyme A (CoA) to succinyl CoA, and in deficiency states methylmalonic acid accumulates and is excreted in the urine.

Vitamin B_{12} deficiency may have many different causes:

1. Pernicious anaemia. This is thought to be caused by autoimmune destruction of gastric parietal cells. This leads to intrinsic factor deficiency and thus malabsorption of vitamin B_{12}. Achlorhydria also occurs in this condition.
2. Postgastrectomy – if surgery has been extensive enough to remove the parietal cell area, or if bacterial overgrowth occurs.
3. Abnormal intestinal flora. Bacterial overgrowth occurs in the gut if there are areas that do not drain normally. This may be because areas of stasis occur, which are associated particularly with strictures, diverticuli or blind loops. Stasis also results from abnormal motility of the gut; this occurs in diabetes mellitus complicated by autonomic neuropathy and scleroderma of the gastrointestinal tract. Whatever the cause, bacterial overgrowth leads to deficiency through utilization of vitamin B_{12}, thereby reducing the amount that passes to the terminal ileum. Vitamin B_{12} deficiency can also occur in patients who harbour the fish tapeworm *Diphyllobothrium latum* because of utilization by the parasite.
4. Small intestinal disease. Conditions which impair the absorptive capacity of the terminal ileum, particularly surgical resection or mucosal changes (e.g. Crohn's disease), may reduce the assimilation of vitamin B_{12}.
5. Dietary deficiency. As vitamin B_{12} is not found in plants, deficiency may occur in very strict vegetarians (vegans).

Vitamin B_{12} deficiency is investigated by measuring serum levels and, occasionally, by estimating methylmalonic acid excretion in urine. The Schilling test, in which vitamin B_{12} absorption is measured before and after the administration of intrinsic factor, is an investigation to determine the pathogenesis of pernicious anaemia. The patient is given radioactive vitamin B_{12} orally, together with an intramuscular injection of the vitamin to saturate tissue stores. As the radioactively labelled vitamin B_{12} will not be bound in tissues, urinary excretion is a measure of the amount absorbed. This is low in pernicious anaemia but excretion will be normal if a second test is performed in which vitamin B_{12} is given together with intrinsic factor. If absorption is still low in the second test the most likely causes are the blind-loop syndrome or ileal disease.

KEY POINTS

VITAMIN B_{12}

- Vitamin B_{12} is absorbed in the terminal ileum after binding with intrinsic factor which is secreted in the stomach

- Deficiency of vitamin B_{12} causes megaloblastic anaemia and subacute combined degeneration of the spinal cord

- Vitamin B_{12} deficiency is caused by pernicious anaemia, bacterial overgrowth in the gut or disease affecting the terminal ileum

---

Ascorbic Acid (Vitamin C). Ascorbic acid is an antioxidant and is also required for the synthesis of collagen. Thus, vitamin C is required for the normal maintenance of connective tissue and for normal wound healing. Deficiency of vitamin C leads to defective hydroxylation of proline and lysine in procollagen, which is unstable as hydroxylation is necessary for the formation of the normal tertiary structure of collagen. It is thought that vitamin C may be important for hydroxylation reactions involved in corticosteroid synthesis because it is found in high concentrations in the adrenal gland. All animals, with the exception of primates and the guinea pig, can synthesize ascorbic acid from glucose; thus, man is dependent on an adequate dietary intake, rich sources being citrus fruits and vegetables.

Clinical deficiency (scurvy) occurs due to inadequate dietary intake, with two peaks of incidence. The first is in infants aged 6–12 months who receive processed milk without supplements containing ascorbic acid. Second, the diet of elderly subjects, particularly those who live alone, may also be deficient in ascorbate-rich foods. The clinical manifestations in adults include skin papules, petichiae, purpura, muscle haemorrhages, poor wound healing, gum disease and anaemia. Osteoporosis also occurs as vitamin C is required for the synthesis of collagen in the organic matrix of bone. Infants may also suffer from intracranial haemorrhage and bleeding into the periosteum of long bones, causing swellings.

Ascorbate has been taken by large numbers of subjects for long periods, as some believe that it reduces the incidence and severity of the common cold without having any ill-effects. There is little evidence to support this, although a high vitamin C intake may reduce the severity of colds. Two problems with large doses of vitamin C are theoretically possible: increased oxalate excretion, since some ascorbate is converted to this end product, and increased iron absorption, ascorbate maintaining iron in the ferrous form in the gut.

Plasma ascorbate levels are a poor indicator of vitamin C deficiency; measurement of tissue stores is more informative. Leukocyte ascorbate contents are sometimes measured for this purpose. An alter-

native approach is to give patients vitamin C supplements and measure urinary excretion (vitamin C saturation test); this is reduced in scorbutic subjects, as deficient tissues take up the vitamin C. Investigations of ascorbate status should be undertaken early if a patient is admitted, as a hospital diet rapidly corrects any deficiency.

Fat-Soluble Vitamins

Retinol (Vitamin A) Vitamin A is present in many animal tissues and carotinoids, which are converted to vitamin A on digestion, occur widely in plants. After absorption, vitamin A is transported by a specific protein, retinol-binding protein, and large amounts are stored in the liver. Retinol contains a terminal alcohol group which may be oxidized to an aldehyde (retinal) or a carboxylic acid (retinoic acid); these forms also have vitamin activity. It is required for visual function, epithelial development and the synthesis of cell membrane glycoproteins. Vitamin A is a weak antioxidant.

Deficiency leads to night blindness, vitamin A being a component of the retinal pigment rhodopsin. Increased keratinization occurs in the skin, blocking sebaceous glands and causing follicular keratosis. The conjunctiva and other epithelia undergo squamous metaplasia, these changes resembling those seen in premalignant conditions. Softening of the cornea, keratomalacia, which may ulcerate and cause blindness occurs in severe cases.

Vitamin A toxicity has been described in Arctic explorers who have eaten rich dietary sources, particularly polar bear or seal liver, or because of excess vitamin ingestion. Symptoms of acute toxicity include drowsiness, headache, abdominal pain, vomiting and skin desquamation. Papilloedema may occur. Hair loss and skin fissuring are additional symptoms in chronic toxicity.

Vitamin A may be measured in plasma although levels are not closely related to tissue stores, as concentrations usually fall only when stores are severely depleted.

KEY POINTS

VITAMIN C

■ Vitamin C is required for hydroxylation reactions, including the synthesis of normal collagen

■ Early signs of vitamin C deficiency include petechiae and purpura

■ Leukocyte ascorbate levels are a better indicator of vitamin C status than plasma levels

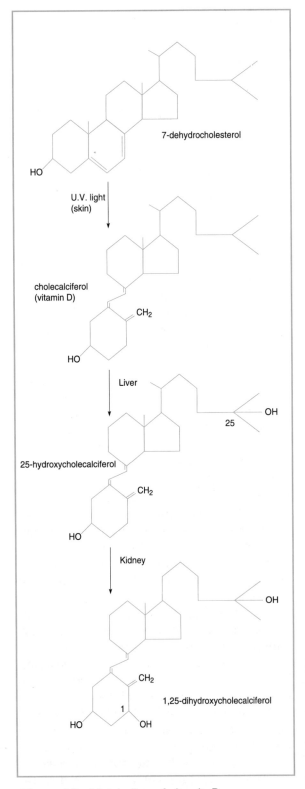

Figure 4.2 Metabolism of vitamin D.

Cholecalciferol (Vitamin D) Vitamin D can be synthesized in the skin by the action of ultraviolet light on the precursor 7-dehydrocholesterol, and is also found in the diet, as it is present in animal fat and fortified margarines. With adequate exposure to sunlight the body's requirements for vitamin D can be met by endogenous synthesis of cholecalciferol in the skin. Dietary vitamin D is absorbed in the small intestine and transported in chylomicrons to the liver, where it is metabolized to 25-hydroxycholecalciferol. This is transported in plasma by a specific α_1-globulin to the kidney, where further hydroxylation occurs in the cells of the proximal tubule, forming a hormone, 1,25-dihydroxycholecalciferol (calcitriol, **Figure 4.2**). Calcitriol is also transported in plasma by vitamin D-binding protein, the main target organs being the intestine and bone. The major physiological role of vitamin D is in the regulation of calcium and phosphate metabolism (see chapter 9). In common with many other steroid hormones, vitamin D acts by regulating the transcription of genes and thus protein synthesis. In the enterocyte, the synthesis of a calcium-binding protein is regulated and in bone osteocalcin is produced.

Vitamin D deficiency leads to rickets in children and osteomalacia in adults; both are conditions in which mineralization of the organic matrix of the skeleton is defective. There are several causes of vitamin D deficiency, which are considered in detail

KEY POINTS

VITAMIN D

- Vitamin D is active in man after conversion to a hormone, 1,25-dihydroxycholecalciferol

- Vitamin D deficiency causes rickets in children and osteomalacia in adults

- Excessive vitamin D intake causes hypercalcaemia

in chapter 9. Excessive intake in the form of supplements is a cause of hypercalcaemia.

Vitamin D deficiency and excess is investigated by measuring concentrations of cholecalciferol and its metabolites in plasma.

Vitamin E Several tocopherols which have vitamin E activity occur in nature, vegetable oils being rich sources. The most potent is α-tocopherol which is an important antioxidant that protects cell membranes and lipoproteins from damage caused by oxidative stress. Deficiency may be due to malabsorption of fat, the most extreme form of which is seem in abetalipoproteinaemia, a rare inherited metabolic disorder in which enterocytes are unable to synthesize apolipoprotein B-48, and thus chylomicron formation is severely impaired. Affected children fail to thrive, have steatorrhoea and develop neurological signs and symptoms that are due to degeneration of the cerebellum and the posterior columns of the spinal cord. Less severe vitamin E deficiency can occur in other causes of malabsorption (see chapter 10). There is interest in the effect of vitamin E supplementation in the prevention of coronary heart disease, the rationale being that oxidative modification of lipoproteins, which would render them more atherogenic, is prevented by vitamin E. Vitamin E status is investigated by measuring levels in plasma.

Vitamin K Vitamin K is a naphthoquinone which occurs in two forms, one being present widely in vegetables, the other being synthesized by intestinal bacteria. Vitamin K is absorbed from the intestine in chylomicrons and transported to the liver where it is physiologically active. It is a cofactor for enzyme systems which process various proteins by γ-carboxylation after they have been synthesized: these include four coagulation factors, prothrombin and factors VII, IX and X. Post-translational modification of these proteins is necessary for their physiological action and this is inhibited by the anticoagulant warfarin.

Neonates tend to be deficient in vitamin K as the gastrointestinal tract is sterile at birth and milk, particularly breast milk, is a poor source. In adults, deficiencies occur due to fat malabsorption or with administration of antibiotics which reduce the intestinal flora. Vitamin K status is investigated by measuring the prothrombin time, this being determined by the activity of dependent clotting factors.

Water and Electrolytes

The requirements for water and the major electrolytes, sodium and potassium, are determined by losses from the body, intake being in excess of needs. Intake is determined largely by social custom and habit, homeostasis being dependent on the kidney, with excretion of excess intake (see chapter 5).

Minerals

Calcium
The body contains approximately 1 kg calcium, which is the most abundant mineral in the body. Most is found in the bones where calcium is a major constituent, although the 1% which is outside the skeleton affects many cellular metabolic processes. The daily intake of calcium varies between 350 and 1200 mg, in European countries approximately half being provided by milk and cheese. Other major sources include nuts, pulses and raw leafy vegetables. Calcium metabolism is described in chapter 9.

Magnesium
The adult body content of magnesium is about 25 g: approximately 80% is present in the skeleton, and most of the remainder is present within cells, where it is required for the activity of many enzymes. Magnesium is

also required for neuromuscular transmission Appreciable amounts of magnesium are present in most foods, the average British intake being 600 mg per day, approximately two-thirds of this being provided by cereals and vegetables. Magnesium metabolism is considered in chapter 9.

Trace Elements

The human body contains approximately 40 elements, and the nine major ones constitute 99% of body weight. The remainder are designated trace elements although many of these are essential for health. Trace elements have important biological properties, although many are toxic if present in excess. Many are complexed with proteins in the body, either for transport, in storage forms, or in enzymes (**Table 4.3**).

Iron

Adult males contain approximately 4 g iron, females a little less. Meat, cereals and vegetables contain iron and most people obtain 10–14 mg per day from the diet. However, the form of iron in the diet is important, absorption being more efficient from haem (Fe^{2+}) in meat than it is from vegetables, in which it occurs largely in the (Fe^{3+}) form. Iron metabolism is considered in detail in chapter 21.

Zinc

The body content of zinc is approximately 2 g (30 mmol) in adults, normal serum concentrations being 10–17 μmol l^{-1} and the erythrocyte content being around 200 μmol l^{-1}. Meats, whole grains and legumes are good dietary sources, the normal intake being about 15 mg per day. Normally, approximately 20% is absorbed, although this fraction is reduced on high-fibre diets, since fibre increases faecal excretion. Not all zinc absorbed by enterocytes enters the body; some is bound by a protein in intestinal cells by a mechanism similar to that which binds iron in the intestinal wall. Metals bound in this manner are lost when effete enterocytes are extruded from the tips of intestinal villi into the lumen of the gut.

Zinc is transported in plasma by albumin, α_2-macroglobulin and transferrin. It is not stored to an appreciable extent within the body. Zinc is present in at least 70 enzymes and deficiency is well described although rare, occurring in acrodermatitis enteropathica, an inherited defect of zinc absorption, and acquired states associated with impaired nutrition. Acrodermatitis enteropathica is characterized by a pustular, bullous dermatitis, loss of hair and diarrhoea; similar skin changes have been described in patients on long-term parenteral nutrition – these responded to zinc supplements. Zinc is essential for optimal wound healing. Deficiency states are

Table 4.3 Protein complexes of essential trace elements (excluding iron)

Element	Protein	Function
Zinc	Albumin, α_2-macroglobulin, transferrin	Transport
	Various enzymes	Nucleic acid, protein and porphyrin synthesis, amino acid and carbohydrate metabolism
Copper	Cytochrome c oxidase	Cellular respiration
	Caeruloplasmin	Various enzyme activities
	Superoxide dismutase	Antioxidant
	Dopamine hydroxylase	Catecholamine synthesis
Selenium	Glutathione peroxidase	Antioxidant
Manganese	Glycosyl transferases	Polysaccharide and glycoprotein synthesis
Molybdenum	Xanthine oxidase	Uric acid metabolism

assessed by measuring plasma rather than serum levels as zinc is released from platelets during clotting. Samples should be taken fasting with minimal venous stasis, and should be free from haemolysis, as erythrocytes contain significant amounts of zinc. It is important to use special collection tubes that are known to be free from contamination.

Copper

An adult contains approximately 150 mg (2 mmol) of copper, larger amounts occurring in the liver than in other organs, although the brain, heart and kidney also contain appreciable quantities. Copper is a component of many enzymes, including cytochrome oxidase, caeruloplasmin and superoxide dismutase. Daily dietary requirements are 2.5 mg and the daily intake is 4 mg, with approximately 50% of this being absorbed. Little is found in urine, biliary excretion being the main route of elimination. The plasma concentration of copper is 12–26 μmol l^{-1}, and over 90% of this is present in caeruloplasmin. Deficiency occurs occasionally in premature infants, in patients receiving total parenteral nutrition, in protein-energy malnutrition and in severe diarrhoea. Clinical findings are anaemia, neutropaenia and, in infants, hair depigmentation. Menkes' syndrome is a sex-linked inherited metabolic disorder in which serum and tissue copper levels are very low due to a defect in absorption. Findings include characteristic hair abnormalities, depigmentation and abnormal structure (kinky hair), defects in connective tissue structure which may cause dissecting aneurysm of the aorta, abnormal bone structure and progressive mental retardation. Wilson's disease is also an inherited metabolic disorder affecting copper metabolism (see chapter 11).

Selenium

Fish and cereals are rich sources of selenium, the daily intake being approximately 1 μmol. Selenium is an essential component of the enzyme glutathione peroxidase which destroys peroxides, particularly hydrogen peroxide, which form in cells. The action of glutathione peroxidase is complementary to that of vitamin E, since tocopherol is active at cell membranes and glutathione peroxidase in the cytoplasm of cells. Deficiency occurs in the Kershan area of China where the soil content of selenium is very low, myocardial changes being a characteristic feature. These include myocardial enlargement and focal necrosis, depending on the severity of the deficiency. Rarely, a similar cardiomyopathy occurs in patients receiving total parenteral nutrition – this responds to selenium supplements.

MALNUTRITION
Protein–Energy Malnutrition

Protein–energy malnutrition (PEM) is a spectrum of disorders in which the intake of energy and protein is insufficient to meet metabolic requirements. Vitamin and mineral intake is also usually inadequate and the clinical features vary depending on the severity of the various deficiencies. In underdeveloped countries PEM is common, due mainly to primary dietary deficiencies, although increased metabolic demands may also contribute. Inadequate intake of both energy and protein causes marasmus, while in kwashiorkor energy intake is adequate but protein is insufficient. Although it occurs in adults, PEM is more common and more severe in children as, in addition to nutrients which are needed for the maintenance of normal metabolic function, there are exacting requirements for growth.

Marasmus occurs in epidemics due to famine, and is also endemic in many areas of Africa, Asia and South America. Children fail to thrive and appear emaciated, with no subcutaneous fat. Secondary infections and dehydration are common. Kwashiorkor often occurs in children who are weaned onto a diet with an inadequate protein content, or is precipitated by an infection or other stress which results in increased catabolism of endogenous protein. Clinical features include failure to thrive, growth failure and oedema, which is usually most marked in the lower limbs. Areas of desquamation and either hypo- or hyperpigmentation are seen in the skin and, particularly in African children, hair changes occur which include loss of curl and altered pigmentation (patches of hair may appear red or blond). Muscle wasting, angular stomatitis, cheilosis and anaemia are common features. Changes in internal organs also occur in PEM, including reduced secretion of digestive enzymes, fatty liver causing impaired hepatic function, myocardial atrophy and impaired immune function.

Associated Nutritional Deficiencies

Vitamin and mineral deficiencies are common in PEM with vitamin A, folate, pyridoxine, vitamin K, iron, magnesium, zinc, potassium, copper, selenium and chromium deficiencies all being described. These are important to consider for two reasons; first, specific deficiencies may cause irreparable damage, e.g. vitamin A deficiency leading to keratomalacia and blindness, and second, although vitamin and mineral supplements are usually given during treatment, these may be insufficient to correct all deficiencies.

Management

Patients cannot immediately accept normal food because there are digestive enzyme deficiencies and they often have gastroenteritis. Rehydration is a priority and oral solutions achieve this in some patients, although intravenous replacement is often necessary. Diluted milk with added sugar is given initially, the strength of this being increased when it is accepted. The supply of energy can cause problems as fat is required to provide calories but is not tolerated if there is maldigestion of fat. Glucose is given initially and vegetable oils are added gradually when these are tolerated; vitamin and mineral supplements are also added.

Nutritional Deficiencies in the Developed World

Both PEM and single-nutrient deficiencies are rare in developed countries although they do occur in specific groups, particularly in neglected children and in elderly subjects, scurvy and osteomalacia being seen not infrequently in the latter. PEM is sometimes seen in hospitalized patients, particularly those with debilitating illnesses accompanied by anorexia. If such a patient suffers trauma, has major surgery or develops an infection PEM may then develop. PEM may also occur in malabsorption, AIDS, chronic renal failure and following gut resection. This trend is particularly important in surgical patients as various assessments of outcome, including the incidence of postoperative infections, wound healing and the length of hospital stay, are associated positively with PEM.

Anorexia Nervosa and Bulimia

These are related eating disorders that mostly affect young middle- and upper-class white women. In a desire to lose weight patients with anorexia diet obsessively, leading to emaciation. In bulimia there is binge eating followed by vomiting and excessive use of laxatives; significant weight loss is unusual. The features of starvation are present in anorexia and secondary amenorrhoea is characteristic.

Assessment of Nutritional Status

This involves dietary history, examination, anthropometric measurements and laboratory investigations. It is important to assess weight before treatment is started and midarm circumference and triceps skinfold thickness are generally measured. Laboratory assessments include haemoglobin and albumin although other proteins, particularly transferrin and retinol-binding protein, are more sensitive indicators of nutritional status as they have shorter half-lives. A useful index of muscle mass is given by the urinary creatinine excretion expressed as a ratio of that expected for normal subjects of the same sex, height and weight. Mineral and vitamin status should be investigated if indicated by specific clinical findings.

Principles of Nutritional Support

Nutritional support in the form of tube feeding is essential therapy for patients who cannot take adequate nutrition orally and who are at risk because of nutritional deficiencies. In enteral feeding nutrients are infused into the upper gastrointestinal tract while intravenous infusion is undertaken in parenteral feeding. The principles of these forms of nutritional support are similar, the type of support being indicated by clinical factors. Whenever possible enteral feeding is preferred because it is cheaper, technically simpler and preserves immunological function better than parenteral nutrition.

Indications

Indications for enteral nutrition include severe PEM, conditions associated with increased protein breakdown, such as full-thickness burns, severe dysphagia, courses of chemotherapy and radiotherapy, in hepatic, renal and pulmonary failure associated with undernutrition, bowel disorders including resection, and postoperatively. Parenteral nutrition is indicated if the gastrointestinal tract is nonfunctional, including massive small intestinal resection, fistulas, hyperemesis gravidarum and intensive chemotherapy. Other indications include severe acute pancreatitis and when enteral nutrition is inadequate. Nutritional support is often undertaken for short periods in hospital but home support is often successful when indicated by chronic conditions, e.g. short bowel syndrome.

Composition of Nutrients

An average patient will require 2000–3000 calories, 60–90 g protein and 2–3 l of fluid; essential minerals, trace elements, vitamins and essential fatty acids should be included. Requirements vary considerably and are greater if there is excessive fluid loss or increased catabolism, e.g. following burns.

Enteral Nutrition In enteral feeding the preparations given depend on whether digestive function is normal, the choice being whole polymeric foods or chemically defined preparations. Regimens containing whole proteins, oligosaccharides and fat preparations are polymeric foods cheaper and avoid the use of hypertonic solutions which would have to be used if glucose was the main energy source. Hypertonic solutions cause fluid fluxes into the intestinal lumen, with the risk of osmotic diarrhoea.

Parenteral Nutrition With intravenous feeding hypertonic fluids must be given to prevent fluid overload. However, concentrated sugar solutions cause thrombophlebitis of small veins and therefore effective parenteral nutrition requires infusion into a central vein. Calories are provided as dextrose and fat emulsions, approximately half the energy requirements being provided by each. This ensures that a supply of essential fatty acids is provided and lessens the risk of metabolic complications from excessive amounts of carbohydrate or fat.

Complications of Nutritional Support

Problems arise from the mechanics of administering fluids and because of metabolic complications (**Table 4.4**). Dehydration or overhydration are relatively common. Diarrhoea during enteral feeding can have several causes including gastroenteritis, fluids being given too rapidly, administration of hyperosmolar fluids, and giving lactose-containing solutions to lactase-deficient subjects. Hyperglycaemia can occur because sick patients often have

Table 4.4 Complications of nutritional support

Mechanical	Metabolic
Misplaced tube	Fluid overload
Aspiration (enteral)	Dehydration
Erosion of gastro-intestinal mucosa (enteral)	Hyperglycaemia
	Hypophosphataemia
	Hyperlipidaemia
Diarrhoea (enteral)	Electrolyte and
Thrombosis (parenteral)	mineral
Infection of cannula (parenteral)	imbalances
	Vitamin deficiency

glucose intolerance. In addition, the liver normally metabolizes glucose postprandially, buffering changes in blood glucose which would otherwise occur. This is bypassed in parenteral nutrition, large amounts of glucose being delivered directly to the systemic circulation. Glucose is metabolized after initial phosphorylation and patients utilizing large amounts of carbohydrate have an increased requirement for phosphate, particularly after a period of starvation. Hyperlipidaemia can occur in parenteral feeding if the rate of infusion exceeds the clearance of lipid.

Monitoring of Patients

Patients receiving nutritional support require close monitoring. Clinical assessments for hospital patients include daily fluid balance charts, periodic weighing, measurement of skinfold thickness and midarm circumference, and checking urine for glycosuria and ketones. Laboratory monitoring includes measurement of urea, creatinine, electrolytes, glucose, osmolality, serum proteins, acid–base status, liver function, blood count, minerals, trace elements and vitamins. In unstable patients or following the introduction of nutritional support glucose and electrolytes are typically measured daily, with measurements reducing in frequency as the patient stabilizes. Vitamins and trace elements are

measured less frequently – often monthly unless there is a specific deficiency.

DISORDERS OF OVERNUTRITION
Obesity

The definition of obesity is somewhat arbitrary and is based the ratio of height to weight. Several methods of calculating this have been used, one that has been widely accepted being the body mass index (BMI). This is:

$$\text{Body mass index} = \frac{\text{weight (kg)}}{\text{height (m)}^2}$$

Health risks associated with weight are lowest for a BMI of 20–25 kg m^{-2} and a BMI > 30 kg m^{-2} is defined as obesity.

Pathogenesis

Obesity occurs when the energy intake is in excess of requirements, although the regulation of eating behaviour is poorly understood. Both environmental and genetic factors are important determinants of body weight, although overeating is the usual cause of obesity. Rarely, obesity may be secondary to an endocrine disorder (**Table 4.5**), although major metabolic abnormalities are not found in the majority of patients. The resting metabolic rate is usually not lower in obese than lean subjects.

Table 4.5 Secondary causes of obesity

Cause	Pathogenesis
Hypothyroidism	Decreased caloric requirements
Cushing's syndrome	Altered fat distribution
Hypothalamic disorders	Overeating

Table 4.6 Diseases complicating obesity

Disease	Pathophysiology
Vascular disease	Hypertension, dyslipidaemia, diabetes
Hypertension	Unclear
Diabetes mellitus	Insulin resistance
Dyslipidaemia	Increased hepatic triglyceride synthesis
Gall bladder disease	Increased biliary cholesterol excretion
Osteoarthritis	Increased wear and tear on joints
Respiratory disorders	Impaired ventilation

Complications

Several diseases occur more commonly in obese subjects (**Table 4.6**). Mortality rates increase as body weight rises owing to an increased incidence of CHD. The distribution of fat appears important; the incidence of CHD and cerebrovascular disease rises with increasing abdominal fat, as measured by the waist:hip ratio ('middle-aged spread'). The reason is unclear but hypertension, dyslipidaemia and diabetes mellitus may all contribute to this additional risk. Increased insulin secretion and tissue insensitivity to insulin occur and the risk of Type 2 diabetes mellitus increases with the degree of obesity.

Management

In principle the management of obesity is simple – eat less. The total caloric intake should be reduced, with careful attention to high calorie foods, particularly fat and alcohol. In practice, weight reduction is often difficult as it requires great resolve. Education and psychological support can be helpful and some patients benefit from keeping dietary diaries. Therapy with anorectic drugs is of limited value as their efficacy is modest and the appetite-suppressing effect usually wears off.

FURTHER READING

Garrow JS. Treatment of obesity. *Lancet* 1992; **340**: 409–13

Garrow JS, James WPT. *Human Nutrition and Dietetics* (9th edn). Edinburgh: Churchill Livingstone, 1993.

Neale G. *Clinical Nutrition*. London: Heinemann, 1988

Ravussin E, Swinburn BA. Pathophysiology of obesity. *Lancet* 1992; **340**: 404–8

Shenkin A. Clinical aspects of vitamin and trace element metabolism. *Baillière's Clinical Gastroenterology* 1988; **2**: 765–98

Sizgal HM. Parenteral and enteral nutrition. *Annual Reviews in Medicine* 1991; **42**: 549–65

Truswell AS. *ABC of Nutrition* (2nd edn). London: British Medical Journal, 1992

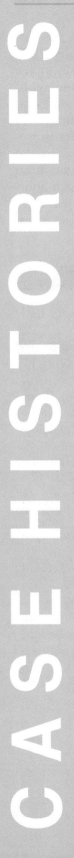

CASE 4.1

The following biochemical results were obtained in a 37-year-old woman with extensive Crohn's disease following the introduction of parenteral nutrition

random blood glucose	9.6 mmol l^{-1}
albumin	28 g l^{-1}
total calcium	1.95 mmol l^{-1}
phosphate	0.3 mmol l^{-1}

Explain these results, all of which are abnormal.

CASE 4.2

A 76-year-old man who lived alone was admitted to hospital following a cerebrovascular accident. On examination he was emaciated and widespread petechial haemorrhages were noted. What nutritional deficiency must be considered?

CASE 4.3

A 45-year-old business executive underwent a health check. The family history revealed that his father had suffered a myocardial infarction at the age of 57, although was still alive at the age of 72. The patient weighed 102.5 kg and his height was 1.76 m; he was a nonsmoker, his blood pressure was 170/100 mmHg and he undertook little regular exercise. Plasma lipid concentrations were:

total cholesterol	6.4 mmol l^{-1}
triglycerides	2.9 mmol l^{-1}
HDL cholesterol	0.8 mmol l^{-1}

Is he obese? What health risks are associated with obesity?

5

SODIUM AND WATER METABOLISM

INTRODUCTION

The total body content of sodium is approximately 3700 mmol in an average man, while water accounts for approximately 60% of body weight. There is less water in women, 55% of body weight, owing to a higher body fat content – adipose tissue contains very little water. The metabolism of sodium and water are closely linked both physiologically and clinically; they are therefore best considered together.

SODIUM AND WATER HOMEOSTASIS

Sodium Distribution

Approximately 2800 mmol of sodium is freely exchangeable while 900 mmol is complexed in bone. Exchangeable sodium is present mainly in the extracellular fluid (ECF) where the sodium concentration averages 140 mmol l^{-1}; the concentration in intracellular fluid (ICF) is around 10 mmol l^{-1}. Potassium, with a concentration of 150 mmol l^{-1}, is the major cation of the ICF, while its extracellular concentration is around 4 mmol l^{-1}. Although sodium diffuses into cells it is actively extruded in exchange for potassium which leaks out into the ECF. Thus, the net effect is that the concentration differences between these cations in the intra- and extracellular compartments are maintained.

Water Distribution in the Body

Water distribution in the body is controlled largely by physical factors, particularly the solute content of intra- and extracellular fluids and the hydrostatic pressure of the vascular system.

Forces Controlling Water and Solute Movement

Osmotic Pressure

The presence of solute modifies the properties of a solvent in a number of ways, including lowering its freezing point, elevating its boiling point and exerting an osmotic pressure. When two solutions with different solute contents are separated by a semipermeable membrane there is a net flow of water across the membrane from the dilute (low osmotic pressure) to the concentrated (high osmotic pressure) solution (**Figure 5.1**). Net transfer of water continues, either until the osmotic pressure on both sides of the membrane is equal, or the difference in osmotic pressure is balanced by an additional force, such as hydrostatic pressure. Since compartmentalization of sodium and potassium between ICF and ECF is main-

tained by active transport processes and cell membranes function as semipermeable membranes, water distribution between cell compartments is controlled by the osmotic pressure within compartments (**Figure 5.2**).

Osmolarity and Osmolality

The osmotic effect of a solute is determined by the number of particles which are formed in solution. Thus, substances of low molecular weight, such as sodium, glucose and urea, contribute more to osmotic pressure than those with a large molecular mass, such as proteins; solutes that ionize at the normal body pH will form twice as many particles as an undissociated solute. Both osmolarity and osmolality are measurements of solute concentration, the units of osmolarity being $mmol\ l^{-1}$ while osmolality is $mmol\ kg^{-1}$ of solvent. The difference between the two is negligible for the range of concentrations found in biological fluids, osmolality having the advantage that it is independent of temperature. Osmolality is used by clinical laboratories to assess solute

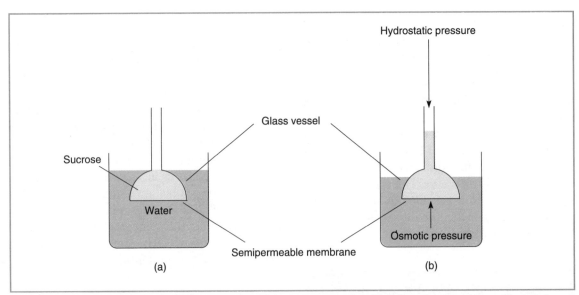

Figure 5.1 The effect of osmotic pressure. The inner vessel, which incorporates a capillary tube at the upper end, contains a solution of sucrose and is closed at the lower end with a semipermeable membrane. This is placed in a beaker of water so that the fluid levels in the two vessels are identical (a). If sucrose cannot cross the semipermeable membrane water is attracted into the inner vessel by osmotic pressure and the fluid level rises in the capillary until the osmotic pressure is balanced by the hydrostatic pressure (b).

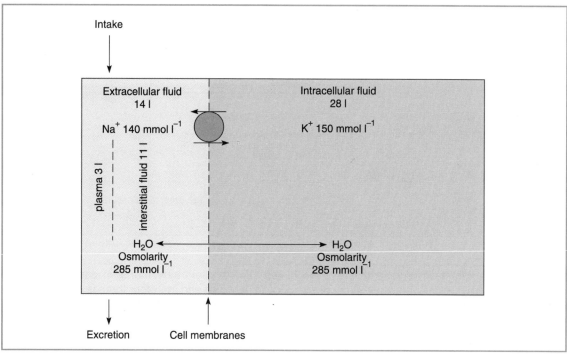

Figure 5.2   Water distribution in the body. There are two major fluid compartments, intracellular and extracellular, the latter consisting of plasma and interstitial fluid. The main cation of the extracellular fluid is sodium while potassium is present in high concentrations within cells. These concentrations are maintained by active cell-membrane pumps, while water diffuses freely across cell membranes. Thus, water distribution between the compartments is determined by their osmotic pressure.

contents, the method of assessment being the determination of the freezing point.

In health, The osmolality of plasma is approximately 285 mmol kg^{-1}. There are various formulae for calculating osmolality, the simplest is:

$$2[Na^+] + 2[K^+] + glucose + urea = osmolality$$

where concentrations are mmol l^{-1}. The cation concentrations are doubled to allow for the associated anions, chloride and bicarbonate, although the formula ignores the contributions of other low molecular weight substances such as calcium, and also proteins. However, sodium is not quite fully dissociated and using 2[Na$^+$] compensates for other constituents. The calculated and measured osmolality are usually in close agreement unless an unmeasured solute

which is osmotically active, such as ethanol, is present in significant amounts.

KEY POINTS

OSMOLALITY

- Osmolality expresses the solute content of a fluid

- The osmolalities of the ICF and ECF determine the distribution of water between the compartments

- Plasma osmolality is approximately 285 mmol kg^{-1}

Colloid Osmotic (Oncotic) Pressure

The ECF consists of two subcompartments, plasma which is contained within the vasculature, and interstitial fluid which bathes tissue cells. These differ in composi-

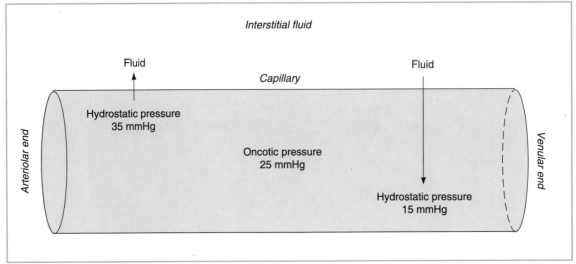

Interstitial fluid

Fluid

Capillary

Fluid

Hydrostatic pressure
35 mmHg

Oncotic pressure
25 mmHg

Hydrostatic pressure
15 mmHg

Arteriolar end

Venular end

Figure 5.3 Diagrammatic representation of the forces affecting fluid movements in capillaries. At the arteriolar end the hydrostatic pressure exceeds the oncotic pressure and therefore there is a net outflow of fluid. Hydrostatic pressure is lower than oncotic pressure at the venular end and net reabsorption of fluid occurs.

tion, mainly owing to differences in their protein content. While water, electrolytes and other low molecular weight substances cross capillary walls relatively freely, plasma proteins are restrained due to their size. Although these proteins contribute little to osmolality because of their large molecular mass, they exert a pressure, the colloid osmotic (oncotic) pressure, as a result of being contained within the vasculature. This is an important determinant of fluid distribution between blood vessels and interstitial fluid.

Hydrostatic Pressure

The mechanical pressure generated by the heart is responsible for hydrostatic pressure in the body. The mean pressure in the larger arteries is approximately 100 mmHg, although this drops as arteries divide. At the arteriolar end of capillaries, hydrostatic pressure is around 35 mmHg, while this falls to approximately 15 mmHg at the venular end. The oncotic pressure exerted by plasma proteins is 25 mmHg – this changes little in the microvasculature. Because intravascular hydrostatic pressure exceeds oncotic pressure at the arteriolar

end of capillaries there is net efflux of fluid to the interstitial space. This is reversed at the venular end as the hydrostatic pressure in capillaries is lower than the oncotic pressure, and thus interstitial fluid is drawn back into the vessels (**Figure 5.3**); some interstitial fluid is also returned to the vascular tree via the lymphatic system. Hydrostatic pressure and plasma oncotic pressure determine the distribution of the water and small solutes of ECF between the vascular compartment and interstitial fluid. Disturbances of these lead to increased accumulation of interstitial fluid and oedema formation.

Sodium Homeostasis

The dietary content of sodium is very variable although intake is greater than inevitable losses, balance being maintained by renal excretion of the excess (**Figure 5.4**). The amount of sodium filtered by the glomeruli is very large, exceeding 25 000 mmol day^{-1}, while less than 1% of this is excreted (100–200 mmol day^{-1}). Approximately 70% of filtered sodium is reabsorbed

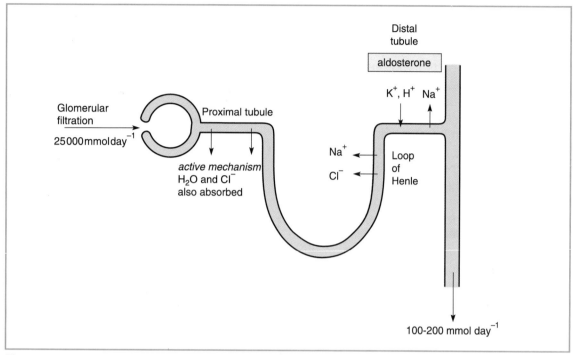

Figure 5.4 Renal control of sodium homeostasis. Approximately 70% of sodium reabsorption occurs in the proximal convoluted tubules, 25% in the loop of Henle and the remainder in the distal convoluted tubules. Reabsorption in the loop of Henle generates an osmotic gradient in the interstitial tissue of the kidney which provides the mechanism for water reabsorption in the collecting duct.

in the proximal convoluted tubule by an active transport process in which chloride and, to a lesser extent, bicarbonate are also absorbed as counter-ions. Water is passively transported with sodium and thus an isotonic fluid is absorbed. The glomerular filtration rate (GFR) influences sodium reabsorption at this site, relatively small fluctuations having great potential for changing sodium excretion. Frequent variations in GFR occur with changes of posture, protein feeding and other factors, although sodium excretion changes little in response to these. There is thus some physiological compensation, as reabsorption increases as GFR increases (glomerulo-tubular balance). Major changes in GFR alter sodium and water reabsorption, these increasing as the GFR falls. This effect may be mediated by other factors which influence sodium reabsorption at the proximal tubular site, particularly the capillary oncotic pressure

and hydrostatic pressure around the tubules. High capillary oncotic pressure and low hydrostatic pressure favour sodium and water reabsorption. The solute content of the glomerular filtrate is also important. If an unabsorbed solute, such as the osmotic diuretic mannitol or excess glucose, is present water is trapped within the lumen of the tubule, also preventing sodium reabsorption. This is the mechanism of sodium and water depletion in diabetic ketoacidosis.

Around 25% of filtered sodium is reabsorbed in the ascending limb of the loop of Henle. This is concentrated within the medulla by the combined effects of active sodium reabsorption and the blood vessels associated with the loops of Henle, the descending vasa recta, generating an osmotic gradient from the cortex to the medulla (countercurrent multiplication). This provides the mechanism for controlling water reabsorption in the collecting duct (countercurrent exchange). Little water is reabsorbed in the loop of Henle and thus the fluid leaving the loop is hypotonic.

Approximately 5% of sodium reabsorption occurs in the distal convoluted tubule in exchange for potassium and H^+ ions. Aldosterone, which is secreted by the zona glomerulosa of the adrenal gland, regulates this process by increasing sodium reabsorption and promoting potassium and H^+ ion excretion. The secretion of aldosterone is controlled mainly by the renin–angiotensin system, renin secretion being increased by hypotension and sodium depletion.

Several naturetic hormones have been described, including one secreted by atria of the heart, atrial natriuretic peptide (ANP). ANP, In response to saline loading, promotes sodium excretion by increasing GFR.

Water Homeostasis

In health, water intake exceeds requirements and balance is maintained by excretion. There are insensible losses through the skin in the form of sweat, through the lungs in expired air, and in faeces (**Table 5.1**). The remainder is removed by renal excretion, normal urine output being considerably greater than the 500 ml required daily for the excretion of water-soluble metabolic waste products that are eliminated from the body by the kidney.

There is regulation of both intake and excretion of water. Intake is controlled by the thirst mechanism, this being dependent on a centre in the hypothalamus which responds to increasing extracellular osmolality. Between 180 and 200 l of fluid are filtered each day by the kidneys, 80% of this being absorbed together with sodium in the proximal convoluted tubule (**Figure 5.5**). The distal reabsorptive mechanisms of water and sodium regulation are dissociated, water balance being controlled by vasopressin (antidiuretic hormone, ADH). The major control of vasopressin secretion

Table 5.1 Water turnover in a healthy adult

	Intake (ml)	Output (ml)
Oral fluids	1500	
Water in food	600	
Endogenous water production	400	
Losses from:		
skin		500
lungs		400
faeces		100
kidney		1500
Totals	2500	2500

Table 5.2 Factors affecting antidiuretic hormone (ADH) secretion

Increased secretion	Decreased secretion
Increased ECF osmolality	Decreased ECF osmolality
Decreased ECF volume	Increased ECF volume
Increased angiotensin II Stress (pain, operation) Exercise Drugs (nicotine, morphine, sulphonylureas barbiturates)	Alcohol

ECF, extracellular fluid.

is exerted by osmoreceptors in the hypothalamus, although other factors also affect secretion (**Table 5.2**). Osmoreceptors respond to differences between extracellular and intracellular osmolality, increasing extracellular osmolality stimulating secretion. Vasopressin acts by increasing the permeability of the collecting duct in the kidney, allowing water to be attracted into the interstitial fluid and thus the ascending vasa recti by the osmotic gradient generated by the countercurrent multiplier mechanism (countercurrent exchange). If extracellular osmolality is reduced there is

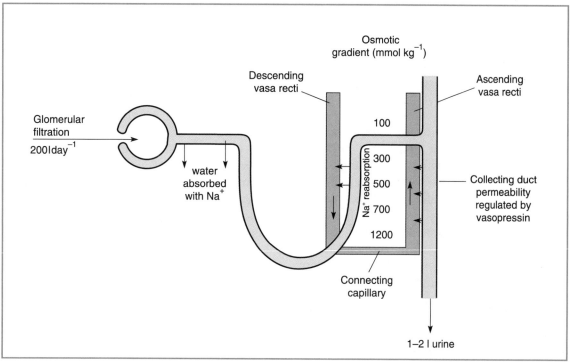

Figure 5.5 Renal control of water excretion. Approximately 80% of water reabsorption occurs in the proximal convoluted tubule in association with sodium transport, the remainder being absorbed in the collecting duct. Water reabsorption at this site is controlled by vasopressin which increases permeability of the collecting duct, allowing water to be absorbed by the osmotic gradient generated by sodium reabsorption in the loop of Henle.

no thirst or stimulation of vasopressin secretion, water reabsorption is inhibited and dilute urine is formed.

The osmotic control of vasopressin secretion is extremely sensitive, osmoreceptors responding to 1% variations in ECF osmolality. Vasopressin secretion also responds to changes in ECF volume, stretch receptors being present in large vessels and the atria.

Decreasing blood volume increases vasopressin secretion, stimulation by volume receptors being reinforced by angiotensin II. In some clinical conditions, volume and other stimuli, such as stress or drugs, may override the osmotic control of vasopressin secretion. Secretion is inhibited by alcohol.

KEY POINTS

WATER HOMEOSTASIS

- 80% of renal water reabsorption occurs in the proximal tubule in association with sodium transport

- Vasopressin regulates water reabsorption in the collecting duct

- The main control of vasopressin secretion is exerted by osmoreceptors in the hypothalamus

Assessment of Sodium and Water Status

Both clinical assessment and laboratory measurements are essential for the evaluation of sodium and water status.

Clinical Assessment

The clinical evaluation includes noting the presence of thirst, dryness of the tongue and mucous membranes, testing tissue turgor and assessing central venous pressure, weight and fluid balance charts.

Laboratory data cannot be interpreted sensibly without these assessments.

Laboratory Assessment

The concentration of sodium in plasma is a product of the relative amounts of extracellular sodium and water. Thus, the concentration may be reduced either because sodium has been lost in greater amounts than water or through water being selectively retained, which reduces the sodium concentration by dilution. The plasma sodium level is therefore a poor indicator of the amount of extracellular fluid sodium present. Plasma potassium concentrations may be reduced or elevated in disorders of sodium and water metabolism, with serious consequences (see chapter 6). Increased haemoglobin, packed cell volume (PCV) and plasma albumin levels often occur in volume depletion, although these may also be affected by the primary disease. A high plasma urea level often occurs in volume depletion owing to reduced GFR, although this can also be due to a variety of other conditions, including impaired renal function. Plasma osmolality is useful in the investigation of hyponatraemia.

Plasma Sodium Measurement Plasma sodium concentrations are determined either by ion-specific electrodes, which determine plasma sodium activity, or flame photometry, which determines concentration. There are two types of ion-selective electrodes: direct-reading, which measure sodium activity in undiluted samples, and indirect-reading, when plasma is diluted prior to analysis. The measurements are essentially similar except when the fractional water content of plasma is reduced, e.g. because the amount of triglyceride or protein in plasma is very large (**Figure 5.6**). If the amount of water per unit volume of plasma is reduced sodium activity is normal if a direct-reading ion-selective electrode is used, whereas a spuriously low value is obtained with an indirect-reading ion-selective electrode because if specimens are diluted a smaller

amount of plasma is sampled. Flame photometry methods, like indirect-reading ion-selective electrodes, use dilutions and therefore give low values under these circumstances. Spuriously low values are also found with these methods in patients with paraproteinaemia, partly because the fractional water content of plasma is reduced and partly because smaller amounts are aspirated by analysers because of the high plasma viscosity. By measuring sodium activity in the aqueous phase of plasma, direct-reading ion-selective electrodes avoid this artefact.

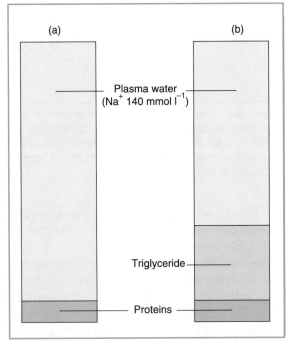

Figure 5.6 Fractional water content of plasma. Each column represents 1 l of plasma. (a) Normal: around 7% of plasma volume is occupied by proteins into which water and thus sodium does not penetrate. (b) Severe hypertriglyceridaemia: the fraction of water in the litre of plasma is reduced as it does not penetrate into circulating triglycerides. If the sodium concentration remains constant in the water phase the apparent sodium concentration in the litre of plasma will be reduced by a factor determined by the volume occupied by the triglycerides. If this is 20% the apparent sodium concentration will be $140/100 \times 80 = 112$ mmol l^{-1}. However, the sodium activity in the aqueous phase will be normal.

DISORDERS OF SODIUM AND WATER METABOLISM

Combined Sodium and Water Depletion

Combined deficiency of both sodium and water is relatively common while pure depletion of either is much rarer. The term dehydration is often used to describe combined depletion but, because sodium is also lost, volume depletion is a better term.

Causes

Combined sodium and water deficiency is almost always caused by increased losses, reduced intake only very rarely being severe enough to cause clinical depletion. There are three major routes of excessive loss of sodium and water from the body: through the skin, from the gastrointestinal tract or through impaired renal reabsorption (**Table 5.3**).

Gastrointestinal Tract   Up to 10 l of fluid are secreted by the gastrointestinal tract each day, these varying in sodium content from 60 mmol l^{-1} (gastric juice) to 140 mmol l^{-1} (small intestinal secretions). Losses lead to volume depletion and since secretions also contain potassium, H^+ and bicarbonate the metabolism of these may also be disordered.

Skin   Sweat is hypotonic, sodium concentrations being 20–60 mmol l^{-1}. Because of this, water is lost in relatively greater

Table 5.3   Causes of combined salt and water (volume) depletion

Gastrointestinal losses
◆ Vomiting, diarrhoea, aspiration, drainage from fistulas
Skin losses
◆ Sweating, burns
Renal losses
◆ Diuretic phase of acute tubular necrosis
◆ Osmotic diuresis
◆ Salt-wasting tubulointerstitial disease
◆ Addison's disease

amounts when sweating is excessive and water depletion may predominate. Considerable losses of sodium and water occur in full-thickness burns, and sequestration of water and sodium can also occur in injured skin owing to increased capillary permeability.

Renal   Extremely large amounts of sodium and water can be lost in the recovery phase of acute renal failure (see chapter 8). While the excretion of excess sodium and water which have accumulated during the oliguric phase is appropriate, true volume depletion also occurs because of delayed recovery in tubular function. Severe losses rarely persist beyond a few days. Excessive losses can also occur, usually for no more than a few days, following relief of urinary tract obstruction. Occasionally, patients with chronic renal failure are prone to large sodium and water losses, particularly where tubulointerstitial disease occurs, e.g. pyelonephritis, polycystic kidneys. Patients with chronic renal failure may develop volume depletion if their intake is restricted, e.g. due to vomiting, because conservation mechanisms are impaired.

Volume depletion occurs with normal renal function under three circumstances:

(i)   diuretic therapy in patients whose oedema has been relieved or where it is sequestered internally and cannot be mobilized, e.g. ascites;

(ii)   osmotic diuresis, as occurs in diabetic ketoacidosis;

(iii)   aldosterone deficiency (Addison's disease).

Clinical Features

The clinical features of volume depletion result largely from the reduced extracellular fluid volume (**Figure 5.7**). Symptoms include weakness, confusion and lethargy, while physical signs include decreased skin turgor, rapid pulse and postural hypotension. In severe cases blood pressure may be reduced and shock can occur. There may also be signs and symptoms

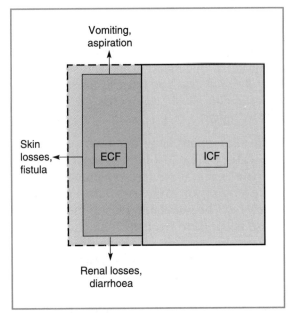

Vomiting, aspiration

Skin losses, fistula

ECF

ICF

Renal losses, diarrhoea

Figure 5.7 Body fluid compartments in volume depletion. The normal extracellular fluid (ECF) volume (pale green area) is reduced (dark green area) but if the fluid loss is isotonic there will be no change in the intracellular fluid (ICF) volume, since there will be no osmotic gradients between the compartments.

caused by the primary abnormality, although this is not always clear from the clinical features. Very little change in intracellular fluid volume occurs, particularly if sodium and water are lost in proportion.

Laboratory Findings

Plasma sodium concentration is often normal although decreased or increased levels can occur, depending on the relative deficits of sodium and water. Thus greater water loss occurs in excessive sweating resulting in hypernatraemia, while hyponatraemia occurs in Addison's disease or where volume depletion is treated with hypotonic solutions. Plasma urea concentration is usually increased, as volume depletion leads to a reduced glomerular filtration rate and thus urea retention. Haematocrit and plasma protein concentrations are usually increased. The homeostatic response to volume depletion is reduced urinary vo-

lume and renal sodium conservation, concentrations dropping to <10 mmol l^{-1}. Concentrations > 20 mmol l^{-1} suggest renal losses.

Management

Modest deficits can often be treated with oral replacement while severe depletion requires intravenous fluids. Isotonic saline is the fluid of choice when the plasma sodium level is approximately normal. The effect of treatment must be carefully monitored by clinical examination, including blood pressure measurement and assesment urine output. Associated metabolic disturbances, e.g. potassium depletion in excessive gastrointestinal losses, may also require treatment.

KEY POINTS	**SODIUM AND WATER (VOLUME) DEPLETION**
	■ Volume depletion is nearly always caused by increased losses which can occur through the gastrointestinal tract, the skin or the kidney
	■ Volume losses are largely restricted to the ECF
	■ The plasma sodium concentration is often normal

Water Depletion

Water loss without sodium depletion is rare but water depletion results where secretions in which the sodium concentration is lower than plasma are lost.

Causes

Causes of water depletion are outlined in **Table 5.4.** Inadequate intake is rarely the sole cause of water depletion since the thirst mechanism will ensure that losses are replaced. However, water intake may be restricted if severe dysphagia is present, e.g. due to a carcinoma of the oesophagus.

Table 5.4 Causes of water depletion

Inadequate water intake
◆ Severe dysphagia
◆ Infancy, the elderly
◆ Coma

Excessive losses
◆ Via the lungs
  hyperventilation
◆ Via the skin
  Sweating
◆ Via the kidney
  Diabetes insipidus
  Osmotic diuresis

Resetting of osmoregulatory centre
◆ Brain injury

Patients with a high fever or those being ventilated may lose water rapidly through increased losses from skin and hyperventilation, in particular infants or comatosed patients who are unable to respond to increasing thirst. Acutely ill elderly subjects who live alone may be physically unable to get themselves fluids, particularly if they are disabled, e.g. by severe arthritis or a stroke. Water loss in diabetes insipidus is caused either by insufficient vasopressin production or a failure of the kidneys to respond to the hormone (nephrogenic diabetes insipidus). Excessive water losses are usually compensated for as the thirst mechanism is intact; however, losses can occur if diabetes insipidus follows a head injury. Occasionally, the thirst centre is destroyed by a cerebral tumour and resetting of the osmoregulatory centre to a higher plasma osmolality has been described following severe head injury. Osmotic diuresis leads to excessive water losses owing to impaired renal reabsorption, glycosuria in diabetes mellitus being one such cause.

Clinical Features

Loss of water without equivalent sodium depletion causes hypernatraemia. This leads to increased extracellular osmolality which induces a shift of water from the intracel-lular to extracellular compartment. Thus, the fluid deficit will be shared by both cellular compartments, rather than being restricted to the extracellular compartment as it is in isotonic sodium and water deficiency (**Figure 5.8**). Because of this, signs of extracellular fluid depletion and peripheral circulatory failure are much less common in water depletion than in volume depletion. Cellular dehydration may result in cerebral dysfunction, leading to confusion, fits and coma. Subdural haemorrhages can occur, due to tears caused by contracting brain volume. Coma is unusual if hyperna-traemia develops slowly, as adaptation occurs which increases intracellular osmolality, possibly owing to increased synthesis of small organic molecules, thus limiting the water shifts. Under these circumstances rapid correction of the extracellular hyper-osmolality by the administration of intravenous dextrose (metabolically equivalent to water) may lead to cellular overhydration.

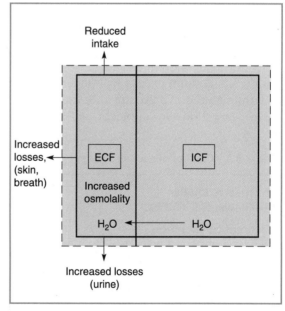

Figure 5.8 Body fluid compartments in water depletion. The normal volume of both the intracellular fluid (ICF) and extracellular fluid (ECF) (grey area) is reduced (green area) as a result of water depletion in the ECF, increased ECF osmolality and transfer of water from the ICF due to an osmotic gradient.

Hypernatraemia

Hypernatraemia is nearly always caused by water depletion, although occasionally it may result from the intravenous administration of sodium-containing solutions, particularly sodium bicarbonate given during cardiopulmonary resuscitation to correct metabolic acidosis. Other causes include sodium-rich feeds in babies. The ECF osmolality is increased, and water shifts occur from the ICF. Except in diabetes insipidus, the urinary sodium concentration is high as the ECF is expanded, leading to inhibition of renal tubular reabsorption. Mild hypernatraemia may occur with mineralocorticoid excess (Conn's syndrome (primary hyperaldosteronism) and Cushing's syndrome), often accompanied by hypokalaemia and metabolic alkalosis. The mechanism responsible is increased renal tubular reabsorption of sodium with increased excretion of potassium and H^+.

Sodium Excess

The causes of sodium excess are outlined in **Table 5.5**. Sodium excess will occur if saline is administered at a greater rate than that of renal excretion. In subjects with normal

Table 5.5 Causes of sodium excess

Excessive intake
◆ Intravenous infusion

Decreased excretion
◆ Excess mineralocorticoids
  Aldosterone (Conn's syndrome)
  Cortisol (Cushing's syndrome)
◆ Reduced glomerular filtration rate
  Acute renal failure
  Chronic renal failure
◆ Oedema syndromes
  Congestive cardiac failure
  Hepatic cirrhosis with portal hypertension
  Nephrotic syndrome
  Idiopathic oedema

renal function this is usually due to excessive intravenous infusion. Sodium retention is common in acute renal failure owing to impaired excretion, and can also occur in chronic renal failure if sodium intake is even slightly in excess of the reduced excretory capacity of the kidney. Increased tubular reabsorption causes sodium retention in the presence of excess mineralocorticoids. The plasma sodium concentration is a poor guide to sodium excess, as it is often normal if water retention also occurs.

Sodium and water retention can cause oedema. Oedema is caused by the accumulation of interstitial fluid, which is recognized clinically as pitting in dependent parts (the ankles in ambulant subjects, the sacrum in supine patients) or puffiness around the eyes (periorbital oedema). Oedema occurs the when the movement of fluid into capillaries at the venular end of capillary beds is less than the movement out at the arteriolar end (**Figure 5.3**). The factors that can cause this include increased capillary hydrostatic pressure, decreased plasma oncotic pressure, increased capillary permeability and decreased lymphatic drainage. In congestive cardiac failure the hydrostatic pressure within venules is increased, less interstitial fluid re-enters the capillary and thus oedema occurs. Severe hypoalbuminaemia, e.g. in nephrotic syndrome, leads to oedema by reducing the plasma oncotic pressure. Patients with hepatic cirrhosis can develop oedema due to hypoalbuminaemia and they may also develop ascites.

Water Excess

Water excess is usually caused by reduced excretion resulting from defective urinary dilution, although excessive intake may be responsible (**Table 5.6**). The normal kidney can excrete 15–20 l of water per day and, very rarely, intake is greater than this excretory capacity (psychogenic polydipsia). A further rare cause of increased

Table 5.6   Causes of water excess

Intake greater than excretory capacity
◆ Psychogenic polydipsia
◆ Water absorption from bladder irrigation

Reduced excretion
◆ Inappropriate antidiuretic hormone secretion
  Tumours
  Trauma, surgery
  Infections
  Pulmonary disease
  CNS disorders
◆ Hypocortisolism
◆ Hypothyroidism
◆ Drug induced
  Sulphonylureas (tolbutamide)
  Psychotropic agents (carbamazepine,
    amitryptilene)
  Cytotoxic and immunosuppressive drugs
    (vincristine, cyclophosphamide)

Increased intake combined with reduced excretion
◆ Postoperative intravenous fluid
  administration

intake is by absorption through an inflamed urinary bladder which is being irrigated by water.

In the syndrome of inappropriate diuretic hormone secretion (SIADH) vasopressin is released despite dilution of body fluids and increased extracellular volume. Urinary osmolality is not maximally dilute (100 mmol kg^{-1}) even when there is marked hyponatraemia and usually exceeds the plasma osmolality; renal function is normal. Tumours, particularly small-cell carcinomas of the bronchus, may secrete ADH or ADH-like molecules with similar biological activity, leading to water retention. Inappropriate secretion of ADH sometimes occurs with pulmonary tuberculosis or other chronic chest infections and has also been described in central nervous system disorders including meningitis, encephalitis, tumours, stroke and acute intermittent porphyria.

Endocrine causes include cortisol deficiency and hypothyroidism. Water reten-

tion in hypopituitarism is thought to be due to cortisol deficiency. The secretion of many hormones, including vasopressin, increases as part of a metabolic response to injury following trauma or surgery, although this is not usually severe enough to lead to water retention unless excess water is administered. Some drugs (**Table 5.6**) exert antidiuretic effects, either by potentiating the action of vasopressin or by stimulating inappropriate ADH secretion.

Clinical Features

Hyponatraemia occurs with water retention and clinical symptoms are likely when values fall below 125 mmol l^{-1}, particularly if the condition develops rapidly. Water retention reduces extracellular osmolality and an osmotic gradient develops across cell membranes. Thus, water flows from the extracellular to intracellular compartment, leading to cell swelling (**Figure 5.9**). This can lead to impaired cerebral function as the

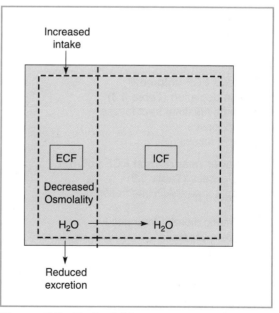

Figure 5.9 Body fluid compartments in water overload. The normal body compartments (green area) are both increased since water excess reduces extracellular fluid (ECF) osmolality, resulting in a transfer of water to the intracellular fluid (ICF) because of an osmotic gradient.

brain is enclosed in a tight box, the cranium, and if cells increase in size sufficiently, they are compressed, causing confusion, headaches, convulsions and coma. Rarely, extreme hyponatraemia (<110 mmol l^{-1}) occurs without symptoms, particularly if the condition develops slowly. Work with animals has suggested that when the onset of hyponatraemia is gradual, a compensatory loss of intracellular potassium occurs, preventing a significant osmotic gradient and thus cell swelling from developing.

Hyponatraemia

The causes of hyponatraemia can be divided into three groups, depending on whether the ECF volume is reduced, normal or increased (**Table 5.7**). Hyponatraemia is not synonymous with sodium depletion since the causes include water excess and oedema states, in which sodium and water retention occur. A scheme for investigating hyponatraemia is outlined in **Figure 5.10**.

Table 5.7 Causes of hyponatraemia

Reduced ECF volume
Volume depletion (**Table 5.3**)
◆ Gastrointestinal tract losses
◆ Skin losses
◆ Renal losses

Normal or near normal ECF volume
Water excess (**Table 5.5**)
◆ Inappropriate ADH secretion
Osmotic
◆ Osmotic diuretic (mannitol)
◆ Hyperglycaemia
Artefactual
◆ Faulty blood sampling
◆ Decreased plasma fractional water content

Increased ECF volume
Sodium and water retention (oedema)
◆ Congestive cardiac failure
◆ Cirrhosis
◆ Nephrotic syndrome

ECF, extracellular fluid; ADH, antidiuretic hormone.

Hyponatraemia with Reduced ECF Volume

This group includes the causes of volume depletion considered above (gastrointestinal tract, skin and renal losses).

Hyponatraemia with Normal or Near Normal ECF Volume

The possibility of a low plasma sodium being an artefact should be considered. This can occur if blood is taken from an arm into which 5% dextrose is being infused or if blood is taken from an indwelling cannula without sufficient flushing. Apparent hyponatraemia may result from a reduction in the fractional water content of plasma owing to hypertriglyceridaemia or hypoproteinaemia (see above). The plasma sodium concentration may also be reduced if a solute is present which is confined to the ECF. Thus the osmotic diuretic mannitol does not cross cell membranes in significant

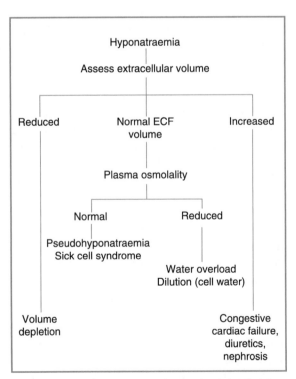

Figure 5.10 Suggested scheme for investigating hyponatraemia.

amounts and, if infused, will increase the osmolality of the ECF. This causes water to transfer to the ECF from the ICF, thus lowering the plasma sodium concentration. Similarly, in diabetes mellitus glucose is limited to the ECF in severe hyperglycaemia because of a lack of insulin action. This may cause water shifts to the ECF, thereby diluting sodium. Hyponatraemia can occur in many acute and chronic conditions in the absence of abnormalities of water and sodium excretion, this being designated the sick-cell syndrome. The causes of this are not clear, resetting of the hypothalamic osmostat being postulated to be one mechanism.

Hyponatraemia with Increased ECF Volume

Hyponatraemia can occur in oedematous states such as congestive cardiac failure. Although the total ECF volume is increased there is redistribution of sodium and water, with interstitial fluid volume being increased and plasma volume decreased. This leads to activation of volume receptors and stimulation of vasopressin secretion. Diuretic therapy, particularly thiazides, can lead to hyponatraemia by interfering with distal tubular sodium reabsorption, which disturbs the mechanism of urinary dilution and thus impairs water excretion.

KEY POINTS

HYPONATRAEMIA

- Hyponatraemia is commonly due to water excess

- Hyponatraemia is dangerous if it occurs rapidly because the water content of intracellular spaces increases

- Hyponatraemia can cause cell swelling leading to cerebral compression

FURTHER READING

Arieff AI. Management of Hyponatraemia. *British Medical Journal* 1993; **307:** 305-8

Gill GV, Flear CTG. Hyponatraemia. *Recent Advances in Clinical Biochemistry* 1985; **3:** 149-76

Maxwell MH, Kleeman CR, Narins RG (eds). *Clinical Disorders of Fluid and Electrolyte Metabolism* (4th edn). New York: McGraw-Hill, 1987

Narins RG, Jones ER, Stom MC, *et al.* Diagnostic strategies in disorders of fluid, electrolyte, and acid–base homeostasis. *American Journal of Medicine* 1982; **72:** 496

Sterns RH, Narins RG. Hypernatremia and hyponatremia: pathophysiology, diagnosis and treatment. In Adroguè HJ (ed.). *Acid–Base and Electrolyte Disorders.* New York: Churchill Livingstone, 1991, pp. 161–91

CASE HISTORIES

CASE 5.1

A 24-year-old woman who was known to have insulin-dependent diabetes mellitus was admitted to casualty with signs and symptoms suggestive of ketoacidosis. The following were the results of the initial blood tests:

sodium	117 mmol l^{-1}
potassium	4.6 mmol l^{-1}
chloride	95 mmol l^{-1}
total CO_2	11 mmol l^{-1}
urea	9.4 mmol l^{-1}
creatinine	180 μmol l^{-1}
glucose	25.6 mmol l^{-1}
osmolality	322 mmol kg^{-1}
plasma sample reported as grossly lipaemic	

Explain the low plasma sodium concentration.

CASE 5.2

A 56-year-old man presented to his general practitioner with breathlessness and was noted to have finger clubbing. The following electrolyte results were obtained:

sodium	121 mmol l^{-1}
potassium	2.9 mmol l^{-1}
chloride	88 mmol l^{-1}
total CO_2	20 mmol l^{-1}
urea	3.2 mmol l^{-1}
creatinine	75 μmol l^{-1}
osmolality	253 mmol kg^{-1}

Explain these results.

CASE 5.3

An 85-year old woman who lived alone was discovered by neighbours in a drowsy, confused state. On admission she was extremely dirty and her tongue was dry. Admission electrolytes were as follows:

sodium	159 mmol l^{-1}
potassium	3.7 mmol l^{-1}
chloride	123 mmol l^{-1}
total CO_2	26 mmol l^{-1}
urea	19.8 mmol l^{-1}
creatinine	145 μmol l^{-1}

What are the possible causes of the electrolyte disturbances?

6

POTASSIUM METABOLISM

INTRODUCTION

Total body potassium in adults is around 3500 mmol, of which only about 70 mmol is present in extracellular spaces; thus, potassium is the major intracellular cation of the body and because of this potassium plays a primary role in the maintenance of intracellular volume. The ratio of extracellular to intracellular potassium is an important determinant of membrane potential in nerves and muscle, including cardiac muscle.

POTASSIUM HOMEOSTASIS

Potassium is widely available in the diet, being present in appreciable amounts in both plants and animals. The average daily intake is 50–100 mmol day^{-1}. Considerable amounts of potassium are secreted by gastrointestinal secretions, although these are largely reabsorbed. Very small amounts are lost in sweat and faeces, the remainder being excreted by the kidney. Potassium is freely filtered by the glomerulus and almost completely reabsorbed in the proximal convoluted tubule (**Figure 6.1**). Urinary excretion of potassium occurs through distal tubular secretion by two mechanisms, active secretion and passive diffusion, together with H$^+$, in exchange for sodium. This latter mechanism is the more important quantitatively, potassium and H$^+$ secretion maintaining electrochemical balance in the tubular lumen. Several factors influence potassium excretion:

1. The relative concentrations of potassium and H$^+$ in the tubular cells. In metabolic acidosis, potassium secretion will be reduced, since hydrogen ion excretion will increase as a result of raised cellular levels of H$^+$. Conversely, increased potassium excretion occurs in metabolic alkalosis, since cellular levels of H$^+$ are

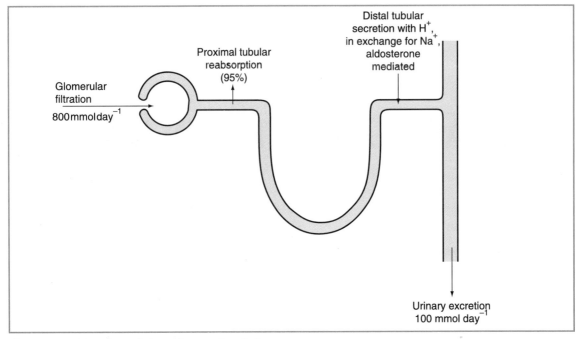

Figure 6.1 Renal regulation of potassium balance.

reduced. In potassium depletion, cellular levels are reduced and increased H^+ secretion occurs.

2. If the tubular secretion of H^+ is impaired potassium secretion is increased. This occurs in type I renal tubular acidosis (see below).

3. The amount of sodium reabsorbed in the distal tubule affects potassium secretion. If sodium reabsorption is increased, an electrochemical gradient occurs, favouring passive potassium secretion. This occurs if increased amounts of sodium are delivered to the distal tubule (e.g. diuretic therapy) and if aldosterone action is increased.

4. Aldosterone stimulates potassium secretion directly, in addition to increasing sodium reabsorption and greater passive potassium secretion.

5. A high rate of flow of fluid within the renal tubule favours potassium secretion.

The kidney responds effectively to increased intake but is less efficient at conserving potassium than sodium. In-creased potassium intake increases aldosterone secretion directly, which enhances excretion.

The intracellular distribution of potassium within the body is maintained by sodium–potassium adenosine triphosphatases (ATPases) in cell membranes. Two other factors influence potassium distribution – plasma insulin and H^+ concentrations. Insulin promotes cellular uptake of potassium, while in the presence of metabolic acidosis increased amounts of potassium leak from cells in exchange for H^+ ions, which are sequestered within cells.

KEY POINTS

POTASSIUM HOMEOSTASIS

- In a 70 kg adult approximately 70 mmol is extracellular and 3500 mmol intracellular

- Homeostasis is maintained by regulation of renal excretion

- Acid–base balance, aldosterone action and sodium metabolism affect renal potassium excretion

POTASSIUM DEPLETION AND HYPOKALAEMIA

Plasma potassium concentrations are 3.3–4.4 mmol l^{-1}, with serum levels being slightly higher owing to release from cells during the clotting process. In practice this difference is unimportant as reference ranges are determined for the type of sample used. Hypokalaemia and potassium depletion are not synonymous because low plasma potassium concentrations can occur owing to redistribution from the extracellular fluid (ECF) to the intracellular fluid (ICF), rather than as a result of losses.

Causes of Potassium Depletion and Hypokalaemia

The causes of potassium depletion and hypokalaemia are outlined in **Table 6.1.**

Table 6.1 Causes of potassium depletion and hypokalaemia

Artefactual
◆ Dilution of blood by intravenous fluid

Reduced intake

Internal redistribution
◆ Alkalosis
◆ Insulin administration
◆ Familial periodic paralysis

Increased losses
◆ Gastrointestinal losses
  Vomiting, diarrhoea, fistula drainage, aspiration
  Villous adenoma
  Purgative abuse
◆ Renal losses
  Diuretics
  Osmotic diuresis
  Excess mineralocorticoids
  Renal tubular acidosis
  Magnesium depletion
◆ Skin losses
  Excessive sweating

Artefactual

There are fewer artefactual causes of hypokalaemia than hyperkalaemia, although venepuncture should be undertaken in the opposite arm from any intravenous infusion to avoid the possibility of diluting the blood sample.

Reduced Intake

Reduced intake rarely leads to depletion since potassium is available from most foods. However, potassium depletion can occur in prolonged starvation and anorexia nervosa, although many patients with the latter condition also take purgatives which can increase faecal loss of potassium. Alcoholic patients may have a diet that is poor in potassium and hypokalaemia can occur, although other factors, such as liver disease and magnesium deficiency, may make more significant contributions to potassium depletion than reduced intake.

Internal Redistribution

Internal redistribution of potassium with increased cellular uptake causes hypokalaemia in the absence of potassium depletion. In alkalotic states, H$^+$ ions move out of cells in exchange for extracellular potassium. The renal excretion of potassium is also increased. However, metabolic alkalosis may occur as a consequence of hypokalaemia, as the renal excretion of H$^+$ ions is increased. Insulin infusion or increased insulin secretion following a glucose load increases potassium cellular uptake, mainly by the liver and muscles, by increasing sodium–potassium ATPase activity. Familial periodic paralysis is a rare inherited disorder, affecting males predominantly, in which episodic shifts of potassium from the ECF to ICF occurs which lead to muscle weakness. The precise aetiology is unclear but this condition is thought to be caused by the production of a mineralocorticoid in addition to aldosterone.

Gastrointestinal Losses

The secretions of the gastrointestinal tract contain a relatively large proportion of ECF potassium and therefore vomiting and aspiration of gut secretions can cause hypokalaemia (**Table 6.2**). Colonic secretions and mucus contain up to $40 \, \text{mmol} \, l^{-1}$ potassium and excessive losses of these are a cause of depletion. A villous adenoma of the rectum may secrete up to 1 l of fluid per day. Gastrointestinal secretions also contain sodium and if this is not replaced adequately hyperaldosteronism will develop. This will have the effect of increasing potassium depletion. Purgative abuse induces potassium loss by increasing faecal excretion.

Renal Losses

Hypokalaemia is a well-recognized complication of diuretic therapy. Potassium excretion is increased by thiazides, loop diuretics and carbonic anhydrase inhibitors. Sodium reabsorption is inhibited proximal to the site of potassium excretion in the renal tubule and therefore the delivery of sodium to the distal tubule is increased, more being available for aldosterone-mediated exchange with potassium. Potassium depletion is often not significant with diuretic therapy but hypokalaemia can sometimes occur, particularly in hypertensive patients, and the elderly appear particularly prone to develop hypokalaemia despite a normal diet. Potassium supplements should be considered in patients receiving both diuretics and digoxin, as the effects of digoxin are potentiated by hypokalaemia. Intercurrent illness, particularly diarrhoea and vomiting, may induce hypokalaemia in patients receiving diuretics.

Osmotic diuretics interfere with potassium absorption in the proximal tubule, leading to increased excretion. Although increased urinary losses occur in diabetic ketoacidosis hypokalaemia is extremely rare and, indeed, hyperkalaemia is relatively common. This is because the metabolic acidosis causes exchange of H^+ ions and potassium across cell membranes, increasing ECF potassium concentrations (see chapter 1). However, when diabetic ketoacidosis is treated with insulin therapy, potassium re-enters the cells and hypokalaemia develops, which usually requires potassium replacement.

There are two main types of renal tubular acidosis (see chapter 7). Because H^+ ions are not secreted normally, increased losses of potassium in exchange for sodium occur in the distal tubule and the unusual combination of hypokalaemia and a metabolic acidosis results.

Mineralocorticoid Excess

Aldosterone is a major factor regulating potassium excretion and increased urinary losses occur in hyperaldosteronism. Hypokalaemia occurs in both primary (Conn's syndrome) and secondary hyperaldosteronism, the latter due to renin-secreting tumours, hyperplasia of juxtaglomerular bodies (Bartter's syndrome) and renal ischaemia. Secondary hyperaldosteronism

Table 6.2 Composition of gastrointestinal secretions

Secretion	24-h volume (l)	Potassium (mmol)	Sodium (mmol)
Saliva	1	20	50
Gastric juice	1–2	15	50–70
Bile	1	5	100
Pancreatic juice	1–2	5	150
Succus entericus	1–2	5–10	140

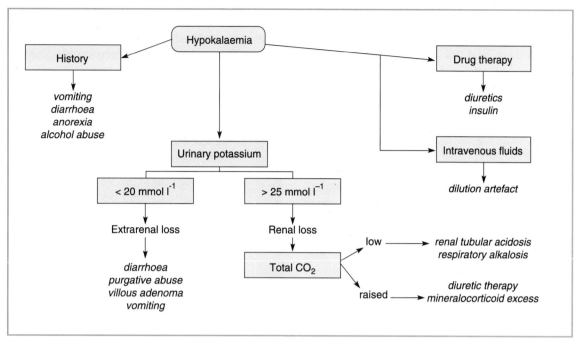

Figure 6.2 Suggested scheme for the differential diagnosis of hypokalaemia.

also occurs for 2–3 days postoperatively owing to increased renin secretion induced by anaesthesia. This is of limited duration and does not usually lead to hypokalaemia unless potassium is also lost by an additional route, such as nasogastric aspiration or vomiting. Glucocorticoids have weak mineralocorticoid activity and potassium depletion sometimes occurs in Cushing's syndrome, particularly if this is due to ectopic adrenocorticotrophic hormone (ACTH) production (see chapter 15). Licorice contains a substance which has mineralocorticoid activity and severe hypokalaemia occurs in subjects who eat large quantities.

Magnesium Depletion

Hypokalaemia has been found in association with magnesium deficiency, this only responding to treatment after magnesium replacement. This may be due to a defect in Na–K ATPase, which is magnesium dependent.

Excessive Sweating

Fluid losses through the skin increase in hot climates and during prolonged severe exercise. Sweat contains 10–20 mmol l[-1] potassium but additional losses can occur if fluid loss causes hypovolaemia, due to increased renin secretion and secondary hyperaldosteronism.

Clinical Features of Potassium Depletion

Moderate degrees of depletion may be asymptomatic, particularly if the condition develops slowly; many patients with more severe or acute depletion complain of muscle weakness, and paralysis can occur in extreme cases. Characteristic ECG changes may be seen, although they are only crude indicators of potassium depletion. These include flattening and inversion of T waves, more marked U waves and ST segment depression. Potassium depletion enhances digoxin toxicity. A further effect of potassium depletion is impaired renal function, particularly impairment of urinary concentration leading to polyuria. Potassium is required for normal insulin secretion and insulin release in response to increasing blood glucose concentrations is impaired in potassium depletion.

Investigation

The cause may be obvious from the clinical features, e.g. vomiting, diarrhoea, drug history (**Figure 6.2**). However, hypokalaemia is found occasionally with no explanation which is immediately apparent and causes such as purgative abuse should be considered. Assessment of acid–base status and urinary potassium excretion may be helpful. The presence of a metabolic acidosis suggests renal tubular acidosis while inappropriately high urinary potassium excretion points to renal losses. Urinary excretion usually falls to < 10 mmol l^{-1} when depletion is due to gastrointestinal losses, while values > 25 mmol l^{-1} suggest a renal cause. It should be remembered that an extracellular alkalosis may cause or result from potassium depletion.

Management

Whenever possible, potassium supplements (usually potassium chloride) should be given by mouth. Intravenous administration is required when hypokalaemia is severe, or if the patient is unable to take oral supplements. The concentration of potassium in intravenous fluids should not exceed 50 mmol l^{-1}, as rapid infusion of more concentrated solutions can cause local pain. The rate of infusion should not exceed 20 mmol h^{-1}, except in severe cases, particularly patients with paralysis, when infusion rates of up to 40 mmol h^{-1} may be considered. The results of treatment are monitored by repeated plasma determinations, evaluation of related symptoms and electrocardiograms (ECGs). In general, im-

provement in ECG abnormalities is a poor guide to potassium status, although such monitoring is important when rapid infusion is undertaken.

> **KEY POINTS**
>
> **HYPOKALAEMIA**
>
> - Hypokalaemia may be asymptomatic, even when severe
> - Plasma potassium concentration is a poor guide to total body potassium
> - Hypokalaemia usually indicates potassium depletion, although internal redistribution may be responsible

HYPERKALAEMIA

Causes

The causes of hyperkalaemia are outlined in **Table 6.3**.

Table 6.3   Causes of hyperkalaemia

Artefactual
- Haemolysis
- Breakdown of leukaemic cells
- Delayed separation of plasma
- Faulty venepuncture technique
- Inappropriate anticoagulant for specimen

Increased intake
- Infusion
- Oral supplements

Increased release from cells
- Tissue damage
- Metabolic acidosis
- Digoxin toxicity

Decreased excretion
- Renal failure
- Mineralocorticoid deficiency (Addison's disease)
- Angiotensin converting enzyme inhibitors
- Potassium-sparing diuretics

Artefactual

Because potassium concentration is very high within cells, plasma concentrations may be increased if cell lysis occurs during sampling. Causes include haemolysis and breakdown of leukaemic cells. Potassium may also leak from cells after venepuncture if cell separation from plasma is delayed. Erythrocyte potassium concentrations are usually maintained for 2–3 h as, until it is exhausted, endogenous glucose will maintain membrane Na–K ATPase activity. Occasionally, an inherited disorder of erythrocyte membrane function causes potassium levels to increase *in vitro* within 2 h.

Blood should be sampled from the opposite arm from infusion sites, as free communication between superficial veins may lead to contamination of a blood sample; this may cause apparent hyperkalaemia if the infusate contains potassium. Some anticoagulants, such as ethylene diamine tetraacetic acid (EDTA), contain potassium and should not be used for electrolyte analysis.

Excessive Intake

Excessive intake rarely causes hyperkalaemia because the normal kidney is able to excrete large amounts. However, potassium supplementation in patients receiving diuretic therapy can cause hyperkalaemia, particularly if mild renal impairment is present. Intravenous potassium administration may lead to hyperkalaemia if the infusion is rapid, this being more severe if tissue uptake is limited, e.g. by insulin deficiency.

Increased Release From Cells

Potassium leaks from damaged cells into the ECF and hyperkalaemia can therefore occur in burns, crush injuries and rhabdomyolysis. Cytotoxic therapy may lead to rapid destruction of cells, particularly in the treatment of haematological malignancies. Acute metabolic acidosis leads to exchange of potassium and H^+ across cell membranes and thus hyperkalaemia. Digoxin inhibits Na–K ATPase activity and in severe toxicity causes hyperkalaemia.

Decreased Excretion

Impaired excretion may cause hyperkalaemia, although this is unusual in chronic renal failure unless oliguria occurs. Hyperkalaemia occurs frequently in acute renal failure and contributing factors include oliguria, metabolic acidosis and increased tissue breakdown. Decreased distal tubular exchange of both potassium and H^+ for sodium result from aldosterone deficiency in Addison's disease – hyponatraemia, hyperkalaemia and metabolic acidosis are characteristic of this condition. Drugs can interfere with aldosterone action by two mechanisms. First, by reducing aldosterone production (angiotensin converting enzyme (ACE) inhibitors, e.g. captopril and enalopril), and second, by competing with aldosterone for binding sites in the distal tubules, inhibiting its action and leading to increased retention of potassium and H^+. Aldosterone antagonists such as spironolactone act in this way.

Clinical Features and Investigation

The most important clinical consequence of hyperkalaemia is cardiac arrhythmias. Tall tented T waves are seen on ECG with plasma potassium concentrations of approximately 6 mmol l^{-1}, while absent P waves, widened QRS complexes and ventricular arrhythmias leading to fibrillation occur progressively at higher concentrations. Muscular weakness leading to flaccid paralysis also occurs in hyperkalaemia.

Hyperkalaemia requires urgent investigation to establish the cause because of the cardiac consequences. The initial investigations will usually include plasma sodium, total CO_2 and urea concentrations and therefore renal failure, Addison's disease and metabolic acidosis can be considered. Artefactual causes should be eliminated and the drug history should be checked. If the cause is still not apparent urinary potassium concentration should be measured; it is inappropriately low in hypoaldosteronism.

Management

Mild hyperkalaemia can usually be managed by treating the cause; progressive or severe abnormalities require specific treatment. Intravenous infusion of 10–20 ml 10% calcium gluconate antagonizes the cardiotoxic effects of hyperkalaemia, although this does not alter potassium levels and thus the effect is of short duration. Infusion of hypertonic glucose solutions causes cellular uptake of potassium by stimulating insulin secretion, thus reducing plasma levels. Insulin is usually administered simultaneously although this is probably only necessary in insulin-dependent diabetic patients. The effect lasts several hours. Sodium bicarbonate infusion (100–200 ml, 8.4% solution) induces an intracellular shift of potassium by causing an extracellular alkalosis, the effect being particularly marked in acidotic patients.

None of these treatments removes excess potassium from the body. This can be achieved by administering a cation-exchange resin orally or as an enema, or by either peritoneal dialysis or haemodialysis.

KEY POINTS

HYPERKALAEMIA

■ Cardiac arrhythmias are an important consequence of hyperkalaemia

■ Artefactual causes of hyperkalaemia must be considered

■ True hyperkalaemia results from impaired excretion or internal redistribution of potassium

FURTHER READING

DeFronzo RA, Bia M, Smith D. Clinical disorders of hyperkalaemia. *Annual Review of Medicine* 1982; **33**: 521-54

Lutarewych MA, Battle DC. Disorders of potassium balance. In: Adrogué HJ (ed.), *Acid–Base and Electrolyte Disorders.* New York: Churchill Livingstone, 1991, pp. 193–232

Maxwell MH, Kleeman CR, Narins RG (eds). *Clinical Disorders of Fluid and Electrolyte Metabolism* (4th edn). New York: McGraw-Hill, 1987

Morgan DB (ed.). Electrolyte disorders. *Clinics in Endocrinology and Metabolism* 1984; **13**: 231–434.

CASE 6.1

A 47-year-old woman underwent cholecystectomy and 2 days later a sample was sent for postoperative electrolyte analysis. The results were as follows:

sodium	142 mmol l^{-1}
potassium	11.3 mmol l^{-1}
chloride	108 mmol l^{-1}
total CO_2	21 mmol l^{-1}
urea	6.1 mmol l^{-1}
creatinine	74 μmol l^{-1}

The specimen was not haemolysed. What are the possible causes of the hyperkalaemia?

CASE 6.2

A 38-year-old woman had been feeling unwell for 3 weeks and had been vomiting intermittently for 6 days. She was sent to the Accident and Emergency Department by her general practitioner who found that she was dehydrated when he was called to see her at home. Urine analysis was negative for glucose and ketones and initial blood tests showed the following:

sodium	119 mmol l^{-1}
potassium	5.8 mmol l^{-1}
chloride	91 mmol l^{-1}
total CO_2	18 mmol l^{-1}
urea	27.8 mmol l^{-1}
creatinine	147 μmol l^{-1}

Explain these results.

CASE 6.3

A 73-year-old man had a history of congestive cardiac failure which was treated with a thiazide diuretic and potassium supplements. On review in outpatients he complained of weakness and unsteadiness when walking and was found to have the following blood results:

sodium	135 mmol l^{-1}
potassium	2.7 mmol l^{-1}
chloride	91 mmol l^{-1}
total CO_2	32 mmol l^{-1}
urea	8.3 mmol l^{-1}
creatinine	126 μmol l^{-1}

Comment on these results.

HYDROGEN ION AND BLOOD GAS HOMEOSTASIS

INTRODUCTION

Acids are produced continuously during normal metabolism, although the blood concentrations of free hydrogen ions (H^+) vary between narrow limits. The concentration of H+ in blood is usually expressed as the negative $logarithm_{10}$ (pH), the pH of extracellular fluid normally being 7.35–7.45. Expressed as a molar concentration this represents 35–45 nmol l^{-1} H^+. Measurements of intracellular pH, which must be indirect in order to preserve cell structure, suggest that this is lower, around 6.9.

Relatively constant H^+ concentrations are important physiologically, as small changes in pH affect enzyme activity and thus metabolism. The immediate defence against changing H^+ concentrations is provided by buffers, while excretion is regulated by adaptive responses in the lungs and kidney.

ACID PRODUCTION

Hydrogen ions are generated during intermediary metabolism from several sources including ATP hydrolysis, respiratory chain

Table 7.1 Acids and potential acids produced in man

Acid	Source	Normal fate	Daily production (mmol)
Carbon dioxide (carbonic acid)	Cellular respiration	Excretion by lungs	20 000
Organic acids			
Lactic acid	Anaerobic glycolysis	Gluconeogenesis	1000
Ketone bodies	Fatty acid oxidation	Tissue oxidation	
Mineral acids			
Sulphuric acid	Sulphur-containing amino acids	Renal excretion	70
Phosphoric acid	Organic phosphorus-containing compounds		

reactions and the reduction of nicotinamide nucleotides. Although 150 000 mmol H^+ are produced by these mechanisms each day, reutilization occurs and therefore there is no net gain of acid. Acidic anions are produced from several sources (**Table 7.1**). The principle product of the oxidation of substrates for energy utilization, mainly carbohydrate and fat, is carbon dioxide. Although carbon dioxide is not an acid it dissolves in water to form carbonic acid and since large quantities are produced, 12 000–20 000 mmol day^{-1}, accumulation of carbon dioxide may lower body pH. However, production of carbon dioxide and its excretion through the lungs are normally in balance. Because carbon dioxide is excreted by the lungs, it can be viewed as being volatile acid.

Nonvolatile acid is of two types, organic and inorganic. Organic acids, mainly lactic acid and ketone bodies, are produced from carbohydrates and lipids. Lactate is produced continuously from the anaerobic metabolism of glucose, particularly in erythrocytes and skeletal muscle. Production by skeletal muscle increases during strenuous exercise, although glycolysis in erythrocytes produces lactate continuously, as these cells do not contain mitochondria or enzymes for the aerobic oxidation of pyruvate. Considerable quantities of lactate are produced normally but these are reconverted to glucose, mainly in the liver. Plasma lactate concentration is normally around 1 mmol l^{-1}, although this rises if production increases or metabolism is impaired. Acidic ketone bodies, acetoacetate and 3-hydroxybutyrate, are produced from the metabolism of fatty acids in the liver and utilized as an alternative fuel to glucose (see chapter 1). Blood concentrations of ketone bodies in the fed state are very low, less than 1 mmol l^{-1}, with only slight increases (0.1 mmol l^{-1}) occurring overnight. However, ketone body production increases with prolonged fasting, with blood levels of up to 3 mmol l^{-1} after three days, and also in diabetic ketoacidosis where levels of 10 mmol l^{-1} may occur. Because organic acids are almost fully metabolized, under normal circumstances they contribute little to net acid excretion.

Inorganic acids arise from two main sources, sulphur-containing amino acids and phosphorus-containing organic compounds. Oxidation of sulphydryl groups in cysteine and methionine results in the synthesis of sulphuric acid while hydrolysis of phosphoesters produces phosphoric acid. Approximately 40–80 mmol of these strong acids are produced daily, although they do not exist in these forms since they are buffered. Inorganic acidic anions must be excreted from the body by the kidney.

ACID PRODUCTION

■ Three types of acid, carbon dioxide (carbonic acid), organic acids, and inorganic acids, are produced during metabolism

■ Carbon dioxide is excreted by the lungs

■ Organic acids (ketones, lactate) are normally utilized by the body

■ Inorganic acids are excreted by the kidney

BODY BUFFERS

An acid is a substance that increases H^+ concentration, thus reducing pH, while a base is a proton acceptor. Bases decrease H^+ concentrations and raise the pH. A buffer is a substance that attenuates changes in pH which would otherwise result from the addition of a strong acid or base to a solution. Buffers are solutions of weak acids or bases which contain both dissociated and undissociated forms. The general equilibrium equation for a buffer system is:

$$H^+ + B^- = HB$$

where HB is the undissociated weak acid and B^- is a base, since it combines with H^+.

If a stronger acid, i.e. one which dissociates more readily, is added to this solution, the change in H^+ concentration is minimized, as the law of mass action will apply and the equilibrium will be shifted to the right. The Henderson–Hasselbach equation is often used to consider pH changes resulting from the addition of acid or base to a buffer system:

$$pH = pK + \log \frac{[B^-]}{[HB]}$$

Where pK is the dissociation constant.

The efficiency of a buffer system in limiting changes in pH is greatest when the amount of free base is equal to the amount of undissociated acid; the pH equals the pK when the concentration of these is equimolar. The capacity of buffers to limit pH changes is also determined by their concentration.

Buffers in Blood and Extracellular Fluid

There are four principal buffers in the ECF and ICF (**Table 7.2**):

(i)   carbonic acid–bicarbonate system,
(ii) proteins,
(iii) haemoglobin,
(iv) phosphate buffer system.

The principal buffers of ECF are the carbonic acid–bicarbonate system and haemoglobin, while proteins and phosphates are the main intracellular buffers.

Carbonic Acid–Bicarbonate

The equilibrium reaction for the buffer pair is:

$$H^+ + HCO_3^- = H_2CO_3$$

The addition of H^+ causes the equilibrium to be displaced to the right. Carbonic acid is a relatively strong acid, the problem that this would otherwise cause being overcome by

Table 7.2 Body buffers

Buffer$^-$ (base)	→	H Buffer (acid)
$H^+ + HCO_3^-$	→	$H_2CO_3 \rightarrow CO_2 + H_2O$
$H^+ + HPO_4^{2}$	→	$H_2PO_4^-$
$H^+ + Hb^-$	→	$H.Hb$
$H^+ + Prot^-$	→	$H.Prot$

the equilibrium of carbonic acid with dissolved carbon dioxide.

$$H_2CO_3 = CO_2 + H_2O$$

As carbon dioxide is rapidly excreted by the lungs, the overall effects of the above two equations is to limit pH changes. This, together with the relatively high concentration of bicarbonate in the extracellular fluid (ECF), also overcomes the other deficiency of this buffer system, the low pK (6.1) compared with the mean pH of blood (7.4). The amount of carbon dioxide in blood is determined by measuring the partial pressure of the gas (P_{CO_2}, see below), the molar concentration being obtained by multiplying the P_{CO_2} in kilopascals by 0.225, the solubility coefficient. The Henderson–Hasselbach equation expresses the relative concentrations of bicarbonate and carbon dioxide thus:

$$pH = 6.1 + \log \frac{[HCO_3^-]}{P_{CO_2} \times 0.225}$$

For the normal body pH of 7.4 log $[HCO_3^-]/P_{CO_2} \times 0.225$ is 1.3, for which the antilog is 20. Therefore the ratio of $[HCO_3^-]/P_{CO_2}$ expressed in molar concentrations is 20:1.

Haemoglobin

Haemoglobin plays an important role in the regulation of H^+ concentration, its buffering capacity being due to the polar groups of the constituent amino acids. Haemoglobin is a more important buffer than other proteins for three reasons: (i) its relatively high molar concentration; (ii) it is relatively rich in histidine, which has a pK of approximately 7, close to blood pH; and (iii) its role in the transport of blood gases (see below).

Proteins

Proteins other than haemoglobin are relatively minor buffers in the ECF but, because of higher intracellular concentrations, they are important cellular buffers.

Phosphate

The phosphate buffer pair mono- and di-hydrogen phosphate (HPO_4^{2-} and $H_2PO_4^-$) is present in low concentrations in the ECF although it is an important urinary buffer.

KEY POINTS

BUFFERS

- Buffers limit the change of pH that would be caused by the addition of strong acid or base

- The major buffers of the ECF are carbonic acid–bicarbonate and haemoglobin

- The major buffers of the ICF are proteins and phosphates

BLOOD GAS TRANSPORT AND ACID–BASE BALANCE

Peripheral Tissues

The erythrocytes supply peripheral tissues with oxygen and also play a key role in carbon dioxide metabolism. Carbon dioxide produced within cells diffuses into the ECF, increasing the P_{CO_2}. It enters erythrocytes, where the enzyme carbonic anhydrase (carbonate dehydratase) promotes the hydration of carbon dioxide and its dissociation into H^+ and HCO_3^- (**Figure 7.1**). Since the partial pressure of oxygen (P_{O_2}) is low relative to arterial blood, oxygen dissociates from haemoglobin and enters the tissues. Deoxyhaemoglobin buffers H^+, this having the effect of causing further oxygen release. Bicarbonate diffuses from red blood cells into the ECF and is replaced within erythrocytes by ECF chloride, maintaining electrochemical balance (chloride shift). Thus, the ECF bicarbonate:carbon dioxide ratio is maintained. A small amount of carbon dioxide combines directly with nitrogen groups in haemoglobin forming carbamino groups.

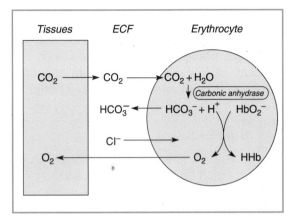

Figure 7.1 Transfer of oxygen and carbon dioxide between peripheral cells and erythrocytes. The oxygen tension in peripheral cells is low and therefore oxygen dissociates from haemoglobin. The CO_2 tension in tissues is low and it therefore diffuses into erythrocytes where it is hydrated, forming bicarbonate. This diffuses into the extracellular fluid (ECF) chloride diffusing in the opposite direction (chloride shift). Hydrogen ions generated during this process are buffered by haemoglobin. HHb, deoxyhaemoglobin; HbO_2, oxygenated haemoglobin.

The Lungs

The process of gas transport is reversed in the lungs (**Figure 7.2**). The $P\text{CO}_2$ is low in the lungs and carbon dioxide therefore diffuses from the ECF into the alveoli, thus creating a concentration gradient between plasma and erythrocytes. Carbon dioxide diffuses from erythrocytes, reversing the carbonic anhydrase reaction and removing H^+ from haemoglobin. Carbon dioxide is also released from carbamino groups. Bicarbonate diffuses down a concentration gradient into the red cells and chloride returns to the ECF. The $P\text{O}_2$ in alveoli is high compared to venous blood and therefore oxygen diffuses into erythrocytes, oxygenating haemoglobin.

The rate of alveolar excretion of carbon dioxide and oxygenation of haemoglobin depends on the rate of respiration, which is controlled by the respiratory centre. This is located in the hypothalamus, where

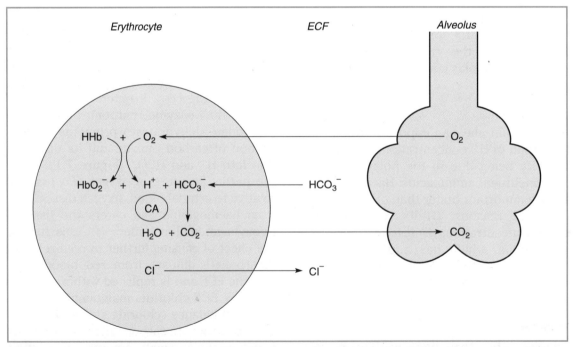

Figure 7.2 Transfer of oxygen and carbon dioxide between erythrocytes and alveolar air. The processes which occurred in peripheral tissues are reversed because the oxygen tension is high and the CO_2 tension is low in alveolar air compared with erythrocytes. ECF, extracellular fluid; HHb, deoxyhaemoglobin; HbO_2, oxygenated haemoglobin CA, carbonic anhydrase.

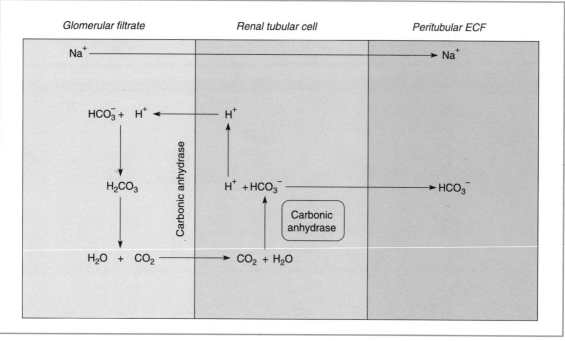

Figure 7.3 Bicarbonate reabsorption in the renal tubule. Bicarbonate cannot cross the tubular luminal membrane and is thus converted to CO_2 by H^+, which is secreted. This depends on membrane-bound carbonic anhydrase. Bicarbonate is generated by the tubular cell which diffuses into the extracellular fluid (ECF).

receptors respond to increasing carbon dioxide and H^+ concentrations. Therefore, the respiratory rate increases if the P_{CO_2} rises or the pH falls. There are also chemoreceptors in the aortic and carotid bodies which respond to changes in oxygen tension.

RENAL FUNCTION AND ACID–BASE BALANCE

The kidney has several important roles in acid–base balance, including bicarbonate reabsorption and generation, and the excretion of hydrogen ions and acidic anions.

Excretion of Acidic Anions

Provided the glomerular filtration rate is adequate, the acidic anions sulphate and phosphate are cleared from the plasma and excreted in the urine.

Reabsorption of Filtered Bicarbonate

Approximately 4000 mmol of bicarbonate are filtered each day by the glomeruli, most of which is reabsorbed in the proximal tubules (**Figure 7.3**). The proximal tubular cells are impermeable to bicarbonate, reabsorption being achieved by converting the bicarbonate to carbon dioxide; this process requires the secretion of hydrogen ions. Carbon dioxide is formed during cellular metabolism and is hydrated, as the cells contain carbonic anhydrase. The resulting H^+ ions are secreted and combine with bicarbonate in the tubular lumen; bicarbonate is then catalysed by carbonic anhydrase located in tubular cell brush borders. The carbon dioxide which is produced

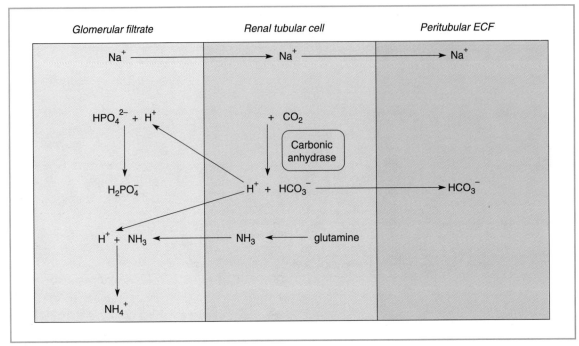

Glomerular filtrate   *Renal tubular cell*   *Peritubular ECF*

Figure 7.4 Net hydrogen ion excretion and buffering in the renal tubule. The major acceptors of H^+ are phosphates and ammonia. ECF, extracellular fluid.

enters the tubular cells and contributes to the bicarbonate regeneration process. The intracellular hydration of carbon dioxide generates bicarbonate which diffuses into the ECF, electrochemical balance being maintained by the simultaneous absorption of sodium. Normally, filtered bicarbonate is reabsorbed completely, although the tubular reabsorptive capacity is exceeded if the plasma bicarbonate concentration is $> 28\,\text{mmol l}^{-1}$. Under these circumstances bicarbonate will appear in the urine.

Hydrogen Ion Excretion and Bicarbonate Regeneration

Phosphate Buffering

Hydrogen ion excretion requires the presence of a buffer in the tubular fluid. In the proximal tubule bicarbonate accepts H^+, although bicarbonate reabsorption does not result in net H^+ excretion. This depends on other acceptors being present – the phosphate buffer system and urinary ammonia (**Figure 7.4**). The concentration of intraluminal phosphate increases in the more distal parts of the tubule because the bulk of water reabsorption occurs in the proximal tubule. Cellular carbon dioxide is hydrated in the distal tubular cells by a mechanism similar to that in the proximal tubule (catalysed by carbonic anhydrase). Hydrogen ions are excreted in exchange for sodium and bicarbonate is generated, which diffuses into the ECF. Secreted hydrogen ions are buffered by phosphate in the tubular luminal fluid. Urinary phosphate buffering accounts for the excretion of approximately $30\,\text{mmol H}^+$ per day.

Urinary Ammonia

Approximately $40\,\text{mmol H}^+$ are excreted each day as ammonium ions. The ammonium ion is produced within distal tubular cells from glutamine. Ammonium ions cannot diffuse out of the tubular cells into the lumen although ammonia is freely diffusible. Ammonium ions are in equilibrium with ammonia and this diffuses into the tubular lumen where it combines with H^+ forming ammonium which cannot then diffuse back into the tubular cell. The net effect of this is to trap H^+ in the tubular lumen,.

Urinary ammonia excretion increases in response to systemic acidosis, with up to 10 times the normal excretion occurring in conditions such as diabetic ketoacidosis.

KEY POINTS

THE ROLE OF THE KIDNEY IN H^+ HOMEOSTASIS

- Reabsorption of filtered bicarbonate

- H^+ excretion and bicarbonate regeneration

- Excretion of the acidic anions phosphate and sulphate

THE GASTROINTESTINAL TRACT AND ACID–BASE BALANCE

The Stomach

Hydrochloric acid is secreted by the stomach although, under normal circumstances, secretions are not lost from the body. In addition to secreting H^+ bicarbonate is generated by the gastric mucosa which diffuses into the ECF. Disturbances of acid–base balance occur if gastric secretions are lost by vomiting or aspiration.

The Small Intestine

Small intestinal enzymes require a pH of approximately 6.5 for optimal activity: therefore, the acidic gastric secretions must be neutralized and to achieve this bicarbonate is secreted by the pancreas, biliary tree and small intestine. Loss of small intestinal secretions thus causes disturbances of acid–base balance.

ASSESSMENT OF ACID–BASE BALANCE AND BLOOD GAS HOMEOSTASIS

Plasma Total Carbon Dioxide and Plasma Bicarbonate

The plasma total carbon dioxide level ($T{CO_2}$) is the most commonly measured indicator of blood acid–base status. Both carbon dioxide and substances capable of forming carbon dioxide are measured, the latter including bicarbonate and carbonic acid. The concentration of carbonic acid is small enough to be ignored and, as discussed above, the ratio of bicarbonate:carbon dioxide is normally 20:1. As the concentration of total carbon dioxide in plasma is 21–30 mmol l^{-1} in health, approximately 1 mmol l^{-1} is carbon dioxide and the remainder is bicarbonate. Both bicarbonate and carbon dioxide levels change in acid–base disturbances and therefore the total carbon dioxide concentration is only an approximation to the true plasma bicarbonate level, albeit a useful one. The true arterial bicarbonate level can be calculated from blood gas analysis, as the pH and $P{CO_2}$ are measured and the pK of the bicarbonate–carbon dioxide buffer pair is known.

Plasma total carbon dioxide and bicarbonate levels fall after blood is taken because carbon dioxide diffuses slowly from the blood into the air space above the specimen, the rate of loss being increased if a large air gap is present.

Blood Gases and pH

Large arteriovenous differences in $P{O_2}$ and $P{CO_2}$ occur which vary according to the tissue being perfused; thus, blood gas analysis is undertaken on arterial blood. For this reason, blood gas analysis is more unpleasant for the patient than determining the $T{CO_2}$ and is not without risk. Under some circumstances arterial puncture may be impractical, particularly for infants or if repeated investigation is required in an adult patient. For such subjects capillary blood is often taken. The composition of capillary blood approximates to that of arterial if the site of sampling is warm and vasodilated.

Blood is drawn into a heparinized syringe without allowing air to enter. Excess heparin should not be used as this will affect the results of analysis. Cellular metabolism continues after the blood is drawn and therefore specimens should be taken on ice and transported rapidly to the laboratory. The tests undertaken are pH, $P\text{CO}_2$ and $P\text{O}_2$, and arterial bicarbonate can be calculated.

Indications for Blood Gas Analysis

The estimation of blood gases is more inconvenient than measuring plasma $T\text{CO}_2$ and it is therefore undertaken less frequently. Indications include: (i) the evaluation of acute respiratory disease; (ii) patients on a ventilator; (iii) uncertainty about the cause of an abnormal $T\text{CO}_2$; (iv) mixed respiratory and metabolic disorders.

Interrelation of $P\text{CO}_2$, pH and Plasma Bicarbonate

The interrelation between bicarbonate, $P\text{CO}_2$ and pH in blood is expressed by the Henderson–Hasselbach equation, from which a graphical presentation can be derived (**Figure 7.5**). The solid line shows the levels of arterial bicarbonate and $P\text{CO}_2$ which will result in a blood pH of 7.4 and the shaded area covers the ranges of bicarbonate and $P\text{CO}_2$ found normally. The dotted line gives pH and H^+ concentrations for given bicarbonate and $P\text{CO}_2$ levels while the dashed lines show values of these at extremes of acidaemia and alkalaemia. The primary disturbances in acid–base disorders are either metabolic, due to a change in bicarbonate concentrations (A and C), or

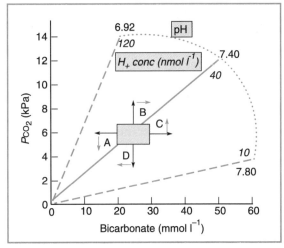

Figure 7.5 Changes in blood hydrogen ion levels, plasma bicarbonate concentrations and arterial $P\text{CO}_2$ which occur in acid–base disturbances. The primary abnormalities are shown by black arrows and compensation by green arrows. A, metabolic acidosis; B, respiratory acidosis; C, metabolic alkalosis; D, respiratory alkalosis. The extremes of pH which occur in disease are shown by the dotted lines and the values of $P\text{CO}_2$ and bicarbonate are shown by the dashed lines.

respiratory (B and D), where changes in $P\text{CO}_2$ are responsible. These are represented by solid arrows while the secondary compensatory changes which limit alterations in the bicarbonate:$P\text{CO}_2$ ratio are depicted by dashed arrows. These will be discussed in the following section on acid–base disturbances.

Anion Gap

Sodium and potassium contribute 90% of the cations in plasma while chloride and bicarbonate account for 80% of the anions. These four ions are estimated by many laboratories. The difference between the sum of the these anion and cation concentrations is termed the anion gap; this is normally 15–20 mmol l^{-1}. Thus (values are in mmol l^{-1}):

Sodium + potassium = chloride +
140   4   102
                    bicarbonate + A^-
                    25   17

where A^- is the anion gap ($17\,\text{mmol}\,\text{l}^{-1}$). Various substances contribute to the anion gap, including negatively charged proteins, phosphate, lactate, and acidic ketone bodies. Increased concentrations of some of these can cause metabolic acidosis and it is sometimes helpful in the evaluation of these conditions to measure the anion gap.

<table>
<tr><td rowspan="5">KEY POINTS</td><td>INVESTIGATION OF ACID–BASE DISORDERS

■ Measurement of venous $T\text{CO}_2$ is the test most commonly used to investigate acid–base status

■ Arterial or arterialized capillary blood is used for blood gas analysis

■ Measurement of the anion gap may be useful in investigating metabolic acidosis</td></tr>
</table>

DISORDERS OF ACID–BASE BALANCE

An increase in the H^+ concentration in blood (reduced pH) is an acidosis (A and B, **Figure 7.5**), while an alkalosis is present if the H^+ concentration is reduced (pH increased) (C and D, **Figure 7.5**). Changes in blood H^+ concentrations lead to compensatory responses which will limit pH changes. Occasionally, these responses restore the blood pH to normal, although the concentrations of body buffers will still be abnormal while the disturbance persists. To differentiate between compensated and uncompensated states, the terms acidaemia and alkalaemia are sometimes used to indicate abnormal blood pH, while acidosis and alkalosis describe any abnormality of H^+ balance, including those in which the pH is within the reference range but the concentration of buffers is abnormal. The last two terms are used in the present text.

Acidosis

Metabolic Acidosis

Metabolic acidosis refers to acid–base disturbances in which the primary abnormality is a reduction in plasma $T\text{CO}_2$ (bicarbonate) concentrations (solid arrow A, **Figure 7.5**). The causes fall into two broad groups, the presence of excess acid, which consumes bicarbonate during buffering, or the loss of bicarbonate from the body. The effect of either process is to reduce the blood bicarbonate:$P\text{CO}_2$ ratio, lowering pH.

Rapid compensation is due to stimulation of the respiratory centre by increased extracellular H^+ concentrations, which reduce the blood $P\text{CO}_2$, thus limiting the change in the bicarbonate:$P\text{CO}_2$ ratio (dashed arrow A, **Figure 7.5**). If the kidney is not the cause of the metabolic acidosis and kidney function is normal, renal acid excretion increases over several days, owing to increased production of ammonia, which buffers urinary H^+. Several hundred mmol of excess acid can be excreted by this mechanism each day. The acidosis is fully compensated if the bicarbonate:$P\text{CO}_2$ ratio is restored to 20:1, although acid–base balance would not be normal under these circumstances if the $P\text{CO}_2$ and bicarbonate concentrations are reduced.

Causes The causes of metabolic acidosis are outlined in **Table 7.3**. These have been divided into two groups, depending on the anion gap. Where this is increased, an acidic anion other than chloride must be present in excess. Such acids include ketone bodies and lactate, which are derived from intermediary metabolism, while others, such as formate and oxalate, arise from exogenous sources.

Ketone bodies are produced more rapidly than they are metabolized in diabetic ketoacidosis and a mild ketosis also occurs in starvation (chapter 1). Severe ketoacidosis, due to the accumulation of 3-hydroxybutyrate, may also occur in alcohol abuse,

Table 7.3   Causes of metabolic acidosis

> **With increased anion gap**
> Increased endogenous acid
> ◆ Ketosis
>   Diabetes mellitus, starvation, alcohol
>   intoxication
> ◆ Lactic acidosis
> Inherited metabolic disease
> ◆ Defects in carbohydrate metabolism
> ◆ Defects in amino acid or fatty acid
>   metabolism
> Increased ingestion of acids or potential acids
> ◆ Poisons
>   Salicylate overdose, methanol ingestion,
>   ethylene glycol poisoning
> Reduced acid excretion
> ◆ Renal failure
>
> **With normal anion gap (hyperchloraemia)**
> ◆ Renal tubular acidosis
> ◆ Carbonic anhydrase inhibitors
> ◆ Therapy with ammonium chloride, arginine
>   hydrochloride or lysine hydrochloride
> ◆ Diversion of urine into the gut
>   Vesico-colic fistula, ureterosigmoidostomy,
>   ileal bladder
> ◆ Diarrhoea

most often following an episode of heavy drinking: starvation and vomiting appear to be contributory factors. Lactic acidosis may also occur in alcoholic patients (see below). Long-chain ketoacids accumulate in some inherited disorders of fatty acid metabolism, such as proprionyl coenzyme A (CoA) carboxylase deficiency and methylmalonic acidaemias, and acidic anions are also present in excess in some amino acid disorders, e.g. maple syrup disease.

Substances which are taken with suicidal intent may cause metabolic acidosis, including ethylene glycol, which is the main constituent of antifreeze, and methanol. These are not themselves acidic but are metabolized to substances that are (ethylene glycol to oxalic acid and methanol to formic acid). These acidic metabolites are toxic and treatment of overdoses is directed at preventing the metabolism to acids, in addition to increasing excretion. The metabolism of these substances may be slowed considerably by infusing ethanol, as this has a higher affinity for the enzyme responsible for the production of the toxic metabolites, alcohol dehydrogenase, than either ethylene glycol or methanol.

Salicylate intoxication may cause a complex acid–base disturbance due to effects on intermediary metabolism and on the respiratory centre. Stimulation of the respiratory centre may lead to a respiratory alkalosis, particularly in adults (see below). Metabolic acidosis may arise because salicylate can uncouple oxidative phosphorylation and inhibit various enzymes which metabolize organic acids. Susceptibility to metabolic acidosis appears to be age-dependent, occurring predominantly in young children and the elderly.

Metabolic acidosis occurs in renal failure through two mechanisms. First, a failure to excrete mineral acids which are produced in the body, and second, a failure to conserve bicarbonate. The former mechanism is largely responsible for metabolic acidosis in uraemic patients, the retained acidic anions leading to an increased anion gap. However, more selective defects in renal function may also cause acid–base disturbances. In renal tubular acidosis (RTA) there is a failure to secrete H^+ ions, without defects in other tubular functions necessarily occurring. Two main types are recognized which occur as isolated defects or as a component of more widespread tubular dysfunction (the Fanconi syndrome). Both types may be hereditary and also result from renal tubular damage caused by hypercalacemia, toxins such as heavy metals, Bence–Jones proteinuria or inherited metabolic disease. In the proximal type (type 2) there is a failure to reabsorb filtered bicarbonate owing to a defect in the carbonic anhydrase mechanism. The distal tubular cells are still able to secrete H^+ and thus the urine can be acidified if a

Table 7.4 Causes of lactic acidosis

Tissue hypoxia present (type A)
◆ Severe hypoxia, e.g. cardiac arrest
◆ Shock, haemorrhage, hypotension
◆ Congestive cardiac failure

No tissue hypoxia (type B)
◆ Liver disease
◆ Biguanide therapy (diabetes mellitus)
◆ Alcohol intoxication
◆ Inherited metabolic disease
glucose-6-phosphatase or fructose-1,6-diphosphatase deficiency

severe systemic metabolic acidosis is present. In distal RTA (type 1) the urine cannot be acidified even if a severe systemic metabolic acidosis is present. This can be tested by administering an oral load of ammonium chloride, which is metabolized as ammonia and hydrochloric acid (**Table 8.4**). Although this increases the degree of metabolic acidosis the urinary pH does not fall below 5.5. The excretion of phosphate and sulphate is unimpaired. Because bicarbonate reabsorption is defective, greater amounts of chloride are reabsorbed as a counterion with sodium, in place of the bicarbonate, which is lost. Thus, hyperchloraemia develops and the anion gap is not increased. Hypokalaemia occurs in both types of RTA, in the distal type because only potassium can exchange for sodium, and in proximal RTA because increased amounts of sodium bicarbonate reach the distal tubule and thus increased sodium absorption occurs at this site, and more potassium is lost.

The oral administration of ammonium chloride constitutes an acid load, as hydrochloric acid is produced from its metabolism. A similar mechanism is responsible for metabolic acidosis which can develop following the administration or arginine hydrochloride or lysine hydrochloride. These amino acid forms are present in some parenteral nutrition solutions because the free amino acids have limited solubility.

Loss of bicarbonate may also have other causes. Drugs that inhibit carbonic anhydrase, such as acetazolamide, increase urinary bicarbonate loss. If urine is diverted into the gut for any reason bicarbonate is exchanged for chloride across intestinal epithelium. Severe diarrhoea may result in bicarbonate losses in liquid stools.

Clinical Features

The primary condition responsible for the metabolic acidosis may produce characteristic features, such as those which occur in diabetic ketoacidosis. In addition to these, characteristic features may result from the acidotic state. Hyperkalaemia is common, except in renal tubular acidosis or diarrhoea, owing to potassium and H^+ exchange across cell membranes. Chronic acidosis, such as occurs in untreated renal tubular acidosis, enhances calcium mobilization from bones and also reduces renal tubular calcium reabsorption. This may lead to osteomalacia, hypercalciuria, nephrocalcinosis and urinary tract stones. Severe metabolic acidosis impairs myocardial contractility and can cause arrhythmias.

Investigation of a Low Plasma Total Carbon Dioxide A metabolic acidosis will cause the plasma $T\text{CO}_2$ concentration to be low, although this will also occur in respiratory alkalosis. While the cause is often apparent from the clinical features, further investigation is sometimes required. A scheme for evaluating a low plasma $T\text{CO}_2$ value is shown in **Figure 7.6**.

KEY POINTS

METABOLIC ACIDOSIS
- Plasma $T\text{CO}_2$ concentrations are reduced in metabolic acidosis
- Metabolic acidosis is caused by excess acid or bicarbonate loss
- Compensation includes reduced plasma $P\text{CO}_2$ and, if renal function is normal, increased acid excretion

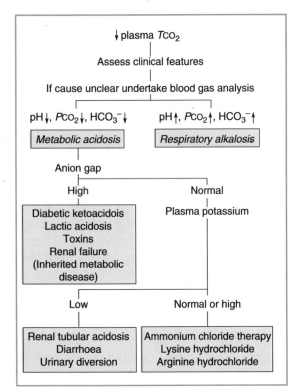

↓ plasma T_{CO_2}

Assess clinical features

If cause unclear undertake blood gas analysis

pH↓, P_{CO_2}↓, HCO_3^-↓	pH↑, P_{CO_2}↑, HCO_3^-↑
Metabolic acidosis	Respiratory alkalosis

Anion gap

High	Normal
	Plasma potassium
Diabetic ketoacidois Lactic acidosis Toxins Renal failure (Inherited metabolic disease)	

Low	Normal or high
Renal tubular acidosis Diarrhoea Urinary diversion	Ammonium chloride therapy Lysine hydrochloride Arginine hydrochloride

Figure 7.6 Suggested scheme for evaluating a low plasma total carbon dioxide concentration.

Lactic Acidosis Large quantities of lactate are produced by erythrocytes and muscle by anaerobic metabolism of pyruvate. Production and utilization are normally in balance and thus lactate does not accumulate unless these processes are impaired. Production increases sharply in strenuous exercise and lactate concentration in blood will rise, although this falls quite rapidly once the exercise has been completed owing to hepatic conversion of lactate to glucose (the Cori cycle). Lactate generation will also increase if oxygen delivery to tissues is insufficient for normal aerobic respiration. Thus, lactate production increases when tissue hypoxia is present, this sometimes being called type A lactic acidosis (**Table 7.4**). Cardiac arrest is probably the most extreme example but increased production also occurs in shock and congestive cardiac failure. Lactate accumulation in blood will also result if removal decreases, even in the absence of tissue hypoxia (type B lactic

acidosis). Since most lactate utilization occurs in the liver, severe hepatic failure can lead to type B lactic acidosis. Biguanides, used as oral hypoglycaemic agents in diabetes mellitus, occasionally cause impaired lactate metabolism and ethanol elevates plasma lactate, although only to a minor degree unless severe liver impairment is also present. Lactic acidosis may also result from inherited defects in gluconeogenesis (see chapter 1).

Respiratory Dysfunction and Blood Gases

Respiratory acidosis is not inevitable in respiratory dysfunction, even if hypoxia (reduced blood P_{O_2}) is present, as carbon dioxide can diffuse from blood into alveolar air approximately 20 times faster than oxygen can diffuse in the reverse direction. However, hypoxia occurs in conditions in which the P_{CO_2} increases (hypercapnia). The mechanisms by which hypoxia occur include impaired diffusion of gases, arteriovenous shunting of blood, ventilation–perfusion inequality (mismatch) and hypoventilation (**Table 7.5**).

Impaired Diffusion Equilibration between alveolar air and pulmonary capillary blood does not occur if the diffusion of gases is impaired. Conditions which interfere with gas exchange do not usually cause hypercapnia unless very severe disease is present. Interference with alveolar gas exchange occurs in pulmonary fibrosis, interstitial pneumonia and connective tissue disorders affecting the lung.

Shunts In shunting, some blood returns to the pulmonary artery without passing through a ventilated area of the lung. Shunts occur in lobar pneumonia, arteriovenous fistulae and adult respiratory distress syndrome. Hypoxia is common in these conditions but the P_{CO_2} is not usually elevated and indeed may be reduced as the rate of ventilation is often increased.

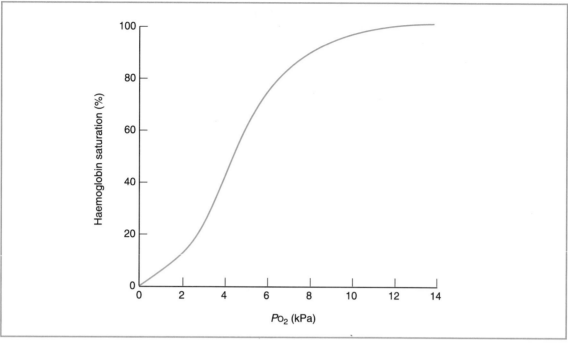

Figure 7.7   Oxygen dissociation curve of haemoglobin.

Ventilation–Perfusion Inequality Ventilation–perfusion inequality occurs because diseases at the alveolar level interfere with normal function, leading to inefficient gas exchange. Causes include chronic obstructive airways disease (chronic bronchitis and emphysema), asthma, pulmonary embolus and interstitial pulmonary disease. Some ventilation–perfusion inequality occurs in the normal lung as, in erect subjects, perfusion at the base of the lung is greater than at the apex. While the apex is also less well ventilated, the differences in ventilation across the lung are smaller than for perfusion. If ventilation is reduced in an area of the lung without vascular perfusion changing, blood Po_2 will not increase in these areas and Pco_2 will not fall. In patchy disease, not all alveoli are affected to the same extent and as blood from affected and unaffected alveoli mix the Po_2 and Pco_2 may be relatively normal, at least initially. With progression, increases in the Pco_2 and decreases in the Po_2 will stimulate respiration, the effect depending on the number of intact alveoli. As the number of affected alveoli increases hypoxia occurs, the excretion of carbon dioxide is impaired and hypercapnia and respiratory acidosis develop. Under normal conditions the arterial Po_2 is 12–14 kPa and haemoglobin is 97% saturated. The oxygen dissociation curve is such that the saturation of haemoglobin only falls to 90% when the Po_2 is 8 kPa (**Figure 7.7**). With lower Po_2 values oxygen saturation of haemoglobin falls steeply and cyanosis develops.

Hypoventilation In hypoventilation, air intake is reduced although the lungs are often normal. Causes include cardiac arrest, flail chest, neuromuscular disorders, and depression of the respiratory centre in the brain by cerebral disease or drugs. Occasionally, hypoventilation may be due to rib cage injuries, ankylosing spondylitis or extreme obesity (Pickwickian syndrome).

Respiratory Acidosis
Respiratory acidosis is caused by impaired carbon dioxide excretion and thus blood Pco_2 increases (solid arrow B, **Figure 7.5**).

Since the primary defect is pulmonary, compensation occurs by renal adaptation – generation of bicarbonate increases, restoring the bicarbonate:carbon dioxide ratio towards normal (dashed arrow B, **Figure 7.5**). The severity of the acidosis is reduced by this compensation, which is more effective in chronic than acute disease. Thus, the $T\text{CO}_2$ concentration may be very high in chronic respiratory disease, limiting the pH change, while the pH will be lower in acute respiratory failure with slight changes in $T\text{CO}_2$ which result from increased buffering by haemoglobin.

Acute respiratory acidosis occurs in cardiac arrest, flail chest, neuromuscular disorders and depression of the respiratory centre in the brain by cerebral disease or drugs. Chronic respiratory acidosis occurs in chronic obstructive airways disease (chronic bronchitis and emphysema) and severe asthma.

Oxygen Therapy Hypoxia is an immediate danger to patients with acute respiratory acidosis and administration of oxygen is often required. However, hypoxia is the major stimulus to respiratory drive in chronic respiratory acidosis, the respiratory centre becoming insensitive to hypercapnia. If oxygen-rich mixtures are administered to such patients the amount carried by haemoglobin increases little, while oxygen dissolved in solution, which is normally very small, increases. This may remove the hypoxic drive to respiration and if oxygen therapy is withdrawn patients may become apnoeic.

KEY POINTS

RESPIRATORY ACIDOSIS

- The primary abnormality is an increase in blood $P\text{CO}_2$

- Renal compensation leads to an increased plasma $T\text{CO}_2$

- Respiratory acidosis is not inevitable in hypoxia

Mixed Acidosis

Both respiratory and metabolic acidoses occur when there is respiratory depression combined with severe hypoxia, leading to increased lactate production. This combination can occur in cardiac arrest, narcotic overdose, severe obstructive airways disease or in respiratory distress syndrome in the newborn. Very low pH values are seen and the $P\text{CO}_2$ is raised, while the $T\text{CO}_2$ is not elevated, as would be expected in respiratory acidosis, but is usually low. The $T\text{CO}_2$ may be normal if the metabolic acidosis is mild.

Alkalosis

Metabolic Alkalosis

The primary abnormality in metabolic alkalosis is a high plasma bicarbonate concentration, the solid arrow C in **Figure 7.5**. Some compensation occurs as a result of respiratory depression with carbon dioxide retention (dashed arrow C), although the scope for this is limited as fully effective compensation would produce hypoxia, which would stimulate respiration. Renal compensation is the inhibition of bicarbonate reabsorption and regeneration, although under some circumstances this does not occur (see below).

Causes The causes of metabolic alkalosis are outlined in **Table 7.6**. In theory, administration of large amounts of sodium bicarbonate could lead to metabolic alkalosis. However, the renal response to elevated plasma bicarbonate, increased excretion, is very rapid and metabolic alkalosis does not occur unless there is renal impairment or huge quantities of bicarbonate are administered ($> 1000\,\text{mmol day}^{-1}$).

Metabolic alkalosis is usually due to increased loss of acid from the gastrointestinal tract or kidney. In many cases, vomiting causes little disturbance in pH or $T\text{CO}_2$ levels since both gastric (acid) and small intestinal

Table 7.5 Causes of hypoxia and respiratory acidosis

Reduced Po_2, normal Pco_2
Impaired gas exchange
◆ Pulmonary fibrosis
◆ Connective tissue disorders
Shunt
◆ Lobar pneumonia
◆ Arteriovenous fistula
◆ Adult respiratory distress syndrome

Reduced Po_2, reduced Pco_2
Ventilation–perfusion inequality
◆ Chronic obstructive airways disease
◆ Severe asthma
◆ Pulmonary embolus
◆ Pulmonary oedema
Hypoventilation
◆ Cardiac arrest
◆ Mechanical injuries
◆ Neuromuscular disorders
◆ Respiratory centre depression
◆ Gross obesity

(bicarbonate) secretions are lost. However, in pyloric stenosis, acid is lost in vomitus while bicarbonate is retained, and severe metabolic alkalosis is characteristic. The severity of this is partly because renal compensation is ineffective since chloride loss and volume depletion also occur. Volume depletion reduces the glomerular filtration rate (GFR) and the kidney responds by retaining sodium avidly. Sodium reabsorption in the proximal convoluted tubule requires the simultaneous cotransport of an anion and since the amount of chloride is decreased and bicarbonate increased in the glomerular filtrate, increased sodium reabsorption leads to bicarbonate retention; bicarbonate loss is required to compensate for the acid–base disturbance. Patients are usually potassium depleted and greater sodium exchange in the distal tubule will lead to increased H^+ excretion, thus generating further bicarbonate. Administration of sodium chloride is required to correct the alkalosis, this increases GFR and provides chloride as a counterion for renal tubular sodium transport. The kidney can then increase bicarbonate excretion.

The other main causes of metabolic alkalosis are mineralocorticoid excess and potassium depletion. Mineralocorticoids stimulate renal H^+ secretion, which enhances bicarbonate reabsorption and generation. This type of metabolic alkalosis does not respond to sodium chloride administration, as patients with mineralocorticoid excess are not volume or chloride depleted. Potassium deficiency, which also occurs in these patients, is a contributory factor, although the relationship between potassium balance and metabolic alkalosis is complex. Metabolic alkalosis occurs in severe potassium depletion due to distal tubular conservation of potassium with increased H^+ ion secretion and bicarbonate generation.

Metabolic alkalosis can develop in hypercapnoeic patients if this is corrected rapidly. Increased plasma Tco_2 is a compensatory response to a chronic respiratory acidosis and if this is relieved by assisted ventilation, the plasma Tco_2 will remain raised until renal compensation increases bicarbonate excretion.

Clinical Consequences Alkalaemia increases the protein binding of calcium, which can lead to reduced plasma levels of ionized calcium and tetany. Hypokalaemia can also occur because of increased cellular uptake of potassium, although potassium deficiency may also be caused by associated abnormalities in potassium metabolism.

KEY POINTS

METABOLIC ALKALOSIS

■ The primary abnormality is increased plasma Tco_2

■ Respiratory compensation occurs to a limited extent, leading to increased blood Pco_2

■ The major causes are pyloric stenosis, mineralocorticoid excess and potassium depletion

Table 7.6 Causes of metabolic alkalosis

Alkali administration
◆ Intravenous sodium bicarbonate
◆ Oral antacids

Loss of hydrogen ions
From the stomach
◆ Vomiting (pyloric stenosis)
◆ Aspiration
Through the kidney
◆ Mineralocorticoid excess
   Cushing's syndrome
   Primary hyperaldosteronism
   Bartter's syndrome
◆ Severe potassium deficiency
◆ Sudden correction of hypercapnia

Table 7.7 Causes of respiratory alkalosis

◆ Hypoxia
◆ Respiratory centre stimulation
   Anxiety, hysteria
   Salicylate overdose
   Cerebral disease (infection, tumour)
◆ Pregnancy
◆ Mechanical ventilation

Respiratory Alkalosis

In respiratory alkalosis the P_{CO_2} is reduced (solid arrow D, **Figure 7.5**), the compensatory response being reduced renal bicarbonate reabsorption and regeneration (dashed arrow D, **Figure 7.5**). The fall in plasma T_{CO_2} levels is usually modest, usually to no lower than 16 mmol l^{-1}. The primary reduction in P_{CO_2} is caused by pulmonary hyperventilation, which may result from several causes (**Table 7.7**). Respiratory conditions in which pulmonary oxygen exchange is impaired can lead to hyperventilation, as can stimulation of the respiratory centre. Tetany and light-headedness can occur, the latter being thought to be caused by cerebral vasoconstriction.

FURTHER READING

Adrogué AJ (ed.). *Acid–Base and Electrolyte Disorders.* New York: Churchill Livingstone, 1991

Kurtzman NA, Batille DC (eds) (1983). Acid-base disorders. *Medical Clinics of North America*, 1983; **57**: 751–932.

Miller AL. Plasma bicarbonate assays – time for a new look? *Annals of Clinical Biochemistry*, 1993; **30**: 233–7

West JB. *Pulmonary Pathophysiology – The Essentials* (4th edn). Baltimore: Williams & Wilkins, 1992.

CASE 7.1

A 35-year-old woman was admitted to hospital unconscious. She had a previous history of alcohol abuse. Initial blood tests showed the following:

sodium	137 mmol l^{-1}
potassium	4.7 mmol l^{-1}
chloride	103 mmol l^{-1}
total CO_2	4 mmol l^{-1}
urea	7.8 mmol l^{-1}
creatinine	84 μmol l^{-1}

What is the differential diagnosis?

CASE 7.2

A 37-year-old man was admitted with a history of persistent vomiting but with no other past medical history. The following results of blood tests were obtained:

sodium	134 mmol l^{-1}
potassium	2.2 mmol l^{-1}
chloride	42 mmol l^{-1}
total CO_2	75 mmol l^{-1}
urea	9.2 mmol l^{-1}
creatinine	108 μmol l^{-1}

What abnormality is present?

CASE 7.3

A 45-year-old woman with a history of chronic bronchitis and asthma was admitted to hospital and the following arterial blood gas results were obtained:

pH	7.07
P_{O_2}	6.8 kPa
P_{CO_2}	10.7 kPa
arterial bicarbonate	19 mmol l^{-1}

What acid–base disturbance is present?

CASE 7.4

The following results were obtained from a patient with glaucoma:

sodium	137 mmol l^{-1}
potassium	4.2 mmol l^{-1}
chloride	112 mmol l^{-1}
total CO_2	13 mmol l^{-1}
urea	5.8 mmol l^{-1}
creatinine	97 μmol l^{-1}

Explain these results.

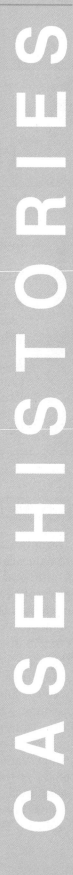

CASE HISTORIES

THE KIDNEY

INTRODUCTION

The internal composition of the body must remain relatively constant for normal health. Continuous excretion of excess water and electrolyte intake, together with the removal of metabolic waste products is required to achieve this. Although there are small contributions from other organs, such as the skin and intestine, the kidney is the major organ regulating body composition of water-soluble constituents. In order to maintain body composition the kidney forms a large volume filtrate of plasma, fine control of excretion resulting from selective conservation of solutes and water. The effect of this selective conservation can be seen by comparing the concentrations of major constituents of plasma and urine (**Table 8.1**). Other functions of the kidney include gluconeogenesis and endocrine secretion (**Table 8.2**).

STRUCTURE OF THE KIDNEY

Each healthy kidney contains approximately one million functional units (nephrons), each of which contains a glomerulus and tubule (**Figure 8.1**). The glomerulus is approximately 200 μm in diameter and consists of a tuft of capillaries that is invaginated into the expanded end of the nephron, Bowman's capsule. The glomerular capillary tuft is formed from an afferent arteriole and drains into an efferent arteriole which then supplies the tubule. Two layers of cells separate blood in capillaries from the glomerular filtrate, capillary endothelium and tubule epithelial cells, between which is a base-

Table 8.1 Comparison of plasma and urinary concentrations

Constituent	Typical concentration (mmol l^{-1})	
	Plasma	Urine
Sodium	140	90
Urea	5	150
Creatinine	0.08	12
Glucose (fasting)	4.3	0

Table 8.2 Functions of the kidney

Excretory and regulatory
◆ Removal of water-soluble waste products (urea, creatinine, urate)
◆ Maintenance of water, electrolyte and acid–base balance
Metabolic
◆ Gluconeogenesis
Endocrine
◆ Renin production
◆ Erythropoietin production
◆ Synthesis of 1,25-dihydroxycholecalciferol
◆ Catabolism of polypeptide hormones (e.g. parathyroid hormone, insulin)

ment membrane (**Figure 8.2**). The endothelium is fenestrated with pores of approximately 100 nm diameter, while the epithelial cells are embedded in the basement membrane by foot processes. The space between foot processes is termed the slit pore. Modified smooth muscle (mesangial) cells are found between capillary loops, and the juxtaglomerular apparatus is located in the angle between afferent and efferent arterioles. The juxtaglomerular apparatus, which also includes a modified region of the tubule, the macula densa, secretes renin.

Bowman's capsule leads into the proximal convoluted tubule which then drains into the loop of Henle. Approximately 85% of

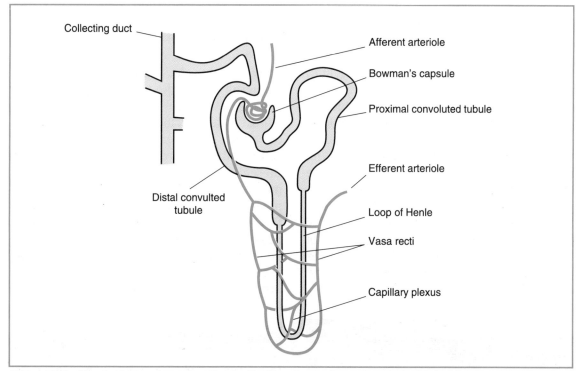

Figure 8.1 Key features of renal anatomy. Outline of a nephron, together with its blood supply. The distal convoluted tubule is closely related to the glomerulus. The peritubular plexus of vessels around the loop of Henle is supplied by the efferent arteriole.

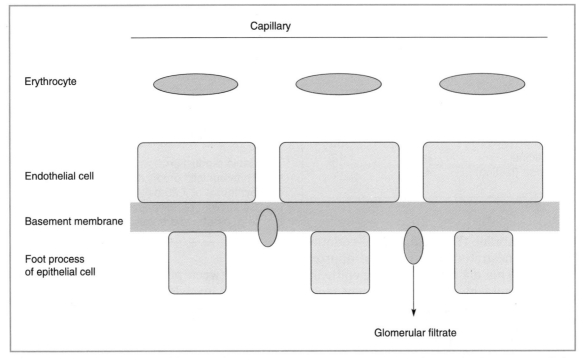

Capillary

Erythrocyte

Endothelial cell

Basement membrane

Foot process
of epithelial cell

Glomerular filtrate

Figure 8.2 Diagrammatic representation of a capillary loop, only one side of which is shown in detail, for clarity.

these are relatively short, remaining within the outer renal cortex, while the other 15% are much longer, extending to the tips of the medulla. The ascending limb of the loop of Henle is thicker than the descending limb and returns to the cortex, where it is apposed to the glomerulus from which it originated. The distal convoluted tubule is shorter than the proximal convoluted tubule and drains into the collecting duct. The blood supply to the tubules arises from the efferent arteriole from which are formed a peritubular capillary network and long loops (vasa recti) which run alongside the loops of Henle. The blood supply of the loops of Henle is a portal system which is at a lower pressure than capillaries supplied by the afferent arteriole.

molecular weight solutes. This high filtration is dependent on the large proportion of the cardiac output, 20–25%, which the kidneys receives, despite constituting only 1% of body weight. An ultrafiltrate is formed: glomeruli permit the free passage of neutral substances up to 4 nm in diameter and almost totally exclude those with a diameter of >8 nm. However, proteins in endothelial cell membranes are negatively charged and therefore the passage of anions is restricted more than neutral molecules, while larger positively charged substances can pass through. Albumin is just small enough to pass through the glomerular 'pores' but does not normally do so to any great extent, as it is negatively charged. Most other proteins are too large to be filtered.

NORMAL RENAL FUNCTION

Glomerular Filtration

Approximately 180–200 l of water are filtered daily by the glomeruli, together with low

Tubular Function

Up to 99% of filtered water and electrolytes are reabsorbed in the tubules (see chapters 5, 6 & 9). Some substances are completely

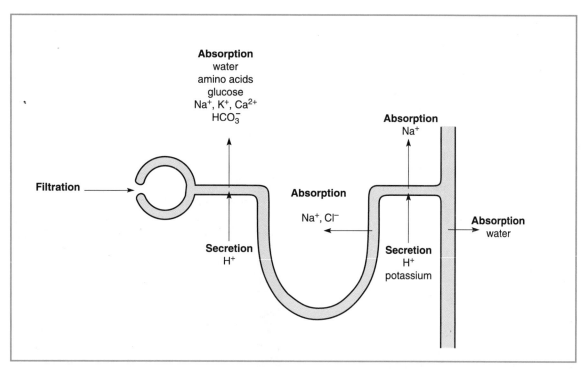

Figure 8.3 Renal tubular absorptive and secretory functions.

conserved under normal circumstances, including bicarbonate, glucose and amino acids. The tubules also excrete H^+ and potassium. The sites of important tubular functions are depicted in **Figure 8.3**.

ASSESSMENT OF RENAL FUNCTION

Glomerular Function

Glomerular Filtration Rate

The glomerular filtration rate is determined by measuring the excretion of a substance which is filtered freely by the glomerulus and not reabsorbed or secreted by the tubules. Historically, inulin was used for accurate measurements, this being administered by constant infusion. Inulin has been superseded by $[^{51}Cr]EDTA$ (ethylene-diamine tetra-acetic acid), as this is much easier to quantify. The need for constant plasma levels of the marker substance during the period of urine collection can be overcome by single time-point injection techniques in which an accurately measured

amount of the marker is infused and plasma levels are sampled at least twice. Using appropriate mathematical procedures, the glomerular filtration rate (GFR) can be calculated from the plasma decay of the marker, the rate of removal from plasma equalling the rate of urinary excretion. Thus, this technique avoids the need for urine collections.

The glomerular filtration rate is 120–150 ml min^{-1} in young adults and decreases slowly but progressively with age, typical values in elderly subjects being 60–80 ml min^{-1}. In children the GFR is usually corrected to a constant body surface area, 1.73 m^2.

Factors controlling the GFR include:

1. The size and permeability of the capillary bed. These are reduced in glomerular diseases.
2. Hydrostatic and oncotic pressure gradients across the capillary wall. The hydrostatic pressure gradient, and thus GFR, is reduced if the intracapillary

hydrostatic pressure decreases; causes of this include ECF volume depletion and intratubular pressure increases, these being due to bladder neck or urethral obstruction. Increases in plasma oncotic pressure, such as occur in multiple myeloma, have a similar effect.

Although measuring [^{51}Cr]EDTA clearance provides an accurate assessment of GFR it is inconvenient, since an infusion is required. An alternative for everyday clinical purposes is to use an endogenous substance, such as creatinine, although urine collections are required. Creatinine clearance is calculated using the formula

$$\text{Clearance (GFR)} = \frac{UV}{P}$$

where U is the urinary concentration, V is the urinary volume and P is the plasma concentration. Plasma creatinine levels are remarkably stable in normal subjects and in those with mild renal impairment and thus a single blood specimen is satisfactory for clearance measurement. A disadvantage of creatinine clearance is that accurately timed urine collections are required. Many patients find it difficult to comply exactly with instructions for 24-h urine collections.

Despite these limitations, creatinine clearance is a reasonably accurate method of determining GFR in subjects in whom renal function is normal or only mildly impaired. However, two difficulties arise with the measurement of creatinine clearance in patients with advanced renal failure. First, when plasma creatinine levels are very high, tubular secretion occurs and creatinine clearance is then an underestimate of GFR. Second, significant day-to-day changes occur in patients with end-stage renal disease. Glomerular function in such patients is assessed more accurately using [^{51}Cr]EDTA, or more conveniently by plasma creatinine concentrations.

Glomerular filtration rate is measured for the following purposes:

(i)   to detect mild renal insufficiency;

(ii) to assess the severity of renal impairment if potentially nephrotoxic drugs are given;

(iii) occasionally, when renal replacement therapy is being considered, although this is usually decided on clinical grounds;

(iv) to monitor changes in renal function.

KEY POINTS

GLOMERULAR FILTRATION RATE

- GFR is determined by measuring the clearance of a substance freely filtered by the glomerulus but not secreted or reabsorbed by the tubules

- GFR is determined by measuring the clearance of creatinine or [^{51}Cr]EDTA

- Creatinine clearance overestimates GFR in end-stage renal disease

---

Plasma Creatinine

Creatinine is a metabolic end-product formed nonenzymatically from creatine phosphate. Because most creatine is found in muscle, creatinine formation and thus plasma levels are related to muscle mass, these being greater in men than in women, and greater in adults than in children. Plasma creatinine concentrations are also affected by the rate of synthesis and total body water content.

Creatinine is filtered by the glomerulus and is not reabsorbed or secreted by the renal tubules in normal subjects. Plasma creatinine concentrations are inversely proportional to the GFR. They increase little until the GFR falls below 30 ml min^{-1} although, as GFR declines further, the increases in plasma creatinine become steep (**Figure 8.4**). Thus, a small decline in GFR will produce a relatively large increase in plasma creatinine concentrations. Because they do not rise significantly with modest reductions of GFR, plasma levels of

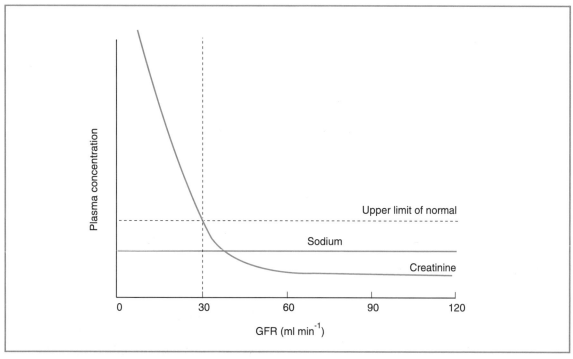

Figure 8.4 The effect of falling glomerular filtration rate on plasma concentrations of sodium and creatinine. Creatinine excretion is determined by glomerular filtration and as this falls, plasma levels rise, although they do not exceed the upper limit of normal until the glomerular filtration rate (GFR) <30 ml min^{-1}. Sodium concentrations are usually normal, even in the presence of advanced renal failure, since tubular reabsorption changes as glomerular filtration falls.

creatinine are insensitive indicators of mild renal impairment.

Plasma Urea

Urea is a metabolic end-product synthesized in the liver from deamination of amino acids. Over 90% of urea is excreted in urine without further metabolism, and it is the major nitrogen-containing waste product. Urea is freely filtered by the glomerulus without tubular secretion, although approximately 50% of filtered urea is reabsorbed passively in the tubules, this fraction increasing at low urine flow rates. Thus, urea clearance underestimates the GFR.

The causes of increased blood urea concentrations are outlined in **Table 8.3**. These include many diseases of the kidney and also several nonrenal factors. The rate of urea synthesis increases in subjects receiving a high protein diet or where there is increased protein breakdown. Protein breakdown is increased in hypercatabolic states in which increased breakdown of tissue proteins occurs, and also with bleeding into the gut, the proteins being digested and the products absorbed. Decreased vascular perfusion of the kidneys causes uraemia, blood urea concentrations being

Table 8.3 Causes of elevated plasma urea concentrations

Prerenal causes
Increased intake
◆ High-protein diet
◆ Bleeding into the gastrointestinal tract
Increased protein breakdown
◆ Hypercatabolic states (trauma, surgery, burns)
Decreased renal perfusion
◆ Volume depletion
◆ Congestive cardiac failure
◆ Renal artery stenosis

Renal causes
Intrinsic renal disease

Postrenal causes
Urinary tract obstruction
◆ Prostatic hypertrophy
◆ Urethral obstruction

---

elevated more than creatinine levels because of increased tubular reabsorption. A similar mechanism leads to greater plasma urea than creatinine elevations in urinary tract obstruction.

Plasma urea and creatinine concentrations are often measured simultaneously. Plasma creatinine levels reflect glomerular function more accurately than urea concentrations, as the latter are affected more by extrarenal factors. However, urea levels are useful because of this, as raised concentrations may suggest clinical problems in addition to impaired renal function. Plasma urea levels also correlate better with uraemic symptoms than creatinine and reflect protein intake, an important factor in the management of chronic renal failure.

Renal Tubular Function

Several procedures for assessing renal tubular function are available, although they are used less frequently in clinical practice than tests of glomerular function.

Urinary Amino Acid Excretion

Amino acids are filtered by the glomerulus but normally are completely reabsorbed by the tubules. They may appear in urine for three reasons:

1. As part of a generalized tubular defect (the Fanconi syndrome.
2. Owing to defective transport of a group of amino acids, e.g. cystinuria (see below).
3. Because of increased concentrations of plasma amino acids, e.g. phenylketonuria (see chapter 19).

These may be differentiated by determining the pattern of amino acid excretion. In the Fanconi syndrome, the pattern of amino acids is generalized, restricted to a characteristic group in transport defects, and to single amino acids in inherited metabolic disorders of amino acid metabolism.

Urinary Glucose Excretion

Glucose is freely filtered by the glomerulus but completely reabsorbed by the tubules under normal circumstances. Glucose can appear in urine for the following reasons:

1. Because the amount being filtered is increased and exceeds the tubular reabsorptive capacity. This is due to hyperglycaemia and occurs commonly in diabetes mellitus.
2. The tubular reabsorptive capacity (renal threshold) is reduced. This occurs in pregnancy.
3. There is a tubular defect which reduces glucose absorption. Glycosuria occurs in the Fanconi syndrome.

Tests of Urinary Concentration and Dilution

For reasons outlined above the concentrating and diluting capacity of the kidney is reduced if renal function is impaired. The water deprivation test, which assesses concentrating ability, is used in the investigation of polydipsia and polyuria but not

Table 8.4   The ammonium chloride test of urinary acidification

- The purpose of the test is to assess H^+ excretion in the presence of a mild metabolic acidosis
- Administration of ammonium chloride is not necessary if a metabolic acidosis is clearly present
- Ammonium chloride capsules (0.1 g kg^{-1} body weight) are administered orally
- The plasma TCO$_2$ is checked. It should have fallen by 4 mmol l^{-1} for metabolic acidosis to have been induced
- Urine is collected hourly for 6–8 h and the pH of urine is tested
- H^+ secretion is normal if the pH falls to ≤ 5.3
- In type 1 (distal) renal tubular acidosis the pH is usually > 6.0
- The pH may fall < 5.3 in type 2 (proximal) renal tubular acidosis

Table 8.5   Causes of proteinuria

Overflow proteinuria
- Normal proteins
  Haemoglobin
  Myoglobin
- Abnormal proteins
  Immunoglobulin fragments (Bence–Jones protein)

Glomerular proteinuria
- Altered renal haemodynamics
  Orthostatic proteinuria, exercise
- Increased glomerular permeability
  Fever
  Glomerulonephritis

Tubular proteinuria
- Tubular damage
  Heavy metal poisoning, drug toxicity
- Interstitial disease
  Interstitial nephritis, pyelonephritis

usually as a general test of renal function, although concentrating ability declines in parallel with GFR. The water deprivation test is considered in chapter 13.

Tests of Urinary Acidification

Both bicarbonate reabsorption and H^+ secretion may be impaired in generalized renal disease. Isolated tubular defects generally affect one of these processes. Impaired H^+ secretion occurs in type 1 renal tubular acidosis. This may be investigated using the ammonium chloride loading test (**Table 8.4**), ammonium chloride behaving metabolically as ammonia and hydrochloric acid. Bicarbonate reabsorption is impaired in type 2 renal tubular acidosis and in the Fanconi syndrome, leading to a low plasma total CO$_2$ (TCO$_2$) and an inappropriately alkaline urine.

Proteinuria

Protein excretion

Normal adult subjects excrete up to 150 mg day^{-1} in urine although rather larger amounts, up to 300 mg 24 h^{-1}, are sometimes excreted by healthy adolescents. Most of this is derived from renal tubular cells, rather than glomerular filtration, the protein present in greatest amounts being a large molecular weight glycoprotein, Tamm–Horsfall protein. Albumin excretion is usually < 30 mg 24 h^{-1}.

Mechanisms of Proteinuria

Proteinuria may result from several mechanisms (**Table 8.5**).

Overflow Proteinuria   This results from elevated plasma concentrations of proteins that are small enough to pass the normal glomerular barrier. The most important cause of this type of proteinuria is multiple myeloma, which produces immunoglobulin light chains. Rarely, haemoglobinuria can result from intravascular haemolysis and myoglobinuria from rhabdomyolysis.

Glomerular Proteinuria   Glomerular dysfunction can lead to proteinuria, either because of altered renal haemodynamics or increased glomerular permeability. Significant quantities of protein may be found in the first specimen passed following strenuous exercise. This is thought to be due to reduced renal blood flow producing stasis of blood in the glomeruli, with increased leakage and decreased absorption of protein in the proximal tubules. Orthostatic proteinuria is a benign condition that affects mainly adolescents and young adults. It occurs when subjects adopt the erect posture and disappears on recumbency. Thus, the first specimen passed in the morning is free of protein in orthostatic proteinuria. Febrile patients often develop transient proteinuria, possibly due to antigen–antibody complexes causing temporary glomerular damage. A number of systemic conditions and primary renal disorders affect glomerular components, increasing permeability and causing proteinuria. This may be of two types, selective and nonselective. Albumin is typically the major protein lost, because of its small molecular mass and its relatively high plasma concentration. Losses are almost exclusively albumin in selective proteinuria, higher molecular weight proteins being retained. Higher molecular weight proteins are lost in nonselective proteinuria; this reflects more severe glomerular damage.

Tubular Proteinuria Polypeptides and low molecular weight proteins are filtered by the glomerulus and reabsorbed by the tubules. Such proteins include β_2-microglobulin and lysosyme, these appearing in the urine in tubular or interstitial damage.

Detection of Proteinuria

Urinary protein is usually detected using a 'dipstick' incorporating a dye that changes colour if proteins are present. Proteins differ in the degree of colour change they produce, sticks being sensitive to albumin, while immunoglobulin fragments such as light chains have little effect. Albumin concentrations of 150 mg l^{-1} or greater are detected.

Determination of proteinuria using dipsticks thus depends on the concentration of urine and early morning specimens, which tend to be more concentrated, are usually studied. More detailed examination of urine is required under some circumstances:

1. If dipstick-positive proteinuria is detected 24-hour protein excretion should be determined.
2. The selectivity of proteinuria gives an indication of the severity of glomerular damage. This is determined by measuring the relative clearances of two proteins of different molecular weight, albumin (69 000) and immunoglobulin G (IgG, 150 000) often being used for this purpose. The ratio of IgG:albumin clearance increases as proteinuria becomes less selective.
3. Microalbuminuria occurs when the excretion of albumin is greater than normal, but not sufficiently high to be detected by conventional dipsticks. It must therefore be investigated using highly sensitive techniques. Microalbuminuria is of interest in diabetic and hypertensive patients, as it appears to predict subsequent cardiovascular disease at an early stage, when medical intervention may be of benefit.
4. Immunoglobulin fragments are detected by more specific techniques such as electrophoresis using a concentrated specimen of urine.

Renal Function in Disease

Impairment of renal excretory function may be acute or chronic, both leading to reductions in GFR. Some types of acute renal failure are reversible but chronic renal failure is often progressive, leading to destruction of nephrons and reduced renal mass. Severely damaged nephrons do not function, the maintenance of urinary excretion depending on unaffected nephrons.

Creatinine and Urea

Progression of renal disease may be very slow. If the production rates of urea and creatinine are constant, increases in plasma levels occur which result in the filtered load (GFR × plasma level) being normal. Thus, production and excretion of nitrogenous waste products is in balance, this being achieved through the 'thermostat' of plasma levels being set higher. Since the number of functioning nephrons is reduced, the amount of solute being filtered and excreted in each individual nephron is much greater than normal.

Sodium

In contrast to nitrogenous waste products, plasma concentrations of sodium are often constant, even in the presence of very severe renal failure (end-stage renal disease). This is because changes in tubular transport compensate for reduced glomerular filtration. As GFR declines, a progressively greater fraction of the filtered load of sodium is excreted, either by reducing reabsorption or enhancing tubular secretion. This further increases the amount of unabsorbed solute in the tubules of surviving nephrons.

Potassium and Phosphate

Phosphate and potassium have a pattern of plasma levels intermediate between those of sodium and creatinine; these are maintained until the GFR falls to less than 25% of normal, but then increases occur.

Water

External water balance is usually maintained in progressive renal failure, although there is reduced functional reserve to adapt to changes such as increased intake or deprivation. The ability to produce concentrated and dilute urine depends on osmotic gradients generated in the interstitial tissue of the kidney by selective tubular transport functions (see chapter 5). The ability to create osmotic gradients is impaired in progressive renal disease. In addition, the amount of unabsorbed solute in individual nephrons is increased, causing a solute diuresis. There is little control over the volume of fluid required for the excretion of this solute.

Hydrogen Ions and Bicarbonate

Metabolic acidosis is commonly seen in renal disease due to impaired secretion of H^+ and reduced reabsorption of bicarbonate.

SYNDROMES OF RENAL DISEASE

Renal disease presents clinically as a number of characteristic syndromes.

Acute Renal Failure

Rapid deterioration in renal function causing retention of urea and creatinine is the hallmark of acute renal failure. It is usually accompanied by oliguria (a urine output of <400 ml 24 h^{-1}), although this is not inevitable. The incidence of acute renal failure is relatively common in high dependency units, such as intensive care wards.

Causes

Acute renal failure may result from prerenal and postrenal causes in addition to intrinsic renal disease (**Table 8.6**), although most cases result from acute tubular necrosis. The commonest cause of acute tubular necrosis is renal ischaemia, which can result from conditions which cause decreased effective blood volume, hypotension, severe volume depletion, and sepsis. Acute tubular necrosis is also a complication of disseminated intravascular coagulation. Nephrotoxic substances which can cause acute tubular necrosis include heavy metals, organic solvents, pesticides and drugs, particularly antibiotics such as aminoglycosides and cephalosporins. Toxins often lead to necrosis of proximal tubular cells.

Table 8.6   Causes of acute renal failure

Prerenal causes
- Volume depletion
- Circulatory failure

Renal causes
- Vascular occlusion
  Large vessel (thrombosis, dissection)
  Small vessel (malignant hypertension, vasculitis, haemolytic-uraemic syndrome)
- Glomerulonephritis
- Acute cortical necrosis
- Acute tubular necrosis
  Vascular
  Toxic
- Acute pyelonephritis
- Acute interstitial nephritis

Postrenal causes
- Obstruction
- Bladder rupture

Prerenal failure is caused by reduced renal perfusion and is readily reversible if appropriately treated; untreated, it can lead to acute tubular necrosis. Postrenal causes are also usually amenable to treatment, bladder neck obstruction (e.g. due to prostatic hypertrophy) being more common than upper urinary tract obstruction (e.g. due to retroperitoneal fibrosis).

Biochemical Features

Oliguric Phase   Oliguria has been considered a characteristic feature of acute renal failure, although urine output does not fall below 400 ml day^{-1} in up to 40% of cases. When it does occur the duration of oliguria varies considerably, although on average it lasts for 10–12 days. If oliguria persists for longer than 4 weeks, causes of acute renal failure other than acute tubular necrosis should be considered, such as cortical necrosis, rapidly progressive glomerulonephritis or vasculitis. In the oliguric phase GFR is very low and urinary excretion of nitrogenous waste products, electrolytes, and H$^+$ is impaired. The daily increments in plasma urea and creatinine average 6 mmol l^{-1} and 60 μmol l^{-1} respectively, although larger increases occur in hypercatabolic patients, particularly those with fever, sepsis, or trauma. Electrolyte imbalance is common, with sodium and water overload and hyperkalaemia occurring. Hyperphosphataemia and hypermagnesaemia owing to retention, and hypocalcaemia, owing to either impaired synthesis of 1,25-dihydroxycholecalciferol or resistance to parathyroid hormone, are also features. Urine is often dark brown, and contains haem pigments and protein. Urinary sodium concentrations are usually >30 mmol l^{-1}, contrasting with those found in oliguria caused by dehydration without intrinsic renal disease. Under these circumstances, tubular function is normal and sodium is avidly retained, urinary concentrations usually being <20 mmol l^{-1}.

Diuretic Phase   The onset of a diuretic phase usually heralds recovery. This may start as an abrupt diuresis, with urinary volume exceeding 4 l day^{-1}, or a gradual increase in urine output. The diuretic phase results from increases in the GFR without accompanying improvement in tubular function. Thus, there is a risk of excessive losses of water and electrolytes. Blood urea and creatinine concentrations no longer increase.

Recovery Phase   Tubular function returns gradually as cells regenerate, although concentrating defects may be detected many months after the oliguric phase and very sensitive tests have shown that most patients do not recover completely normal function. However, residual impairment is usually not clinically significant.

Management

The mortality of acute renal failure is high, but recovery is possible in many cases and appropriate management has resulted in mortality rates falling from >90% to <50%. Prerenal and postrenal causes should be sought and managed appropriately. Defects in intravascular volume should be corrected and fluid intake then determined by losses. Plasma potassium should be monitored carefully and hyperkalaemia treated when indicated. To minimize protein catabolism adequate carbohydrates should be given, where possible by mouth. Rigorous infection control measures are required. Conservative measures may be adequate in patients with short olgiuric phases, but many will require haemodialysis.

KEY POINTS

ACUTE RENAL FAILURE

- Oliguria is a common but not inevitable feature of acute renal failure

- The commonest cause of acute renal failure is acute tubular necrosis

- Recovery from acute tubular necrosis is heralded by a diuretic phase

---

Chronic Renal Failure

While recovery is possible in many cases of acute renal failure, sustained chronic renal injury leads to permanent destruction of nephrons, reduction of renal mass and chronic renal failure. There are many causes of chronic renal failure, the most common being diabetic nephropathy, hypertension, glomerulonephritis and polycystic disease. Although the histological features and rate of progression of the various causes of chronic renal failure differ, they lead to a syndrome with common clinical features, end-stage renal disease.

Pathophysiology

As the number of functioning nephrons decreases, hypertrophy of remaining nephrons occurs, increasing their functional capacity. Although the excretory capacity of individual surviving nephrons is increased, reduction in nephron numbers leads to impaired excretory reserve and eventually

to impaired excretion. Changes occur in ECF composition which first affect solutes that are regulated primarily by glomerular filtration, retention of urea and creatinine occurring when the GFR falls to approximately 30% of normal (**Figure 8.4**). As the disease progresses, solutes that are partly regulated by tubular transport in addition to glomerular filtration are also retained; these include phosphate, urate and magnesium. Adaptive responses lead to increased excretion of sodium and potassium per nephron, and balance is usually maintained until relatively late in the disease. The ability to concentrate and dilute urine is impaired early in chronic renal failure and there is thus a reduced ability to cope with increased fluid intake or losses. A urine output of approximately 2 l is required for obligatory solute excretion.

The clinical features of chronic renal failure (the uraemic syndrome) are thought to be caused by toxic retained metabolites, although the major nitrogenous metabolite, urea, is not thought to be responsible. Candidates include other nitrogenous end-products such as guanidine compounds and amino acid metabolites. A toxic role has been postulated for larger nitrogenous compounds of molecular mass approximately 1500 Da. It is also possible that toxic substances may accumulate owing to decreased renal metabolic rather than excretory function. The kidney normally metabolizes proteins and peptides, including various hormones, and excess parathyroid hormone has been postulated to be an important toxin.

Clinical Features

The uraemic syndrome is a multisystem disorder, many of the features of which are outlined in **Table 8.7**.

Metabolic Complications

Sodium and Water Balance Patients often complain of polyuria which occurs because of loss of renal concentration mechanisms. Signs of extracellular fluid (ECF) expansion

Table 8.7 Clinical features of chronic renal failure

Nervous system
◆ Sleep disturbance
◆ Peripheral neuropathy
Cardiovascular system
◆ Hypertension
◆ Congestive cardiac failure
◆ Pericarditis
Musculoskeletal system
◆ Impaired growth (children)
◆ Weakness
◆ Osteodystrophy
Skin
◆ Pigmentation
◆ Pruritis
Haemopoietic system
◆ Anaemia
◆ Bleeding tendency
Genitourinary
◆ Reduced libido, infertility
◆ Polyuria, nocturia

are not apparent in most patients with stable chronic renal failure, although excessive ingestion of salt may precipitate congestive cardiac failure, fluid retention and hypertension. Hyponatraemia may occur if water intake is excessive. Volume depletion may result if an extrarenal source of fluid loss is present, such as vomiting or diarrhoea.

Potassium Balance Most patients maintain normal plasma potassium levels until advanced disease occurs, when hyperkalaemia may become apparent (see chapter 6).

Hydrogen Ion Balance Acid excretion falls with advancing disease, metabolic acidosis resulting (see chapter 7).

Calcium and Phosphate Metabolism There is a tendency to develop hypocalcaemia because of reduced synthesis of 1,25-dihydroxycholecalciferol (chapter 9). Hyperphosphataemia contributes to this by facilitating calcium deposition in soft tissues (ectopic calcification). Hypocalcaemia sti-

mulates increased parathyroid hormone secretion, parathyroid hyperplasia and secondary hyperparathyroidism resulting. As a result, calcium salts are mobilized from bone, metabolic acidosis contributing to this process. This leads to renal osteodystrophy in which a number of histological changes occur, including osteomalacia. The deposition of aluminium salts in bone contributes to this process, the sources of aluminium being dialysate water and salts administered orally as phosphate-binding agents.

Carbohydrate Metabolism Mild glucose intolerance is common due to resistance to the peripheral effects of insulin.

Lipid Metabolism Triglyceride levels are increased and high-density lipoprotein cholesterol levels are reduced, largely owing to reduced clearance of triglyceride-rich lipoproteins. The incidence of atherosclerosis is increased in chronic renal failure and this may be at least partly due to dyslipidaemia.

Gonadal Function Impaired spermatogenesis and reduced testosterone levels occur in men while menstrual dysfunction, loss of libido and impaired fertility occur in women.

Management

Conservative management includes dietary measures and the control of hypertension. Restriction of protein, salt and water are important. Oral administration of phosphate-binding agents helps to prevent secondary hyperparathyroidism. Conservative measures often help to control symptoms, although renal replacement therapy, either dialysis or transplantation, is required in many patients. Biochemical monitoring in patients receiving haemodialysis should include regular measurement of plasma aluminium concentrations. Careful monitoring of patients following transplantation is important for two reasons: first, acute tubular necrosis may develop immediately after transplantation, particularly when the donor has been hypotensive; second, to detect biochemical evidence of rejection. This leads to increases in plasma creatinine levels and reduced urinary sodium excretion. Some centres monitor urinary proteins that are normally reabsorbed by the renal tubule, such as β_2-microglobulin, or excretion of an enzyme which originates in the renal tubule, usually N-acetyl-β-D-glucosaminidase (NAG).

KEY POINTS

CHRONIC RENAL FAILURE

- Chronic renal failure is caused by a permanent reduction in the number of nephrons

- Biochemical features include uraemia and a loss of the ability to concentrate and dilute urine

- Complications of chronic renal failure include secondary hyperparathyroidism

---

Nephrotic Syndrome

The hallmark of nephrotic syndrome is heavy proteinuria, arbitrarily defined as exceeding 3.5 g day^{-1}, this degree of proteinuria rarely being seen in other renal syndromes. Proteinuria of this magnitude is often accompanied by hypoalbuminaemia, which develops if hepatic synthesis is unable to replace renal losses. If hypoalbuminaemia is severe enough to reduce the plasma oncotic pressure, the third feature of nephrotic syndrome, oedema, develops. A reduction in the effective plasma volume can result, leading to activation of the renin–angiotensin system and increased vasopressin secretion. The reduction in plasma oncotic pressure also appears to stimulate hepatic lipoprotein synthesis and hyperlipidaemia may result. Plasma concentrations of other low molecular weight proteins such as IgG may be low if a nonselective proteinuria is present. Deposits of immuno-

globulins and complement are found in the kidney in several types of nephrotic syndrome.

Causes

The syndrome results from pathological processes which disrupt the normal size and charge barriers; these barriers normally retain serum proteins within the capillaries during glomerular filtration (**Table 8.8**). In minimal change disease there are no demonstrable changes on light microscopy although fusion of epithelial foot processes (**Figure 8.1**) is seen on electron microscopy. The condition is common in children and most patients respond to steroid therapy. There is usually no antecedent illness and the cause is unclear. The proteinuria is usually highly selective. In membranous glomerulonephritis basement membrane thickening occurs due to deposits which contain IgG. These are thought to occur because immunoglobulins either bind to glomerular basement antigen, or attach to circulating antigens which locate at this site by charge–charge interactions with glomerular components. Membranous glomerulonephritis is common in adults and is usually idiopathic, although it can occur in association with malignancies, systemic lupus erythematosis, infections, and also with some drugs. The prognosis is variable, some patients recovering while others progress to end-stage renal disease. Urinary protein selectivity is also variable. In mesangial proliferative glomerulonephritis increased cellularity of the mesangium occurs and deposits of immunoglobulins are often found, suggesting that the condition is an

Table 8.8 Causes of nephrotic syndrome

Minimal change disease
Membranous glomerulonephritis
Proliferative glomerulonephritis
Membrano-proliferative (mesangiocapillary) glomerulonephritis
Focal glomerulosclerosis

immune complex disease. Proteinuria is usually nonselective. In membranoproliferative (mesangiocapillary) glomerulonephritis increased cellularity of the mesangium extends into capillary walls. In many cases, the complement component C3 is found in the lesions. Focal glomerulosclerosis may be superimposed on other types of nephrotic syndrome such as minimal change disease or membranous glomerulonephritis. Focal and segmental increases in the mesangial matrix and basement membrane are seen which often contain immunoglobulins. Proteinuria is usually nonselective.

KEY POINTS

NEPHROTIC SYNDROME

- Urinary protein excretion is >3.5 g day^{-1} in nephrotic syndrome

- Nephrotic syndrome results from disruption of the normal size and charge barriers of the glomerulus

- Selective proteinuria has a better prognosis than nonselective proteinuria

---

Renal Tubular Disorders

Abnormalities of tubular function occurs in acquired disorders (tubulointerstitial disease) and in inherited metabolic diseases. However, particularly in tubulointerstitial disease, secondary damage to the glomeruli may occur, leading to reductions in the GFR. Major causes of tubulointerstitial disease are outlined in **Table 8.9**. Proteinuria is common although rarely exceeds 2 g day^{-1}. It is of a tubular pattern, β_2-microglobulin and lysozyme being found in urine. Generalized or selective defects of other tubular functions occur, including in the proximal tubule, potassium, sodium, amino acid, phosphate, bicarbonate and glucose reabsorption, and urate excretion, while distal tubular dysfunction may lead to defects of urinary acidification or concentration

Table 8.9 Causes of tubulointerstitial diseases of the kidney

Infections
◆ Pyelonephritis
Neoplasia
◆ Multiple myeloma
Toxins
◆ Analgesic nephropathy
◆ Heavy metal poisoning
Metabolic disorders
◆ Uric acid nephropathy
◆ Hypercalcaemia
◆ Hypokalaemia
Immunological disorders
◆ Sjörgren's syndrome
◆ Transplant rejection
◆ Acquired immunodeficiency syndrome
Vascular
◆ Atherosclerotic disease
◆ Sickle cell nephropathy
Inherited diseases
◆ Polycystic renal disease
◆ Urinary tract obstruction
Miscellaneous
◆ Vesicoureteric reflux

(**Figure 8.3**). Generalized defects in proximal tubular function constitute the Fanconi syndrome which, in addition to occurring in acquired tubulointerstitial disease, can occur in inherited disorders. In inherited disorders the Fanconi syndrome may be a primary tubular disorder, or secondary to other conditions which lead to renal tubular damage, such as galactosaemia, glycogen storage disease, inherited fructose intolerance, cystinosis, or Wilson's disease. Selective disorders of tubular transport also occur, such as cystinuria (cystine, ornithine, arginine and lysine transport), renal tubular acidosis (H$^+$ or bicarbonate transport, see chapter 7), and nephrogenic diabetes insipidus (water reabsorption, see chapter 13).

Renal Tract Stones

Renal calculi affect up to 1% of the population and are often recurrent. Several

Table 8.10 Major causes of renal tract stones

Type	Prevalence
Calcium stones	80%
Struvite ($MgNH_4PO_4$) stones	14%
Uric acid stones	5%
Cystine stones	1%

different types of stones occur although approximately 80% contain calcium (**Table 8.10**). Most occur in the upper urinary tract although bladder stones are also found.

Causes

Urine is supersaturated with regard to some constituents, stone formation being inhibited in most subjects owing to the presence of inhibitors of crystallization. Several of these have been identified including pyrophosphate, magnesium, citrate and glycoproteins.

The factors which lead to stone formation include:

1. Increased urinary concentration of a constituent. This can occur because of either abnormally high excretion or concentrated urine resulting from inadequate fluid intake.
2. Reduction in the concentration of inhibitors.
3. A urinary pH that favours stone formation.
4. Stasis of urine.
5. Nucleation. Stone formation may begin because of seeding by a substance with a different composition from the stone. The presence of a seed such as a crystal may lead to deposition of supersaturated urine components and stone growth. This phenomenon is known as epitaxy.

Calcium Stones The majority of calcium-containing stones consist of calcium oxalate, although some are composed of calcium phosphate. Both of these salts are relatively

insoluble, and stones occur when urine output is low and concentration is high; this occurs in hot climates in particular when water intake is restricted. Increased excretion of one of the stone constituents is a more common predisposing cause in temperate climates. Hypercalciuria (excretion of >7.5 mmol day^{-1}) is found in all forms of hypercalcaemia (see chapter 9). Hypercalciuria without hypercalcaemia occurs because of increased intestinal calcium absorption or impaired renal tubular reabsorption of calcium.

Hyperoxaluria also predisposes to calcium-containing stone formation. This occurs either as an inherited metabolic disease of oxalate synthesis (primary hyperoxaluria) or secondary to some other cause (secondary hyperoxaluria), the most common being increased intestinal absorption of oxalate. This is usually secondary to fat malabsorption, malabsorbed fat in the gut binding free calcium in the lumen which would otherwise bind to dietary oxalate, preventing its absorption.

Uric Acid Stones Uric acid stones occur in primary gout or secondary causes of hyperuricaemia (see chapter 20), uric acid excretion being increased. Uric acid stones are more likely to form in acid than alkaline urine.

Struvite Stones Struvite stones occur as a result of urinary tract infections caused by bacteria, mainly *Proteus* species, which split urea, thus producing ammonia. Urinary ammonium concentrations increase, leading to precipitation of magnesium ammonium phosphate.

Cystine Stones Cystine stones occur in cystinuria, an inherited defect of amino acid transport. Ornithine, arginine and lysine are transported by the same renal tubular carrier as cystine, and all are excreted in excess. The solubility of cystine in urine, unlike the other amino acids, is very limited and therefore stones occur when concentrations are high. The transport defect also affects the gastrointestinal tract, although amino acid deficiency does not occur because sufficient is absorbed by alternative mechanisms to supply requirements.

Clinical Features

Small stones may be passed, many patients experiencing severe loin pain due to ureteric colic, often accompanied by haematuria, as the stones pass to the bladder. Large stones can occur in the renal pelvis (staghorn calculi) without major clinical symptoms necessarily being noted, although infection and tubulointerstitial disease are common complications.

Investigation

Analysis of any calculus passed should be undertaken, while plasma calcium, phosphate and uric acid levels should be determined. Urinary excretion of calcium and oxalate, and a test for the presence of cystine, together with urinary pH and culture should be undertaken.

KEY POINTS

URINARY TRACT STONES

- Factors leading to urinary tract stone formation include increased excretion of a constituent and low urine output

- Urinary tract infection with organisms which split urea predispose to stone formation

- Clinical features include loin pain and haematuria

FURTHER READING

Davison AM. *Nephrology*. London: Heinemann, 1987

Espinall CH. Differential diagnosis of acute renal failure. *Clinical Nephrology* 1980; **13**: 73–7

Mandal AK, Herbert LA (eds). Renal disease. *Medical Clinics of North America* 1990; **74**: 859–1083

Quitanilla AP. Renal tubular acidosis. *Postgraduate Medicine* 1980; **67**: 60–73

Winocour PH. Microalbuminuria. Worth screening for in early morning urine samples in diabetic, hypertensive, and elderly patients. *British Medical Journal* 1992; **304**: 1196–7

CASE 8.1

The following results were obtained from a patient known to have chronic renal failure:

sodium	141 mmol l^{-1}
potassium	5.7 mmol l^{-1}
chloride	107 mmol l^{-1}
total CO_2	14 mmol l^{-1}
urea	46 mmol l^{-1}
creatinine	495 μmol l^{-1}

Explain the total CO_2 and potassium results. Is the anion gap normal or abnormal?

CASE 8.2

A 75-year-old man was seen in outpatients three months after discharge from hospital following admission for congestive cardiac failure. He complained of feeling generally unwell and breathlessness. The results of his blood tests were as follows:

sodium	131 mmol l^{-1}
potassium	2.7 mmol l^{-1}
chloride	90 mmol l^{-1}
total CO_2	32 mmol l^{-1}
urea	9.5 mmol l^{-1}
creatinine	132 μmol l^{-1}

Explain these results.

CASE 8.3

A 42-year-old man who had been suffering from type 1 diabetes mellitus for a number of years was found at review to have ankle swelling. The following blood test results were obtained:

sodium	142 mmol l^{-1}
potassium	3.9 mmol l^{-1}
chloride	107 mmol l^{-1}
total CO_2	29 mmol l^{-1}
urea	17.2 mmol l^{-1}
creatinine	190 μmol l^{-1}
albumin	27 g l^{-1}
total protein	55 g l^{-1}

What further investigations are required?

CASE 8.4

A child of 5 years was investigated for right loin pain and was found on X-ray to have a radio-opaque renal stone.

What types of stone could be present and what further investigations should be undertaken?

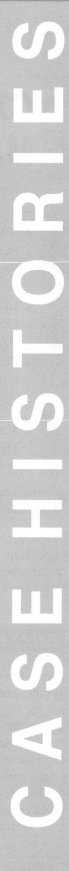

CASE HISTORIES

CALCIUM, PHOSPHATE AND MAGNESIUM METABOLISM

INTRODUCTION

Calcium, phosphorus and magnesium are important constituents of bone and their metabolism is interrelated; they are therefore best considered together.

CALCIUM HOMEOSTASIS

The adult body contains 1–1.5 kg (25 000–37 000 mmol) calcium, over 98% of this being found in the skeleton, where it has an important structural function. In bones, calcium occurs mainly as hydroxyapatite – crystals composed of calcium and phosphate with small amounts of hydroxide and carbonate. Only a minor proportion of skeletal calcium (*c.* 1%) is rapidly exchangeable with plasma, although remodelling of bone results in the turnover of nearly 20% of skeletal calcium each year. Approximately 1% of body calcium is present in the extracellular fluid, where functions include the regulation of neuromuscular excitability, and acting as a cofactor for clotting enzymes. The gradient of extracellular to intracellular free calcium is around 10 000:1, although cellular calcium is also found as insoluble complexes. Within cells, free calcium ions (Ca^{2+}) regulate the activity of various enzymes directly and also exert second messenger hormonal functions by interacting with calcium-binding proteins, such as troponin C and calmodulin.

Regulation of Calcium Metabolism

Normal daily calcium exchange is represented in **Figure 9.1**. Calcium in the gastrointestinal tract originates from the diet and also from secretions. Approximately half is absorbed, mainly in the upper small intestine, by active transport. Up to 250 mmol calcium is filtered daily by the kidney, the majority being reabsorbed in the proximal tubule and loop of Henle; urinary excretion is normally 2.5–7.5 mmol l^{-1}, depending on intake. Small amounts are lost in sweat, these being insignificant unless profuse sweating occurs for a prolonged period.

Parathyroid Hormone

Parathyroid hormone (PTH) is a key regulatory hormone of calcium metabolism whose secretion is stimulated by low plasma Ca^{2+} concentrations and by low plasma magnesium concentrations. The physiological importance of regulation by magnesium is unclear although magnesium depletion can cause hypocalcaemia. The secretion of PTH is inhibited by increased Ca^{2+} levels.

Within the parathyroid glands PTH is transcribed as an 115 amino acid polypeptide and processed to form an 84 amino acid polypeptide, in which form it is stored prior to secretion. The biological activity of PTH is contained within a 32–34 amino acid fragment of the molecule, located at the N-terminal end. Following secretion, PTH is cleaved, mainly in the liver, to produce two fragments, one of which is inactive (C-terminal fragment). PTH is usually measured in blood by assays which depend on immunoreactivity rather than biological activity (immunoassays). In renal failure the rate of metabolism of the C-terminal fragment is reduced, as this is normally removed by the kidney. If assays for measuring PTH are based on the immunoreactivity of the C-terminal end of the molecule, levels may appear higher than would be apparent if biological activity were determined. This is important, since renal failure causes secondary hyperparathyroidism.

The main effect of PTH is to raise plasma Ca^{2+} concentrations through actions on

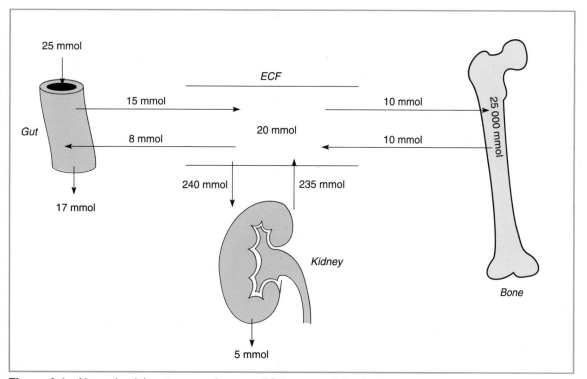

Figure 9.1   Normal calcium turnover in man. ECF, extracellular fluid.

bones, the kidney and, indirectly, the gastrointestinal tract (**Figure 9.2**). In the bones, PTH stimulates osteoclast activity, while in the kidney it increases the reabsorption of calcium and reduces the rate of transport of phosphate and bicarbonate. PTH also stimulates the hydroxylation of 25-hydroxycholecalciferol to form calcitriol, which then acts on the gut to increase calcium and phosphate absorption.

KEY POINTS

PARATHYROID HORMONE

- PTH secretion is regulated by ionized calcium concentrations in plasma

- PTH increases plasma calcium levels by actions on the kidney, bone and gut

- PTH decreases renal tubular phosphate and bicarbonate reabsorption

---

1,25-Dihydroxycholecalciferol (Calcitriol)

Vitamin D is converted to its biologically active form, 1,25-dihydroxycholecalciferol (calcitriol), by successive hydroxylations in the liver and kidney (chapter 4). Calcitriol stimulates intestinal absorption of calcium and phosphate by regulating the synthesis of a protein that transports calcium across the enterocyte. In addition, calcitriol is required for normal mineralization of bone, this being defective in deficiency states. Weakness of skeletal muscles also occurs in vitamin D deficiency, which responds to supplements, suggesting that vitamin D is important for normal skeletal function, although the basis of this is not understood.

Calcitonin

Calcitonin is a 32 amino acid peptide secreted by the *C*-cells of the thyroid gland. It lowers plasma calcium concentrations by inhibiting bone resorption and

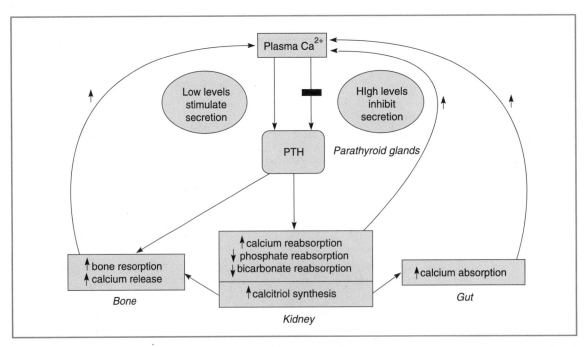

Figure 9.2 Hormonal control of calcium metabolism. Parathyroid hormone (PTH) secretion is stimulated by low plasma Ca^{2+} concentrations and stimulates directly bone resorption and renal calcium reabsorption. PTH also stimulates the kidney to synthesize calcitriol, which in turn promotes bone resorption and also calcium absorption from the gut. The effect of PTH action is to raise plasma Ca^{2+} levels – these inhibit PTH secretion by negative feedback.

renal tubular calcium reabsorption. However, its physiological role is unclear, since no disturbance in calcium metabolism occurs following removal of the thyroid gland.

Plasma Calcium

Three forms of calcium occur in the circulation, almost 50% as free ions (Ca^{2+}), a similar quantity bound to plasma proteins, particularly albumin, and the remainder complexed to other ions (phosphate, citrate and bicarbonate). In health, plasma total calcium concentrations are 2.15–2.55 mmol l^{-1}, while ionized calcium levels are 1.20–1.37 mmol l^{-1}. Protein-bound calcium increases if plasma protein concentrations, particularly albumin, are high. Proteins are thus an important determinant of plasma calcium levels, although the physiologically active fraction is Ca^{2+}. Various formulae have been proposed to correct for the effect of albumin. One that is widely used is:

Corrected calcium = measured calcium

$$+ 0.02[40 - albumin] \text{ mmol } l^{-1}$$

However, corrected formulae give only an approximation of Ca^{2+} levels and for an accurate assessment of this, ionized calcium determination is required. For measurement of total plasma calcium, it is important to take blood without venous stasis, as this causes redistribution of fluid from the occluded vein to extravascular spaces; haemoconcentration affects albumin concentrations and thus total calcium levels more than those of lower molecular weight substances. Ionized calcium levels are affected by blood pH, particularly if changes in H^+ concentrations are acute. Hydrogen ions compete with calcium for binding sites on albumin, ionized Ca^{2+} increasing with high H^+ levels and decreasing if these fall, although there is no change in total calcium levels. The distribution of calcium between proteins and the ionized fraction is usually normal in chronic acidosis and alkalosis.

DISORDERS OF CALCIUM HOMEOSTASIS

Hypercalcaemia

Hypercalcaemia is relatively common, occurring in up to 3% of hospital patients, although it is found in less than 0.5% of a healthy ambulatory population. Hypercalcaemia is usually discovered:

(i) coincidentally when blood is tested for another reason,
(ii) because calcium is monitored in conditions associated with disordered calcium metabolism, or
(iii) because clinical features of hypercalcaemia are present.

Plasma total calcium levels above 3.0 mmol l^{-1} are usually, although not inevitably, associated with symptoms, these including fatigue, depression, anorexia, vomiting and constipation. Defects of renal tubular function, particularly polyuria, occur and ECG abnormalities are also seen – characteristically, a short QT interval. If hypercalcaemia is chronic, soft tissue calcification and renal tract stones develop.

Causes

The causes of hypercalcaemia are outlined in **Table 9.1**. The commonest cause of hypercalcaemia is primary hyperparathy-

Table 9.1   Causes of hypercalcaemia

Hyperparathyroidism
◆ Primary hyperparathyroidism
◆ Tertiary hyperparathyroidism
◆ Multiple endocrine neoplasia
Malignant disease
◆ Tumours with metastases
◆ Tumours producing humoral factor
Excess vitamin D
◆ Vitamin D intoxication
◆ Overproduction by granulomas
◆ Idiopathic hypercalcaemia of infancy
High bone turnover
◆ Thyrotoxicosis
◆ Paget's disease (if immobilized)
◆ Thiazide diuretics
Other causes
◆ Familial hypocalciuric hypercalcaemia
◆ Milk-alkali syndrome

trol of Ca^{2+} levels. Hypercalcaemia develops occasionally in severe renal failure, due to PTH secretion escaping from control by Ca^{2+} levels and becoming autonomous (tertiary hyperparathyroidism). Hyperparathyroidism may also occur in association with other endocrine adenomas, multiple endocrine neoplasia (MEN). Two distinct patterns are recognized, MEN I in which parathyroid adenomas are associated with tumours of the pituitary gland and pancreas, while parathyroid adenomas, phaeochromocytomas and medullary carcinomas of the thyroid occur in MEN II.

Characteristic bone changes may be found in hyperparathyroidism which include loss of bone density, periosteal erosions (osteitis fibrosa cystica), and reabsorption of bone in the phalanges and skull.

roidism, the second most frequent being malignant disease; together, these are responsible for over 90% of cases of hypercalcaemia in adults.

Hyperparathyroidism

Primary hyperparathyroidism is usually caused by a solitary adenoma, although occasionally it results from a carcinoma or from hyperplasia affecting all four glands. Excess PTH secretion leads to hypercalcaemia: hypophosphataemia, due to the phosphatosuric effect of the hormone, is often present, although this is not inevitable. Plasma PTH levels may be within the normal range but such a finding is abnormal in hypercalcaemia since PTH secretion is inhibited by increased Ca^{2+}; thus PTH concentrations should be low.

Secondary hyperparathyroidism results from parathyroid hyperplasia occurring as an appropriate physiological response to hypocalcaemia, this most often being caused by either renal failure or malabsorption of vitamin D. The hypocalcaemia is usually corrected by parathyroid hyperplasia but hypercalcaemia does not occur as hormone secretion remains under the con-

Malignancy-related Hypercalcaemia Hypercalcaemia is a relatively common complication of malignancy, occurring particularly in multiple myeloma and tumours which metastasize to the bone (lung, breast, kidney). The mechanism of hypercalcaemia in these malignancies is extensive bony reabsorption, this being thought to be due to local cytokine secretion or prostaglandin production. A second major mechanism by which hypercalcaemia occurs is as the result of the production of a humoral factor by the tumour, particularly peptides with PTH activity (PTH-related peptide), these being produced characteristically by squamous cell carcinomas of the bronchus.

Other Causes Hypercalcaemia may result from excess vitamin D action, either because of excessive intake, or owing to abnormal metabolism of vitamin D. Excessive intake is often iatrogenic, resulting from treatment of hypoparathyroidism, or is sometimes the result of accidental ingestion. In granulomatous diseases, particularly sarcoidosis, there is increased conversion of 25-hydroxycholecalciferol to calcitriol, this being inhibited by corticosteroid therapy.

Idiopathic hypercalcaemia of infancy is caused by increased sensitivity to vitamin D, but the actual mechanism for this is unclear. Mild hypercalcaemia is common in thyrotoxicosis, increased bone reabsorption being responsible. Immobilization may produce hypercalcaemia if a condition associated with increased bone turnover, particularly Paget's disease, is present. Thiazide diuretics interfere with renal calcium excretion and occasionally induce hypercalcaemia, particularly in patients with increased bone turnover. Familial hypocalciuric hypercalcaemia is inherited as an autosomal dominant trait and the condition is often asymptomatic. The levels of PTH are usually normal and no parathyroid adenoma is found at surgery. The basis of the condition is not understood. Hypercalcaemia may occur in patients who ingest large quantities of milk together with alkali antacids to alleviate symptoms of peptic ulceration. An alkalosis occurs which is thought to reduce urinary calcium excretion. The condition has become very rare since the use of H-2 receptor antagonists for treating peptic ulceration.

Investigation

It is often recommended that blood samples for plasma calcium concentrations should be taken fasting, although there is little evidence that levels rise significantly following a meal. Prolonged venous stasis should be avoided, for reasons outlined above. Plasma total calcium concentrations must be interpreted with knowledge of plasma protein levels. If there is doubt concerning the effect of these, ionized calcium levels should be determined.

Diagnosis of tumour-related hypercalcaemia is not difficult in many cases, as there are often clinical features or radiological findings suggestive of the diagnosis. Clinical features due to the cause of hypercalcaemia may be lacking, however, asymptomatic hypercalcaemia being more common in hyperparathyroidism than malignancy. Plasma phosphate is usually low in primary hyperparathyroidism but may also be reduced in malignancy. Alkaline phosphatase activity may be increased owing to malignancy or hyperparathyroidism. The presence of hypercalcaemia with normal or above normal levels of PTH suggests hyperparathyroidism, since secretion of the hormone should be suppressed in hypercalcaemia if the normal feedback mechanisms are intact. Urinary calcium levels are elevated in most causes of hypercalcaemia; low levels suggest familial hypocalciuric hypercalcaemia.

Management

Specific causes of hypercalcaemia require appropriate treatment but hypercalacemia itself, particularly if severe, may require management. Dehydration is often present and should be corrected, if necessary using intravenous saline. Frusemide is often administered following rehydration: this inhibits tubular reabsorption of calcium. Intravenous and oral phosphate supplements are effective at reducing calcium levels but carry the risk of producing metastatic calcification or renal failure. Calcitonin inhibits bone reabsorption in the short term and is effective in treating hypercalcaemia associated with immobiliza-

---

KEY POINTS

HYPERCALCAEMIA

- The commonest causes of hypercalcaemia are primary hyperparathyroidism and malignancy

- Primary hyperparathyroidism is usually caused by a solitary adenoma

- Malignant disease causes hypercalcaemia by resorption of bone or through the effect of a humoral factor

- Measurement of urinary calcium excretion is rarely useful in investigating hypercalcaemia

tion; biphosphonates also inhibit bone turn-over. Mithramycin is effective in treating hypercalcaemia although its usefulness is limited by toxicity. High-dose glucocorticoids sometimes inhibit hypercalcaemia complicating malignancy.

Hypocalcaemia

Hypocalcaemia in infancy is considered in chapter 18. In older patients, hypercalcaemia may be accompanied by increased neuromuscular excitability with tetany, parasthesiae and muscle cramps occurring. Chvostek's and Trousseau's signs may be positive. Prolonged hypocalcaemia is also associated with cataracts, mental retardation, psychosis and increased intracranial pressure, which may lead to papilloedema.

Causes

The causes of hypocalcaemia are outlined in **Table 9.2**. Blood taken into tubes which contain ethylene diamine tetra-acetic acid (EDTA) as an anticoagulant will have spuriously low calcium levels since calcium is chelated by EDTA, this being the basis of its anticoagulant effect. Hypoproteinaemia causes hypocalcaemia because almost 50% of blood calcium is bound to albumin,

Table 9.2 Causes of hypocalcaemia in adults

Spurious
◆ Chelation by EDTA
Hypoalbuminaemia
Reduced parathyroid hormone action
◆ Hypoparathyroidism
◆ Pseudohypoparathyroidism
◆ Hypomagnesaemia
Defect in active vitamin D
◆ Rickets, osteomalacia
◆ Vitamin D-resistant rickets
◆ Malabsorption
◆ Chronic renal failure
◆ Liver disease
◆ Anticonvulsant therapy
Pancreatitis

although this may not be important physiologically, as the ionized fraction is not affected.

Hypoparathyroidism Several different patterns of hypoparathyroidism are recognized. Congenital absence of the parathyroid glands may occur as an isolated defect or in association with absence of the thymus, facial abnormalities and impaired cellular immune responses which lead to severe, recurrent infections (DiGeorge syndrome). Hereditary hypoparathyroidism with impaired cell-mediated immunity also occurs as part of an autoimmune syndrome, and is often associated with adrenal and primary ovarian failure. Recurrent candidiasis is common. The onset of hypoparathyroidism with an inherited basis usually occurs in childhood, although some cases occur in adults. Hypoparathyroidism may also follow thyroidectomy or other neck surgery, some cases being transient while others are permanent. Removal of parathyroid tissue or ischaemia are thought to be precipitating causes. Pseudohypoparathyroidism is characterized by excessive PTH secretion; hypocalcaemia occurs because of decreased responsiveness of target organs. The condition is sex-linked, males being twice as likely to be affected as females. Skeletal abnormalities occur, leading to short stature, short metacarpals and short metatarsals. Cataracts, mental retardation and testicular atrophy are also features of pseudohypoparathyroidism. Hypocalcaemia often accompanies hypomagnesaemia, this being associated with impaired secretion of PTH.

Abnormal Vitamin D Metabolism Deficiency of vitamin D results from inadequate dietary intake or reduced cutaneous synthesis. This sometimes occurs in elderly subjects who have limited exposure to sunlight. Malabsorption of fat-soluble vitamins may occur in intestinal diseases. Vitamin D deficiency causes rickets in children and osteomalacia in adults. Congenital deficiency of 1α-hydroxylase is the cause of vitamin D-dependent rickets. In chronic renal failure synthesis of calcitriol is defective owing to reduced 1α-hydroxylation of 25-hydroxycholecalciferol, although hyperphosphataemia also contributes to the hypocalcaemia which can occur. Impaired synthesis and secretion of bile salts is thought to lead to impaired digestion and absorption of fats, including vitamin D, in liver disease. Increased metabolism of vitamin D due to increased hepatic microsomal enzyme activity induced by anticonvulsant drug therapy has been described, although low vitamin D intake contributes to osteomalacia in many patients receiving such agents.

Pancreatitis Hypocalcaemia can occur in patients with acute pancreatitis. Release of activated lipases into the peritoneal cavity saponifies fats and released fatty acids can bind calcium. It is likely that other mechanisms also contribute to hypocalcaemia, including hypoalbuminaemia and hypomagnesaemia.

Investigation

The cause of hypocalcaemia may well be apparent from the clinical features. Hyperphosphataemia occurs in both hypoparathyroidism and pseudohypoparathyroidism, plasma PTH being undetectable or very low in the former while levels are elevated in pseudohypoparathyroidism. Occasionally, determination of plasma magnesium and vitamin D levels are required to elucidate the cause. Characteristic radiological features of osteomalacia and rickets include skeletal deformities in children and bands of decalcification in adults, affecting particularly the pelvis, femur and scapula (Looser's zones).

PHOSPHATE HOMEOSTASIS

The total body content of phosphate in the average male is around 25 000 mmol. Approximately 80% of this is in bone, 15%

in intracellular fluid and 0.1% in extracellular fluid. The plasma level of inorganic phosphate is 0.8-1.4 mmol l^{-1}, of which 15% is protein bound and 85% is free. Functions include maintenance of cell wall structure, energy metabolism, enzyme regulation, oxygen transport and buffering of H^+. Phosphate is the most abundant intracellular anion, concentrations being in the order of 100 mmol l^{-1}, mostly in the form of organic phosphates, these including intermediates of glycolysis, adenosine phosphates and creatine phosphate. It is thus a key substance in energy metabolism. Dietary intake is approximately 1 g phosphorus per day, although the availability of phosphates for absorption from different foods varies. Meat and dairy produce contain soluble phosphate which is absorbed easily, while phosphorus in cereals is partly bound to inositol as phytate and thus less is available. Absorption is at least partly controlled by vitamin D, while PTH regulates excretion by decreasing tubular phosphate reabsorption. Urinary excretion also depends on the amount absorbed and the range of urinary phosphate in health is thus very wide.

Hypophosphataemia and Phosphate Depletion

Plasma phosphate concentrations are not always a reliable indicator of intracellular phosphate levels. This is illustrated by finding hyperphosphataemia occurring in diabetic ketoacidosis, although there are often considerable total body deficits, this being analogous to disordered potassium metabolism in ketoacidosis (see chapter 1). While low plasma phosphate levels usually indicate phosphate depletion they may be reduced without depletion in water retention.

Causes of Hypophosphataemia

Causes are outlined in **Table 9.3**. Decreased dietary intake is an unusual cause as phosphate occurs widely in foods, although ingestion of excessive quantities of antacids may cause hypophosphataemia by binding dietary phosphate. Mild hypophosphataemia may occur owing to malabsorption. Both respiratory and metabolic acidosis lead to shifts in phosphate from extracellular to intracellular compartments, most probably because an elevated intracellular pH increases the activity of phosphofructokinase, thus increasing glycolysis and the utilization of phosphate. Treatment of diabetic ketoacidosis with insulin promotes cellular glucose and phosphate uptake; increased glycolysis also occurs, further reducing plasma phosphate levels. Excessive utilization of phosphate occurs during hyperalimentation and refeeding starved patients; if phosphate supplements are not given, profound hypophosphataemia may develop. Increased PTH secretion and hypomagnesaemia lower plasma phosphate concentrations by reducing renal tubular phosphate reabsorption. Primary renal tubular defects of phosphate reabsorption also occur.

Chronic alcohol abuse is an important cause of hypophosphataemia and the pathogenesis is complex. Reduced absorption probably plays a role, due to poor diet, vomiting and diarrhoea. In addition, magnesium deficiency is common in alcoholic patients. Plasma phosphate levels often fall sharply during withdrawal from alcohol, increased carbohydrate intake being a precipitating factor.

Consequences

Phosphate depletion has widespread metabolic effects. Clinical consequences of hypophosphataemia occur mainly with severe depletion associated with a pre-existing wasting illness, the most important causes being alcohol abuse, hyperalimentation and refeeding starved patients. Haemolysis may result from depletion of erythrocyte 2,3-diphosphoglycerate levels and muscle weakness is common; in critically ill patients this sometimes leads to respiratory failure. Rhabdomyolysis is a rare complication, possibly caused by a deficiency of adenosine triphosphate (ATP). Leukocyte and platelet dysfunction are also thought to result from ATP depletion. Various central nervous system features have been described including parasthesiae, ataxia and even coma. Demineralization of the skeleton can occur.

Hyperphosphataemia

Hyperphosphataemia may be artefactual, and result from haemolysis occurring during venepuncture. The main causes of true hyperphosphataemia are chronic renal failure, hypoparathyroidism, untreated acromegaly, excessive phosphate administration and hypercatabolic states. Chronic persistent hyperphosphataemia may result in metastatic calcification.

METABOLIC BONE DISEASE

In the healthy adult remodelling of bone is a continuous process, the constituent parts of which, resorption and new bone formation,

---

Table 9.3 Causes of hypophosphataemia

Reduced absorption
◆ Dietary deficiency
◆ Oral phosphate-binding agents
◆ Malabsorption
Increased cellular uptake
◆ Alkalosis
◆ Diabetic ketoacidosis (recovery phase)
◆ Hyperalimentation
◆ Refeeding starved patients
Increased excretion
◆ Hyperparathyroidism
◆ Hypomagnesaemia
◆ Renal tubular defect
◆ Dialysis
Dilution
◆ Volume expansion
Chronic alcohol abuse

are in balance. New bone formation involves the production of bone matrix (osteoid) by osteoblasts, followed by mineralization. Osteoclasts are responsible for bone resorption. Imbalances in these processes lead to metabolic bone disease, including osteoporosis, osteomalacia and rickets, Paget's disease of the bone and renal osteodystrophy.

Osteoporosis

Osteoporosis is the most common metabolic bone disease; it is characterized by a reduction of bone mass which is not accompanied by changes in the ratio of mineral to osteoid. Histologically, a decrease in the cortical thickness of bone occurs and the number and size of trabeculae in cancellous bone is reduced. Slow loss of bone occurs in both sexes after 40–50 years, this being greater in females than males, and the loss accelerates after the menopause, particularly in trabecular bone. Such bone loss can lead to primary osteoporosis which is often asymptomatic, although bone pain may occur due to fractures, particularly of the vertebrae. Loss of height may also result. Osteoporosis may also be secondary to a variety of diseases, these being outlined in **Table 9.4**.

Biochemical tests are generally unhelpful in osteoporosis, calcium, phosphate and alkaline phosphatase usually being normal, although alkaline phosphatase activity may be increased following a fracture. The urinary excretion of hydroxyproline, an amino acid which occurs in high concentrations in collagen, may be increased if there is rapid bone loss but is often normal. There has been considerable interest recently in pyridinium cross-links – products formed during the maturation of extracellular collagen – as markers of bone resorption. Urinary excretion of these is increased in osteoporosis and in other conditions in which increased bone resorption occurs,

Table 9.4   Causes of osteoporosis

Primary
- Post-menopausal
- Senile

Secondary
- Endocrine
  Cushing's syndrome
  Hypogonadism
  Hyperthyroidism
  Hyperparathyroidism
  Diabetes mellitus
- Gastrointestinal
  Malabsorption
  Chronic liver disease
- Drugs
  Corticosteroids
  Prolonged heparin administration
- Others
  Immobilization

including Paget's disease, primary hyperparathyroidism, and osteomalacia.

Osteomalacia and Rickets

These conditions are characterized by defective mineralization of the organic matrix of bone, most often resulting from vitamin D deficiency. Rickets affects children in whom the epiphyseal plates of the long bone have not fused, resulting in skeletal deformities. These are extremely rare in osteomalacia, the adult form of the disease. Several factors are required for normal mineralization of bone, including sufficient calcium and phosphate at calcification sites and normal osteoblast function. No direct effect of calcitriol on calcification has been demonstrated in man; vitamin D deficiency probably reduces calcification by its effect on plasma calcium and phosphate levels. Rickets and osteomalacia are seen most commonly in the UK in South Asians and the elderly, reduced exposure to sunlight and dietary deficiency of vitamin D being important aetiological factors. Malabsorption may also cause vitamin D deficiency. Defects in renal tubular phosphate reabsorption, occurring either as an isolated abnormality or as part of the Fanconi syndrome, may cause vitamin D-resistant rickets or osteomalacia. In osteomalacia and rickets the most common biochemical features are hypocalcaemia, hypophosphataemia (if renal function is normal) and increased alkaline phosphatase activities.

Paget's Disease of the Bone

In Paget's disease excessive reabsorption of bone occurs, together with new bone formation, this being structurally abnormal (very dense in advanced disease). The condition is usually focal but may be widespread. The disease, the cause of which is unclear, affects less than 1% of the adult population, the incidence increasing with age. Plasma calcium and phosphate levels are usually normal although hypercalacemia may occur if patients are immobilized. Plasma alkaline phosphatase activities are often elevated, reflecting increased osteoblastic activity.

Renal Osteodystrophy

A number of skeletal abnormalities occur in chronic renal failure, particularly osteomalacia and osteitis fibrosa cystica. Osteomalacia appears to be caused by two factors: reduced synthesis of calcitriol, and deposition of aluminium in bones (see chapter 8). Osteitis fibrosa cystica is caused by secondary hyperparathyroidism. The plasma calcium concentration is slightly reduced or goes towards the lower limit of the reference range, plasma phosphate is increased and plasma alkaline phosphatase activity is also elevated.

MAGNESIUM HOMEOSTASIS

The average adult contains 750–1000 mmol magnesium of which approximately 67% is found in bones, 31% within cells and 1% in ECF. Plasma magnesium concentrations are normally $0.7–1.0$ mmol l^{-1}. Most magnesium within cells is bound to ATP, is a component of magnesium-containing enzymes, or is sequestered within mitochondria. The daily intake of magnesium is 8–17 mmol, the richest sources being cereals and vegetables. Approximately 40% of the amount ingested is absorbed, mainly in the jejunum and ileum. Absorption is regulated partly by vitamin D. There is also effective renal regulation of magnesium metabolism, urinary excretion being negligible in deficiency states, but rising significantly when plasma concentrations exceed 0.85 mmol l^{-1}. Renal excretion increases in hypermagnesaemia, hypercalcaemia and if the extracellular fluid volume is increased.

Magnesium Deficiency

Deficiency can exist in the presence of normal plasma levels and therefore hypomagnesaemia is, at best, only a rough indicator of tissue levels. Some recommend the measurement of erythrocyte magnesium levels to investigate deficiency but these are specialized investigations that are not widely available. Magnesium deficiency usually results from decreased absorption or increased excretion, although internal redistribution can also occur (**Table 9.5**).

Magnesium depletion rarely occurs as an isolated deficiency; specific signs and symptoms are few. Patients are usually weak and lethargic and degeneration of muscle fibres has been described. Hypomagnesaemia is often associated with hypocalcaemia, and tetany with positive Chvostek and Trousseau's signs may occur. Magnesium is required for normal PTH secretion. Hypokalaemia is also found frequently with hypomagnesaemia, deficiencies of both being caused by the same conditions, although magnesium depletion also appears to enhance renal excretion of potassium. Mild depletion is usually treated by oral replace-

Table 9.5 Causes of magnesium deficiency

Nutritional deficiency
◆Inadequate intake
◆Parenteral nutrition
Gastrointestinal
◆Malabsorption
◆Diarrhoea
Endocrine
◆Hyperaldosteronism
◆Diabetic ketoacidosis
Alcohol abuse
Increased renal excretion
◆Diuretic therapy
◆Cisplatin therapy
◆Amphotericin B therapy
◆Recovery phase of acute tubular necrosis

ment but since magnesium salts cause diarrhoea, intravenous replacement is often required in severe deficiencies, and when depletion is due gastrointestinal disease.

Hypermagnesaemia

Hypermagnesaemia is usually caused by renal failure, the normal kidney having considerable capacity to excrete excess magnesium. Magnesium can act as a central nervous system depressant and reduce neuromuscular transmission. Hypotension, bradycardia, respiratory paralysis and coma have been described with plasma levels exceeding 5 mmol l^{-1}.

FURTHER READING

Annotation. Pyridinium crosslinks as markers of bone resorption. *Lancet* 1992; **340**: 278–9

Bilezikian JP. Management of acute hypercalcaemia. *New England Journal of Medicine* 1992; **326**: 1196–203

Knochel JP. The clinical status of hypophosphataemia. *New England Journal of Medicine* 1985; **315**: 447–9

Mundy GR. Hypercalcaemia of malignancy revisited. *Journal of Clinical Investigation* 1988; **82**: 1–6

Selby PL, Adams PH. The investigation of hypercalcaemia. *Journal of Clinical Pathology* 1994; **47**: 579–84

CASE 9.1

A 49-year-old woman complained of loin pain which proved to be ureteric colic. Investigations showed the following:

total calcium	2.98 mmol l^{-1}
phosphate	0.69 mmol l^{-1}
albumin	39 g l^{-1}
alkaline phosphatase	180 U l^{-1}
sodium	141 mmol l^{-1}
potassium	3.9 mmol l^{-1}
chloride	113 mmol l^{-1}
total CO_2	19 mmol l^{-1}
urea	7.1 mmol l^{-1}
creatinine	114 μmol l^{-1}

Explain these results.

CASE 9.2

A 45-year-old woman with hyperparathyroidism had been treated by parathyroidectomy and developed hypocalcaemia postoperatively. For this she had received vitamin D and 1α-hydroxycholecalciferol. She was seen in outpatients complaining of feeling unwell and vomiting. The following results of blood tests were obtained:

total calcium	3.95 mmol l^{-1}
phosphate	1.22 mmol l^{-1}
albumin	42 g l^{-1}
alkaline phosphatase	75 U l^{-1}

Why was she hypercalcaemic?

CASE 9.3

A 79-year-old man who lived alone was admitted to hospital having developed progressive weakness over several months. No specific findings were seen on examination. Blood tests showed the following:

total calcium	1.74 mmol l^{-1}
phosphate	0.71 mmol l^{-1}
albumin	39 g l^{-1}
alkaline phosphatase	390 U l^{-1}

What is the most probable diagnosis?

CASE 9.4

A 24-year-old man complained of muscle cramps and parasthesiae. The following blood tests results were obtained:

total calcium	1.41 mmol l^{-1}
phosphate	1.61 mmol l^{-1}
albumin	47 g l^{-1}
alkaline phosphatase	72 U l^{-1}
urea	5.2 mmol l^{-1}
creatinine	86 μmol l^{-1}

What are the possible causes for these abnormalities?

THE GASTROINTESTINAL TRACT

INTRODUCTION

The principal function of the gastrointestinal tract and its associated organs is the digestion and absorption of nutrients. The major foods are ingested as macromolecules which must be broken down to smaller components for absorption. This is achieved by enzymes secreted by the gastrointestinal tract, together with the mechanical processes involved in digestion, chewing, mixing, swallowing, gastric emptying and intestinal transit. During digestion, considerable fluxes of water and electrolytes across gut mucosae occur in addition to major changes in pH in the lumen of the stomach and small intestine. The digestive sequence is controlled by neural and hormonal factors, and the gut is an active endocrine organ.

THE MOUTH AND OESOPHAGUS

During chewing, food is mixed with saliva which has a lubricant function and also contains amylase. Amylase hydrolyses starch to smaller dextrins although the salivary enzyme contributes little to carbohydrate digestion, as it is inactivated by acid in the stomach.

THE STOMACH
Normal Gastric Function

Distension of the stomach and the presence of protein in the lumen stimulate the secretion of gastrin, a peptide hormone produced by the G-cells of the antral mucosa. Alcohol, vagal stimulation and Ca^{2+} also promote gastrin secretion. Gastrin stimulates the secretion of acid by the parietal cells of the stomach, promotes gastric and intestinal motility and also initiates pancreatic secretion. Secretion of gastrin is inhibited by negative feedback from excess intraluminal acid in the pylorus. The low pH in the stomach activates the proteolytic enzyme pepsin, which is secreted as a precursor enzyme, pepsinogen, by the chief cells. Other secretions of the stomach include intrinsic factor, which is essential for the normal absorption of vitamin B_{12} (see chapter 4). Gastric juice also contains a lipase which hydrolyses triglycerides containing short and medium chain fatty acids.

Disordered Gastric Function

Hypersecretion
Duodenal Ulceration Hypersecretion of acid occurs in patients with duodenal ulceration. However, there is marked overlap in the rates of secretion between normal subjects and patients with ulcers and studies of acid secretion have no place in diagnosis or management.

Zollinger–Ellison Syndrome The Zollinger–Ellison syndrome is caused by gastrin-secreting tumours, gastrinomas. Approximately 90% of these are found in the pancreas, the remainder occurring in the duodenum, stomach or spleen. Occasionally, gastrinomas are a component of a multiple endocrine adenomatosis syndrome (MEA-1). Excessive secretion of gastrin causes expansion of the parietal cell mass and hypersecretion of hydrochloric acid. This leads to recurrent peptic ulceration which is resistant to medical treatment.

Hyposecretion
Reduced acid secretion occurs in gastric ulcer and carcinoma. Pernicious anaemia results from autoimmune destruction of parietal cells which causes achlorhydria and a deficiency of intrinsic factor secretion. This leads to impaired vitamin B_{12} absorption.

Assessment of Gastric Function

Endoscopic and radiological investigations are the principal diagnostic procedures used to investigate gastric function. Biochemical function tests are of limited value and are largely restricted to investigations of acid secretion.

Acid Secretion Studies
Studies of acid secretion are occasionally undertaken to investigate pernicious anaemia, the Zollinger–Ellison syndrome or the completeness of vagotomy. Acid secretion is assessed in the resting state and following stimulation.

Pentagastrin Test Pentagastrin is a synthetic peptide with the same amino acids as the terminal sequence of gastrin which is responsible for its physiological actions. The patient, who is fasting, is intubated and the gastric secretions aspirated (resting juice). Secretions are collected for the next hour to determine basal secretion. Pentagastrin (6 μg kg^{-1} body weight) is then injected intramuscularly and secretions are collected for the next hour. No acid is produced in achlorhydria, while both resting and basal acid secretion are high in Zollinger–Ellison syndrome.

Insulin-Induced Hypoglycaemia Hypoglycaemia stimulates acid secretion via the vagus nerve and insulin-induced hypoglycaemia may be used to test the completeness of vagotomy.

Serum Gastrin

Serum gastrin is a labile hormone and careful precautions are needed for its collection and preservation. Blood should be preserved with aprotinin, a protease inhibitor, to prevent degradation. Serum levels are reduced in duodenal ulceration, when gastrin secretion is inhibited by increased H^+ secretion, and fasting levels are increased greatly in Zollinger–Ellison syndrome. Levels are also increased in pernicious anaemia, particularly after a meal, when normally they would be expected to fall as a result of acid secretion.

THE PANCREAS

Normal Pancreatic Function

Exocrine pancreatic secretions have two major components, bicarbonate and enzymes. Pancreatic secretion is stimulated by food in the stomach and duodenum, and the presence of H^+ in the duodenum. Gastrin is a weak stimulus for secretion, hormonal control being due mainly to cholecystokinin-pancreozymin (CCK-PZ) and secretin. CCK-PZ is secreted by the upper small intestine, its secretion being stimulated by peptides, fatty acids and H^+ entering the duodenum. The carboxy-terminal pentapeptide is identical to that of gastrin. Actions of CCK-PZ include stimulating pancreatic enzyme secretion and increasing motility of the small intestine. Secretin is found in the duodenum and upper jejunum and has some amino acid sequences in common with glucagon. The major stimulus for secretion is H^+ and the main action of secretin is to enhance pancreatic bicarbonate secretion, thus neutralizing H^+ in the small intestine. This adjusts the pH of the small intestine to approximately 6.5, the optimum for the activity of pancreatic and small intestinal

enzymes. Pancreatic enzymes include amylase, lipases and proteases, the proteases being secreted as inactive precursors and converted to active species in the gut. The products of pancreatic digestion are oligosaccharides and disaccharides, small peptides and amino acids, fatty acids and free cholesterol.

Disordered Pancreatic Exocrine Function

Several diseases cause disordered exocrine pancreatic function including cystic fibrosis, acute and chronic pancreatitis, and carcinoma of the pancreas.

Cystic Fibrosis

Cystic fibrosis is the most common inherited metabolic disease which is lethal in children, its frequency being 1/2500 live births (see chapter 19). It is a recessive condition in which defective epithelial chloride transport causes viscous secretions that block secretory ducts and alveoli. Pulmonary dysfunction is the most common cause of death and pancreatic insufficiency occurs in approximately 85% of cases. Cystic fibrosis is usually first diagnosed in childhood but occasionally presents in adults.

Acute Pancreatitis

Acute pancreatitis occurs when pancreatic enzymes are activated within the gland. A number of factors predispose to acute pancreatitis (**Table 10.1**) although how these lead to enzyme activation is unclear.

Table 10.1 Causes of acute pancreatitis

Alcohol abuse
◆ Acute
◆ Chronic
Gallstones
Trauma
◆ Blunt abdominal injuries
◆ Postendoscopic retrograde
  cholangiopancreatography
◆ Postabdominal surgery
Metabolic
◆ Severe hypertriglyceridaemia
◆ Hypercalcaemia
◆ Renal failure
Infections
◆ Mumps
Drugs

The activated enzymes digest surrounding tissue and cause oedema, proteolysis, fat necrosis, vascular damage and haemorrhage within the gland. Activated enzymes can also be released from the gland causing injury in the peritoneal cavity. Abdominal pain is the major presenting feature.

Chronic Pancreatitis

Chronic pancreatitis is most often caused by alcohol abuse in Western societies, although other causes of acute pancreatitis may also lead to the chronic condition. In less affluent countries severe protein energy malnutrition is an important aetiological factor. Inflammation with subsequent fibrosis in the pancreas often leads to exocrine insufficiency. Some patients present with abdominal pain, which may be continuous, while others have malabsorption. Impaired glucose tolerance can occur but frank diabetes mellitus is rare.

Carcinoma of the Pancreas

Patients with carcinoma of the pancreas usually present with abdominal pain, weight loss or jaundice. Malabsorption caused by exocrine insufficiency resulting from blockage of the pancreatic duct may be a contributory factor to weight loss.

Assessment of Pancreatic Function

Biochemical pancreatic function tests include measurement of enzymes in body fluids and dynamic function tests. These are direct, where the small intestine is intubated and pancreatic secretions are collected (secretin/CCK-PZ and Lundh tests), or indirect, where assessments are made without intubation (PABA and fluorescein dilaurate tests).

Serum Amylase

Amylase is a small protein (molecular mass 45 kDa). Most serum amylase in normal subjects arises from the salivary glands and therefore the investigation is of little value in detecting reduced pancreatic exocrine mass, as occurs in chronic pancreatitis. Very high serum levels occur in acute pancreatitis, although activities may also be raised in a number of other conditions (see chapter 12). Values greater than 10 times the upper limit of normal are virtually diagnostic of acute pancreatitis and values greater than five times the upper limit of normal are suggestive but not diagnostic of the condition. Maximal activities occur within 24–48 h after an attack and these fall rapidly, often returning to normal within 72 h.

Because of its molecular mass amylase is cleared from the circulation through the kidney. Amylase clearance increases in acute pancreatitis and urinary excretion rates may be increased when plasma activities have returned to normal.

Other Pancreatic Enzymes

Lipase activity may remain elevated longer than amylase in plasma following acute pancreatitis, although it is a less sensitive indicator of pancreatic damage. Immunoreactive trypsin (trypsin enzyme activity in serum being inhibited by antiproteases) is low in pancreatic insufficiency but often high in cystic fibrosis as a result of leakage of trypsin from blocked pancreatic ductules.

Secretin/CCK-PZ Stimulation Test

Following an overnight fast patients are intubated with a double-lumen tube positioned so that gastric and small intestinal secretions can be aspirated separately. Resting secretions are collected and then secretin administered intravenously, followed 30 min later by CCK-PZ. It is thus possible to study the effect of each hormone, measuring the volume of secretion, its bicarbonate content and enzyme activity. In chronic pancreatitis the bicarbonate and enzyme contents of secretions fall while the volume is maintained. Low volumes of secretions are found in patients with carcinoma of the head of pancreas.

Lundh Test Meal

This is a simpler intubation procedure in which a single lumen tube is passed and resting duodenal juice aspirated. A meal of 40 g dextrose, 15 g milk protein and 18 g corn oil is then given and the duodenum aspirated for 2 h. Reduced tryptic activity indicates pancreatic exocrine insufficiency.

PABA Absorption

This test involves the oral administration of a synthetic peptide, BT-PABA (*N*-benzoyl-L-tyrosyl-*p*-aminobenzoic acid) which is split by chymotrypsin to yield PABA (*p*-aminobenzoic acid). PABA is absorbed, conjugated with glycine in the liver and excreted in the urine (**Figure 10.1**). The patient is given BT-PABA with a meal, in order to stimulate pancreatic secretion. Excretion of PABA is reduced in chronic pancreatitis and also in small intestinal and liver disease. In the last two conditions excretion is affected by factors other than digestion of the

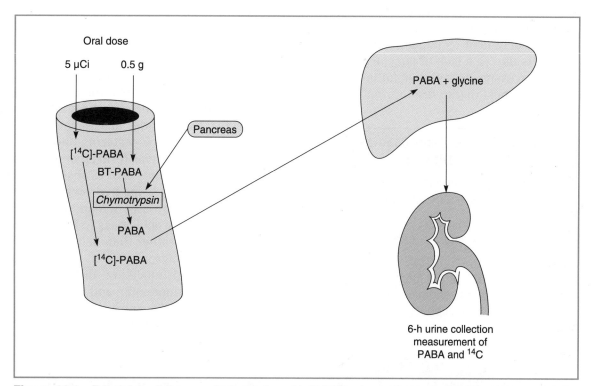

Figure 10.1 Principles of the *p*-aminobenzoic acid (PABA) absorption test. *N*-benzoyl-L-tyrosyl (BT)-PABA is a synthetic peptide which is split by chymotrypsin produced by the pancreas, free PABA being released and absorbed. After conjugation in the liver, PABA is excreted in urine and therefore, if variations resulting from conjugation are corrected by administering radioactively labelled PABA simultaneously, PABA excretion is a test of pancreatic function.

peptide and inclusion of $[^{14}C]$PABA in the test, which does not require hydrolysis, corrects for these.

Fluorescein Dilaurate (Pancreolauryl) Test

Fluorescein dilaurate is a synthetic substrate which is hydrolysed by pancreatic cholesterol esterase. Fluorescein is released and absorbed and, following conjugation in the liver, excreted in urine where it can be measured. To correct for factors other than substrate hydrolysis, free fluorescein is given orally on a second day and the ratio of fluorescein derived from the dilaurate to the excretion of free dye is calculated. The test is less convenient than measuring PABA absorption because a second procedure is necessary.

Impaired Digestion in Pancreatic Disease

Pancreatic exocrine insufficiency, particularly in chronic pancreatitis or cystic fibrosis, may lead to impaired digestion of nutrients due to a lack of enzymes. Steatorrhoea, excessive excretion of fat in stools, is the commonest digestive abnormality which may result.

KEY POINTS

BIOCHEMICAL ASPECTS OF PANCREATIC DISEASE

- Acute pancreatitis occurs as a result of the release of activated enzymes

- Impaired digestion leading to malabsorption occurs in chronic pancreatitis

- The PABA and fluorescein dilaurate tests are investigations of pancreatic exocrine function

---

THE SMALL INTESTINE

Normal Intestinal Function

Small intestinal function includes the final stages of digestion and absorption of the products. Oligosaccharidases are found at the brush border. Sucrose and maltose are hydrolysed rapidly, as more than one enzyme has activity with each of these sugars. Lactose is split more slowly, lactase activity being lower than that of the other disaccharidases. Glucose and galactose are absorbed by a common active transport mechanism, while fructose is transported by independent facilitated diffusion.

Peptidases are found both at the brush border and within the cytoplasm of cells of the mucosa. There are a group of transporters to absorb amino acids and some dipeptides also cross the brush border. These are hydrolysed within the enterocytes.

Most fat digestion occurs in the small intestine, although lingual and gastric lipases hydrolyse approximately 10% of ingested lipid. Fat is emulsified by a mixture of bile salts and polar lipids, particularly phospholipids, to form micelles. Pancreatic colipase displaces emulsifying agents from the surface of these particles, allowing pancreatic lipase to attach to them and hydrolyse triglyceride to monoglycerides and fatty acids. These are absorbed from micelles by diffusion through the mucosa. In enterocytes, triglycerides are resynthesized and together with cholesterol, phospholipids and apolipoproteins form chylomicrons (see chapter 2). Cholesterol is absorbed as the free form, esters being hydrolysed in the lumen of the gut by a pancreatic esterase. Medium-chain fatty acids pass to the liver in the portal blood, rather than being incorporated into chylomicrons.

Most of the products of digestion are absorbed in the duodenum and jejunum but there are specific transport mechanisms in the terminal ileum for the transport of vitamin B_{12} and bile acids.

Malabsorption Due to Small Intestinal Disease

The term malabsorption is used in two senses, the first to describe a condition in which the processes of absorption fail, due specifically to intestinal disease. The second usage, the malabsorption syndrome, is more general and refers to a failure to assimilate nutrients owing to either impaired digestion (disorders of the stomach, liver, biliary tract or pancreas) or defective absorption (small intestinal disease). Several different mechanisms may be responsible for small intestinal malabsorption which are outlined in **Table 10.2**. Illustrative examples of diseases are also given, although malabsorption may result from more than one mechanism. It is important to bear in mind that patients with small intestinal disorders may not suffer from the generalized malabsorption syndrome but may have selective or isolated absorptive defects.

Loss of Small Intestine

Extensive ileal resection is most commonly undertaken because of vascular or Crohn's disease and may result in the short bowel syndrome. Whether malabsorption occurs depends on the length of bowel and the areas which are removed. Resection of up to 50% of the small intestine is usually well tolerated, provided the proximal intestine and terminal ileum are intact. If resections are extensive or the proximal or distal segments are removed malabsorption can result and severe diarrhoea occurs.

Malabsorption is sometimes induced surgically, jejunoileal bypass having been used previously to treat morbid obesity. Bypassing the terminal ileum is sometimes used to treat severe familial hypercholesterolaemia. The resulting bile acid malabsorption reduces serum cholesterol because of increased hepatic synthesis of primary bile acids from cholesterol to compensate for losses.

Mucosal Abnormalities

Coeliac disease is caused by intolerance to gluten, a protein found in wheat. This causes atrophy of intestinal villi, most probably due to local immunological reactions. Gliadin, a fraction of gluten, is thought to enter to the

Table 10.2 Causes of the malabsorption syndrome

Malabsorption
Loss of small intestine
♦ Resection
♦ Jejunoileal bypass
Mucosal abnormalities
♦ Villous atrophy
  Coeliac disease (gluten-sensitive enteropathy), AIDS, tropical sprue
Inflammatory or infiltrative disorders
♦ Regional enteritis (Crohn's disease)
♦ Amyloidosis
♦ Infective (e.g. salmonellosis)
♦ Small bowel lymphoma
Vascular disease
♦ Mesenteric vascular insufficiency
♦ Vasculitis
Endocrine and metabolic disorders
♦ Diabetes mellitus
♦ Carcinoid syndrome
♦ Abetalipoproteinaemia

Maldigestion
Pancreatic exocrine insufficiency
♦ Chronic pancreatitis
♦ Pancreatic carcinoma
♦ Cystic fibrosis
Inactivation of pancreatic enzymes
♦ Zollinger–Ellison syndrome
Reduced intestinal bile salt concentration
♦ Liver disease
♦ Biliary tract obstruction
♦ Bacterial overgrowth
♦ Interrupted enterohepatic circulation
  Ileal resection
  Regional enteritis
♦ Drugs
  Cholestyramine
  Broad spectrum antibiotics
♦ Reduced transit time
  Postgastrectomy

mucosa and activate T-lymphocytes, these producing cytokines (tumour necrosis factor, interleukin-2, γ-interferon) which damage the mucosa. Villous atrophy is also found in patients with acquired immune deficiency syndrome (AIDS). Secondary infection often occurs in such patients, although this is not essential for the development of villous atrophy. Subtotal villous atrophy occurs in tropical sprue, a condition which is probably caused by an infectious agent. Malabsorption in villous atrophy results from reduced absorptive surface area and also because of deficiencies in small intestinal enzymes.

Inflammatory or Infiltrative Disorders

Crohn's disease is a chronic inflammatory disorder of uncertain aetiology which affects segments of the bowel which are often discontinuous. Malabsorption in Crohn's disease may result from several mechanisms. The terminal ileum is often affected, causing interruption to the enterohepatic circulation of bile salts and impaired vitamin B_{12} absorption. Inflamed areas of bowel may adhere together, with fistula or stricture formation. This can cause blind loops in which bacterial overgrowth occurs – a cause of bile salt deconjugation. Inflammation or resection of the small bowel can lead to reduced absorptive surface area and extensive inflammation often causes protein loss into the gut (protein-losing enteropathy).

Vascular Disease

Intestinal ischaemia and bowel infarction lead to malabsorption in some cases.

Endocrine and Metabolic Disorders

Malabsorption occurs in various endocrine and metabolic disorders, including diabetes mellitus. In some diabetic patients malabsorption is caused by pancreatic exocrine insufficiency or coexistent coeliac disease, while in others it appears to result from autonomic neuropathy. Abetalipoproteinaemia is a rare inherited metabolic disorder in which enterocytes cannot synthesize apolipoprotein B (apoB). Large amounts of dietary triglyceride are trapped in the mucosa because they cannot be secreted into lacteals in the absence of apoB synthesis. The intestinal wall becomes distended with fat and this interferes with absorptive processes.

Maldigestion

In addition to pancreatic disease (see above) maldigestion of food may have other causes.

Stomach

Excessive acid secretion may cause maldigestion by inactivating pancreatic enzymes. Steatorrhoea may complicate partial gastrectomy, particularly if the duodenum is bypassed (Billroth II). Several factors are responsible, including reduced pancreatic enzyme secretion owing to decreased release of secretin and CCK-PZ, inadequate mixing of enzymes and bowel contents, stasis in the afferent loop of the duodenum and reduced intestinal transit time as a result of loss of the reservoir function of the stomach.

Liver and Biliary Tract Disease

Steatorrhoea may result from reduced secretion of bile acids into the intestine and vitamin D deficiency can also occur, leading to osteomalacia (see chapter 9).

Bacterial Overgrowth

Gastric acid secretion, peristalsis and intestinal secretion of immunoglobulins ensure that the small intestine is normally sterile or contains few bacteria. Bacterial overgrowth may occur because one of these processes fails, because bile loops of bowel are formed or as a result of diverticuli being present in the intestinal wall. Bacterial overgrowth can cause bile salt deconjugation, interfering with fat digestion and may also result in vitamin B_{12} deficiency owing to utilization by microorganisms.

Defects in Specific Absorption Mechanisms

Specific absorptive mechanisms may be defective in conditions that can also cause the generalized malabsorption syndrome.

Thus, either bile salt or vitamin B_{12} deficiency sometimes occur in the blind loop syndrome. In addition, deficiencies of specific nutrients may be found. Anaemia, caused by iron deficiency or impaired folate absorption, may result from conditions in which there is disease of the small intestinal mucosa. Deficiencies in minerals such as magnesium and zinc can also occur.

Disaccharidase Deficiency

Disaccharidase deficiency may have genetic causes or may occur secondarily to acquired disease (**Table 10.3**). Sucrase and isomaltase deficiencies coexist while alactasia is often an isolated defect. Infantile disaccharidase deficiency causes severe diarrhoea until the offending sugar is removed from the diet. Diarrhoea occurs because the undigested sugar is fermented in the colon by bacteria, producing many small molecules, including the gases carbon

Table 10.3 Causes of disaccharidase deficiency

Congenital (primary)	Neonatal
	Constitutional (ethnic)
Secondary	Jejunal mucosal defects

dioxide, methane and hydrogen, together with organic acids, which lower the faecal pH (**Figure 10.2**). As many small molecules are produced, intraluminal osmotic activity is increased and water enters the lumen from the extracellular space. Hydrogen is absorbed but not metabolized; it is excreted by the lungs and can be detected in the breath. Hydrogen is not produced during intermediary metabolism and therefore breath levels reflect production by enteric bacteria. Some basal hydrogen excretion occurs owing to breakdown of nondigested dietary carbohydrates (fibre).

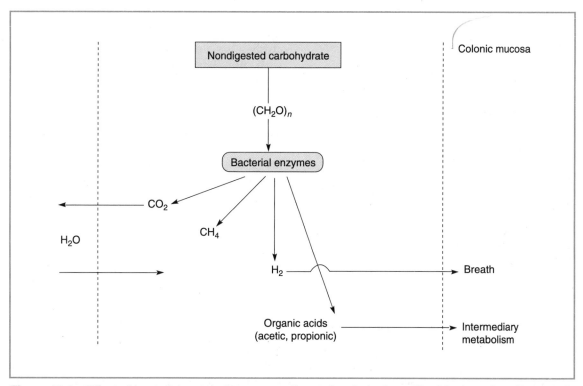

Figure 10.2 Effect of bacterial metabolism on nondigested carbohydrate (fibre) in the colon. Short-chain fatty acids and gases are produced, some of which are absorbed. These include hydrogen, which is not metabolized further but excreted by the lungs: it may be quantified in breath.

Hypo- or alactasia is much more common than other disaccharidase deficiencies, occurring in 90% of the adult population of many ethnic groups. Indeed, it should perhaps be regarded as the norm since Caucasians appear to be the only ethnic group who retain lactase activity in adult life. In constitutional alactasia the enzyme is present in infants but lost after weaning. Most lactase-deficient patients avoid milk and consequently have few symptoms. If lactose is administered bloating, flatulence, abdominal pain and occasionally diarrhoea occur. Disaccharidase deficiency often occurs secondary to small intestinal disease, particularly mucosal defects such as coeliac disease.

Disaccharidase deficiency is diagnosed either by intestinal biopsy and measuring disaccharidase activity directly in biopsy specimens of small intestinal mucosa, or noninvasively by demonstrating increased excretion of breath hydrogen following the ingestion of the relevant sugar. Lactose tolerance tests (measuring blood glucose or galactose concentrations in response to lactose ingestion) are less specific and sensitive than the hydrogen breath test.

KEY POINTS

DISACCHARIDASE DEFICIENCY

- Infantile disaccharidase deficiency is life threatening

- Disaccharidase deficiency in adults is common in all ethnic groups except for Caucasians

- Clinical features include bloating and diarrhoea following ingestion of the relevant sugar

Investigation of the Malabsorption Syndrome

Assessment of Fat Absorption

Fat absorption may be impaired in both small intestinal disease and in maldigestion.

Many techniques have been described for assessment of fat absorption including staining the stools for lipid and measuring the absorption of a fat-soluble substance, e.g. vitamin A. The two most widely used techniques are the direct measurement of fat in stools and a breath test of fat absorption.

Faecal Fat Determination The fat content of faeces is determined by collecting stools for 3–5 days in patients who have been on a normal diet for at least 48 h. Normal subjects excrete less than 18 mmol fat 24 h^{-1}, this being derived largely from the turnover of intestinal cells. There is usually no difficulty with collections if significant steatorrhoea is present since such stools are bulky. However, there is often uncertainty over the period of dietary intake a stool collection represents in normal subjects, or in those with borderline abnormalities, because of variations in bowel habit. The most accurate method of determining fat excretion is a fat balance study in which these factors are controlled. Fat balance studies are undertaken in a metabolic ward with nonabsorbable markers being given orally with each meal (**Table 10.4**). Quantification of these indicates the dietary period represented in the stool collection. The quantitative determination of fat in stools is the most reliable method of determining fat absorption although it is unpleasant, time-consuming and expensive, particularly if fat balance is determined. For these reasons, alternative tests have been developed which can be undertaken in outpatients.

Triolein Breath Test The principle of this investigation is that a test meal is given which contains isotopically labelled triolein, generally [^{14}C]triolein. Normal subjects digest, absorb and metabolize the fat, $^{14}CO_2$ being produced which can be measured in the breath. Excretion of $^{14}CO_2$ is reduced in malabsorption and also in obese subjects who store the fat in adipose tissue.

Table 10.4 Tests measuring stool fat content

Faecal fat	Fat balance
Normal dietary intake for 48 h	Admission to a metabolic ward for a controlled diet; nonabsorbable markers (e.g. chromium oxide pellets) given with meals during the test
Measurement of stool fat	Stool collection for 3–5 days; measurement of stool fat + quantification of nonabsorbable markers

However, this false-negative result does not cause diagnostic confusion.

Several variations of the fat breath test have been described. Because the label is radioactive, the investigation is not suitable for pregnant women or children. Using the stable isotope [^{13}C]triolein overcomes this difficulty although very expensive equipment (mass spectrometer) is required to quantify $^{13}CO_2$ and therefore the investigation is restricted to specialist centres. Various modifications have also been described which attempt to differentiate between fat malabsorption due to pancreatic and intestinal disease. These involve the simultaneous administration of triglyceride and nonesterified fatty acids labelled in different ways. Fatty acids should be absorbed normally in pancreatic disease as only lipase is deficient, while impaired absorption of both fatty acids and triglycerides occurs in intestinal disease because of the mucosal defect. However, such tests are not sensitive enough to discriminate between the different causes of fat malabsorption.

D-Xylose Absorption

In theory, intestinal absorptive capacity could be investigated by estimating nutrient assimilation, e.g. by measuring glucose tolerance. However, glucose is absorbed by a transport mechanism which has a high affinity for its substrates and considerable functional reserve. Impaired glucose absorption will thus only occur in profound malabsorption. In addition, glucose is subject to postabsorptive metabolism, a confounding factor if blood levels are being measured to assess intestinal absorption. D-Xylose absorption is more satisfactory for investigating intestinal absorptive capacity as it is transported passively and is metabolized only to a limited extent. Early tests used 25 g but false-positive results occurred in healthy subjects as a result of unabsorbed xylose causing intestinal hurry, thus reducing absorption. Improved results are obtained if 5 g of D-xylose is used, this being near the limit of the amount that normal adults can absorb. Reduced D-xylose absorption occurs if the absorptive surface area is decreased, e.g. in coeliac disease. Measuring blood levels is more sensitive than assessing urinary excretion, as they are affected less by variations in renal clearance. False-negative results are caused by bacterial overgrowth or an increased extracellular fluid volume, e.g. due to ascites, which increases the space in which xylose is distributed in the body.

Breath Tests

In addition to being used to investigate fat absorption and disaccharidase deficiency

---

KEY POINTS

STEATORRHOEA

- Stool fat excretion is normally <18 mmol day^{-1}

- Steatorrhoea may result from conditions affecting the small intestinal mucosa, the pancreas, the liver, and the biliary tract

- Stool fat excretion is assessed accurately by fat balance studies and conveniently by the fatty acid breath test

breath tests are used to assess intestinal transit time and bacterial overgrowth.

Transit Time Transit time can be measured using a hydrogen breath test in which lactulose, a disaccharide which is not hydrolysed by small intestinal enzymes, is given orally. Lactulose is broken down by colonic bacteria, producing hydrogen. The time between ingestion of lactulose and the increase of breath hydrogen is the mouth-to-caecum transit time.

Bacterial Overgrowth Bacterial overgrowth in the small intestine may result in early breakdown of carbohydrate in the hydrogen breath test (**Figure 10.3**). An alternative investigation is the [^{14}C]glycocholate breath test in which a bile salt (the glycine conjugate of cholic acid) is given orally, a radioactive label being incorporated in the glycine moiety. Normally, bile salts are reabsorbed in the terminal ileum and therefore little breakdown of the conjugate occurs in the bowel. In the presence of bacterial overgrowth, deconjugation leads to release of glycine which is absorbed and metabolized to $^{14}CO_2$. Positive results also occur if the terminal ileum is diseased. If glycocholate is not absorbed by the terminal ileum, bacterial breakdown of the conjugate occurs in the colon.

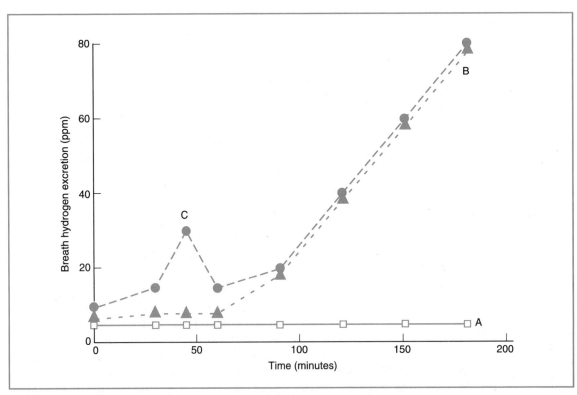

Figure 10.3 Principles of the hydrogen breath test. Under basal conditions (curve A) there is a low level of hydrogen excretion, which results from the colonic breakdown of dietary fibre. Breath hydrogen excretion increases approximately 90 min following the administration of lactulose, a sugar which is not hydrolysed by small intestinal enzymes: this is the mouth-to-caecum transit time. A similar increase in breath hydrogen excretion occurs in hypolactasic subjects following the ingestion of lactose. Early excretion of hydrogen is seen in curve C, resulting from the breakdown of lactulose by bacterial overgrowth in a diverticulum (ppm=parts per million).

Differentiation of Pancreatic and Intestinal Malabsorption

The differential diagnosis of intestinal and pancreatic causes of the malabsorption syndrome depends on clinical findings and investigations which include endoscopy, biopsy and radiology. Biochemical investigations are of value in detecting specific deficiencies and for monitoring the response to treatment. They are not sufficiently specific to replace other more invasive investigative procedures, although they may be helpful in suggesting the cause of malabsorption.

THE LARGE INTESTINE

The contribution of the normal large intestine to digestion and absorption is minimal, although water, electrolytes and short-chain fatty acids (produced from nondigested carbohydrates by bacteria) are absorbed by the colon.

FURTHER READING

Laker MF, Bartlett K. Tubeless tests of small intestinal function. *Recent Advances in Clinical Biochemistry* 1985; **3**: 195–219

Lawson N, Chesner I. Tests of exocrine pancreatic function. *Annals of Clinical Biochemistry* 1994; **31**: 305–14

Misiewicz JJ, Pounder RE, Venables CW (eds). *Diseases of the Gut and Pancreas* (2nd edn). Oxford: Blackwell, 1994

Sleisenger MH (1983). Malabsorption and nutritional support. *Clinics in Gastroenterology* 1983; **12**: 323–610

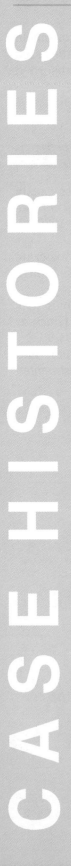

CASE 10.1

A 39-year-old woman was investigated for tiredness and weight loss over the course of the last year. On direct questioning she indicated that she had suffered from diarrhoea for approximately 18 months. On examination she was extremely thin, weighing 49.9 kg (height 1.61 m) and appeared anaemic. The following results were obtained:

albumin	32 g l^{-1}
total calcium	1.81 mmol l^{-1}
phosphate	1.30 mmol l^{-1}
alkaline phosphatase	180 u l^{-1}
haemoglobin	8.7 g dl^{-1}
blood film	macrocytosis

What could be going on here? What is this woman's body mass index (BMI)?

CASE 10.2

A 45-year-old man with chylomicronaemia syndrome was seen in outpatients complaining of diarrhoea of recent onset. He had previously had seven attacks of acute pancreatitis. The results of a [^{14}C]triolein breath test showed that excretion of the radioactive label was only 20% of the lower limit of normal. Explain this result.

THE LIVER AND BILIARY TRACT

INTRODUCTION

The liver plays a key role in the intermediary metabolism of carbohydrates and fats. It is also the major organ of detoxification and excretion of lipid-soluble substances, including the major metabolite of haem metabolism, bilirubin. Other roles include the synthesis of plasma proteins which have a variety of functions, including transport of other molecules and the maintenance of plasma oncotic pressure (see chapter 3). Bile acids, necessary for fat digestion and absorption, are also synthesized and excreted by the liver.

STRUCTURE OF THE LIVER

The liver contains two major cell types, hepatocytes or parenchymal cells which comprise about 60% of the liver, and Kupffer cells which form part of the reticuloendothelial network and comprise approximately 30% of the liver mass. The liver contains functional units, which consist of cords of hepatocytes radiating between portal tracts and small branches of the hepatic vein. These functional units are termed acini if the centre is considered to be the portal tracts or lobules if the centre is the hepatic vein (**Figure 11.1**). The portal

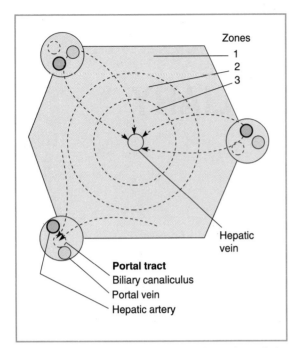

Figure 11.1 Diagrammatic representation of the structure of an hepatic lobule. Blood drains from the portal tracts to the hepatic veins and bile flows in the opposite direction. There are different biochemical functions in the zones of the lobule (see text).

tracts contain portal vein, hepatic artery and bile canaliculus. Because of pressure differences, blood flows from the portal veins and hepatic arteries through sinusoids towards the hepatic veins. Blood in the sinusoids is separated from hepatocytes by Küpffer cells and the space of Disse (**Figure 11.2**). The bile canaliculi are grooves in hepatocytes lined by microvilli into which bile is secreted. These drain in the opposite direction to blood flow, into bile ducts (**Figure 11.1**).

Lobules are divided into three zones, zone 1 being nearest to the portal tract, while zone 3 is nearest to the hepatic vein and zone 2 has an intermediate position. The blood supplying zone 1 has the highest and zone 3 the least oxygen and nutrient contents. Zone 1 is more active in gluconeogenesis and has a greater content of alkaline phosphatase and transaminases than other areas. Zone 3 has the highest concentrations of drug-metabolizing enzymes; it is the area most susceptible to viral, toxic and anoxic liver damage.

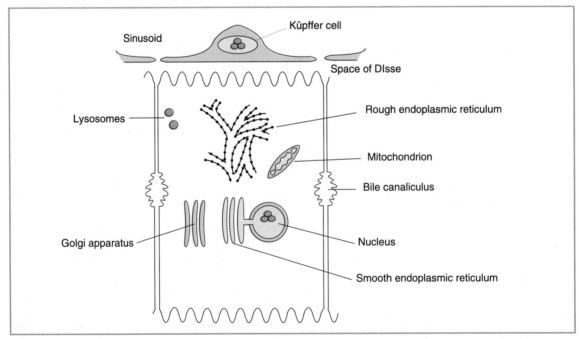

Figure 11.2 Structure and cellular relationships of the hepatocyte. Bile flows in canaliculi, grooves between hepatocytes. Blood flows at right angles to these in the sinusoids

NORMAL HEPATIC FUNCTION

Functions of the liver and methods for assessing these are outlined in **Table 11.1**.

Carbohydrate Metabolism

Hepatic glucose output maintains blood sugar levels between meals, the principal sources of glucose being hepatic glycogen (glycogenolysis) and gluconeogenesis (from lactate, alanine and glycerol). The liver also converts galactose and fructose to glucose (see chapter 1).

Amino Acid and Protein Metabolism

Amino acids derived from the diet and the breakdown of tissue proteins are transported to the liver. Some are transaminated or deaminated to keto-acids, while others are metabolized to urea and ammonia. The liver also synthesizes most proteins found in plasma, the exception being immunoglobulins which are produced by lymphoid tissue. Proteins measured in the investigation of disease are listed in **Table 11.2** (see also chapter 3).

Lipid Metabolism

The liver plays an active role in lipid metabolism (see chapter 2). It removes chylomicron remnants from the circulation and synthesizes very-low-density lipoproteins (VLDL). Intermediate-density lipoprotein (IDL) is converted to low-density

Table 11.1 Functions of the liver and methods of assessment

Function	Assessment
Carbohydrate metabolism	
Gluconeogenesis	Blood glucose level, hepatic glucose production
Lactate utilization	Blood lactate level
Galactose metabolism	Galactose elimination capacity
Protein and amino acid metabolism	
Plasma protein synthesis	Plasma protein concentrations
Urea	Serum urea level
Ammonia metabolism	Blood ammonia level
Lipid metabolism	
Lipoprotein metabolism	Serum lipid and lipoprotein levels
Vitamin D hydroxylation	25-Hydroxycholecalciferol levels
Bile acid synthesis	Serum bile acid levels, tests for fat malabsorption
Detoxification and excretion	
Bilirubin metabolism	Serum bilirubin levels, urinary bilirubin and urobilinogen
Excretion of foreign compounds	Bromosulphthalein excretion indocyanine green excretion, aminopyrine excretion,
Hormone metabolism	Measurement of hormones, assessment of electrolyte balance

Table 11.2 Plasma proteins synthesized by the liver

Protein	Clinical utility
Albumin	Decreased in chronic liver disease
α_1-Antitrypsin	Decreased in α_1-antitrypsin deficiency
Caeruloplasmin	Decreased in Wilson's disease
Coagulation factors	Decreased in chronic liver disease
α-Fetoprotein	Increased in hepato-cellular carcinoma
Haptoglobins	Decreased in haemolysis
Transferrin	Saturated with iron in haemochromatosis

lipoprotein (LDL) by hepatic lipase and there is a high density of LDL receptors on hepatocytes. Precursor particles of HDL are synthesized in the liver, as is lecithin:cholesterol acyl transferase (LCAT), the enzyme which converts precursor to functional HDL particles. Further hepatic roles in lipid metabolism include the production of ketone bodies from nonesterified fatty acids (NEFA), cholesterol excretion into bile and hydroxylation of vitamin D to form 25-hydroxycholecalciferol (see chapter 8).

Bile Acid Metabolism

The primary bile acids are cholic acid and chenodeoxycholic acid which are synthesized only in the liver, from cholesterol. They are secreted in bile and most are reabsorbed through enterohepatic circulation, hepatic synthesis of bile acids being regulated by the amount returning to the liver. Gut bacteria dehydroxylate the primary bile acids producing the secondary acids, deoxycholic and lithocholic acids (**Figure 11.3**). Deoxycholic acid is reabsorbed and enters the enterohepatic circulation, while most lithocholic acid is excreted in the stools.

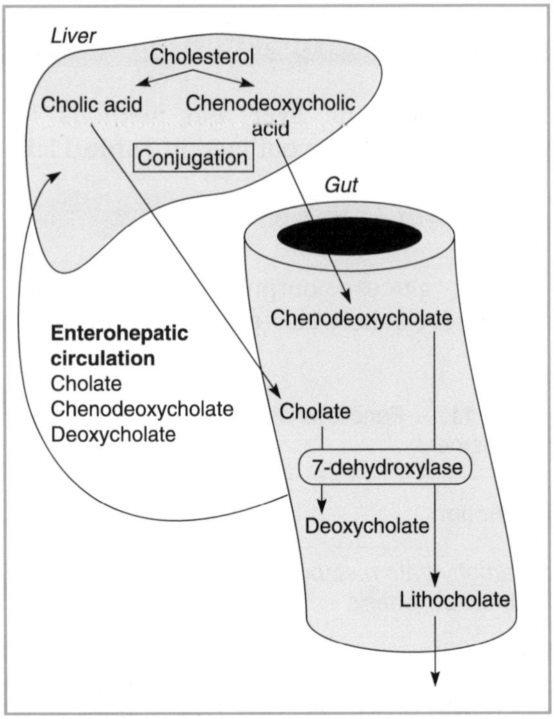

Figure 11.3 Metabolism of bile acids. The primary bile acids cholic acid and chenodeoxycholic acid are synthesized in the liver and excreted into the gut following conjugation with glycine or taurine. Dehydroxylation of some of these occurs in the gut by the action of bacterial enzymes, secondary bile acids being formed. The primary bile acids and deoxycholic acid are largely reabsorbed, undergoing an enterohepatic circulation, while lithocholic acid is mostly excreted in stools.

Conjugation and Detoxification

Bilirubin conjugation and excretion is considered in detail below. Other substances metabolized and excreted by the liver include steroid hormones and drugs.

ASSESSMENT OF HEPATIC FUNCTION

It is possible to investigate many of the functions of the liver in detail (**Table 11.1**). Thus, hepatic carbohydrate metabolism can

be assessed by measuring blood galactose removal following injection, and glucose output can be quantified by using isotope dilution techniques. However, such procedures are complex and time-consuming, involving infusions and repeated blood sampling. For this reason, many of these investigations of hepatic function are carried out only in specialized liver or metabolic units. The assessment of liver function in daily clinical practice is usually performed by measuring serum levels of bilirubin, hepatic enzymes and proteins, with other tests being done occasionally.

Bilirubin Metabolism

Synthesis

Bilirubin is an end-product of haem metabolism and may thus originate from haemoglobin, myoglobin and haem-containing enzymes. Approximately 250–300 mg are produced each day in the reticuloendothelial system, 80% arising from the breakdown of effete erythrocytes. The remaining 20% is produced from myoglobin, enzymes, particularly respiratory chain cytochromes, and the breakdown of erythrocyte precursor cells in the bone marrow.

Unconjugated Bilirubin

Bilirubin is lipophilic and must be conjugated by hepatic enzymes before it can be excreted. Unconjugated bilirubin is transported in plasma bound to protein, mainly albumin. Under normal circumstances this binding is tight although hydrogen ions, fatty acids and some drugs (e.g. salicylates and sulphonamides) may compete for the same binding sites. Owing to its solubility characteristics, unconjugated bilirubin is not filtered by the glomerulus and therefore does not appear in urine.

Conjugated Bilirubin

Protein binding of bilirubin in plasma prevents it being taken up readily by tissues, although it is extracted by the liver, possibly after binding to a hepatic receptor. The intracellular protein ligandin shuttles bilirubin to the rough endoplasmic reticulum where most is conjugated with glucuronic acid by uridyl diphosphate (UDP) glucuronyl transferase, forming bilirubin diglucuronide. Excretion of conjugated bilirubin into the biliary canaliculi is thought to be an energy-dependent process.

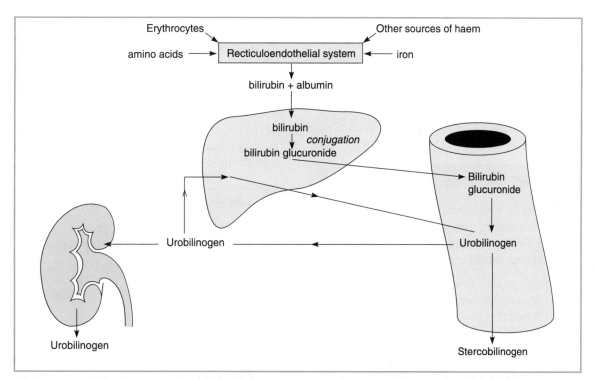

Figure 11.4   Bilirubin metabolism. Bilirubin is a product of haem metabolism which is insoluble in water. It is conjugated prior to excretion in the liver and undergoes metabolism by bacterial enzymes in the gut to form urobilinogen. Some of this is reabsorbed, undergoing an enterohepatic circulation, a small amount being excreted by the kidney.

Enteric Metabolism of Bilirubin

Conjugated bilirubin is polar and thus it is not absorbed in the small intestine. In the colon it is deconjugated by bacteria and converted to a group of colourless products, urobilinogens, which are oxidized readily to coloured uro- (or sterco-) bilins, these being responsible for the characteristic pigmentation of stools. Most urobilinogen is excreted in the stools although small amounts are absorbed across the colonic mucosa. Absorbed urobilinogen undergoes enterohepatic circulation, as most is taken up by the liver and re-excreted in the bile; it is water-soluble, and so some urobilinogen is also filtered by the glomeruli and excreted in urine (**Figure 11.4**).

KEY POINTS

BILIRUBIN

- Bilirubin is formed by the breakdown of haem in the reticuloendothelial system

- Bilirubin is transported bound to albumin in blood for conjugation and excretion by the liver

- Unconjugated bilirubin is insoluble and conjugated bilirubin is soluble in water

---

Jaundice

Bilirubin is a yellow pigment which causes discoloration of the skin and sclerae when serum levels exceed 35–40 μmol l^{-1}. Concentrations may increase for three reasons:

(i) the production rate bilirubin is increased, exceeding the excretory capacity of the liver (prehepatic jaundice);

(ii) conjugating and/or excretory functions are reduced, and the capacity of the liver to metabolize bilirubin produced at normal rates is exceeded (hepatic or hepatocellular jaundice);

(iii) biliary obstruction interferes with the flow of bile and thus bilirubin excretion

(posthepatic, obstructive or cholestatic jaundice).

Pathogenesis of Jaundice

The causes of jaundice are outlined in **Table 11.3**.

Prehepatic Jaundice Prehepatic jaundice is caused most often by increased destruction of erythrocytes – either mature cells or precursors (ineffective erythropoiesis). The breakdown of mature cells can be caused by haemolysis, or as a result of the metabolism of blood following internal haemorrhage, e.g. into a soft tissue injury or fracture. Ineffective erythropoiesis occurs in conditions such as pernicious anaemia, where the maturation of red cells is impaired, or thalassaemia, where the structure of haemoglobin is abnormal.

Hyperbilirubinaemia in prehepatic jaundice results from the accumulation of unconjugated bilirubin; this is not excreted by the kidney. Jaundice occurs because the conjugating capacity of the liver is saturated, although the capacity of the liver for conjugation is greater than the normal rate of bilirubin production. This is not impaired in prehepatic jaundice and increased fluxes of bilirubin through the liver into the gut therefore occur. Greater amounts of urobilinogen are produced, with increased urobilinogen excretion in urine.

KEY POINTS

PREHEPATIC JAUNDICE

- Prehepatic jaundice is most commonly caused by haemolytic disease

- Bilirubin is not excreted in urine

- Urinary urobilinogen concentration is increased

Hepatic Jaundice Congenital disorders of bilirubin transport lead to jaundice because of defective uptake, reduced conjugation or impaired excretion of bilirubin. Generalized hepatocellular dysfunction may occur in

Table 11.3   Causes of jaundice

Type	Mechanism	Cause
Prehepatic	Ineffective erythropoiesis	Pernicious anaemia
		Thalassaemia
	Increased erythrocyte breakdown	Haemolysis
		Internal haemorrhage
Hepatic	Immature conjugating enzymes	Neonatal jaundice
	Inherited bilirubin transport defects	Gilbert's disease
		Crigler–Najjar syndrome
		Rotor syndrome
		Dubin–Johnson syndrome
	Generalized hepatocyte dysfunction	Hepatitis
		Portal cirrhosis
	Drug-induced	Paracetamol
		Isoniazid
Cholestatic	Intrahepatic	Hepatitis
		Biliary cirrhosis
		Anabolic steroids
		Phenothiazines
		Hepatic malignancy
	Extrahepatic	Gallstones
		Bile duct tumour
		Bile duct compression
		Carcinoma head of pancreas

hepatitis and decompensated hepatic cirrhosis. The pathogenesis of jaundice in these conditions is complex, reduced hepatic uptake, decreased conjugation and impaired intracellular transport of bilirubin all contributing. Drugs may cause hepatocellular damage, either due to dose-dependent hepatoxicity (e.g. paracetamol), or to idiosyncratic sensitivity (e.g. isoniazid).

When hyperbilirubinaemia is caused by impaired conjugation bilirubin is unconjugated and there are no increased fluxes of bilirubin through the liver. Therefore, bilirubinuria does not occur and urinary urobilinogen is not increased. If generalized hepatocyte dysfunction is present, uptake of urobilinogen by the liver is reduced and therefore more is excreted through the kidney. Serum bilirubin may be unconjugated or conjugated, as UDP glucuronyl transferase and intracellular transport may be defective. If the rate of conjugation exceeds excretory capacity, conjugated hyperbilirubinaemia will occur and bilirubin may be excreted in urine. This is sometimes seen in recovery from acute viral hepatitis.

Cholestatic Jaundice Cholestatic jaundice results from interference to biliary flow between the sites of secretion by the hepatocyte and drainage into the duodenum. It may therefore be caused by lesions within the liver (intrahepatic cholestasis), or in the biliary tree or head of the pancreas (extrahepatic cholestasis); therefore the term cholestatic is preferable to posthepatic to describe this pattern of jaundice. Intra- and extra-hepatic cholestasis can be differentiated by ultrasound examination or liver biopsy, but not by liver function tests.

Intrahepatic cholestasis may result from generalized hepatocellular dysfunction, such as occurs in hepatitis and decompensated hepatic cirrhosis, and is also a feature of primary biliary cirrhosis. Hepatic malignancies may block branches of the biliary tree. Some drugs, such as anabolic steroids, phenothiazines and sulphonylureas, may cause intrahepatic cholestasis.

Extrahepatic obstruction may be due to tumours in major branches of the biliary tract, head of pancreas or in lymph nodes in the porta hepatis. Gallstones or sclerosing cholangitis may obstruct biliary flow.

Jaundice is due to impaired excretion and accumulation of conjugated bilirubin which can be filtered by the kidney and appear in urine. However, urinary bilirubin may not detected in advanced disease, possibly because changes in bilirubin conjugation occur which produce a less water-soluble conjugate which is bound to albumin. If obstruction is complete bilirubin does not reach the gut; therefore, urobilinogen is not produced and is absent from the urine. Under such circumstances the stools are pale. However, obstruction may be intermittent and therefore urobilinogen may be found in the urine and the stools may be pigmented.

KEY POINTS

CHOLESTATIC JAUNDICE

■ Cholestasis may be caused by lesions within or outside the liver

■ Jaundice is due to conjugated bilirubin

■ Bilirubin is found in urine

Serum Enzymes in Liver Disease

Small amounts of enzymes leak from their intracellular location into serum and cellular dysfunction often causes increased leakage. The measurement of enzymes in serum may therefore be useful in the investigation of organ dysfunction (see chapter 12). Many enzymes in serum originate from the liver and measuring the activities of a small number of these which have different locations helps to differentiate patterns of disease (**Table 11.4**).

Aminotransferases

Aminotransferases are involved in amino acid metabolism. Aspartate aminotransferase (AST) occurs in both the cytosol and mitochondria of cells while alanine aminotransferase (ALT) is a cytosolic enzyme. Increased amounts of both transaminases leak from inflamed or damaged hepatocytes and measurement of one of these enzymes is included in liver function tests. Alanine aminotransferase is more specific for liver disease than AST, while the latter is more sensitive because the liver contains larger amounts.

Lactate Dehydrogenase

Lactate dehydrogenase (LDH) is often raised in hepatocellular dysfunction although it is rarely measured for this purpose since it lacks specificity owing to the wide distribution of LDH in the body.

Table 11.4   Serum enzymes in liver disease

Abnormal mainly in hepatocellular disease
◆ Alanine aminotransferase (transaminase) (ALT)
◆ Aspartate aminotransferase (transaminase) (AST)
◆ Lactate dehydrogenase (LDH)

Abnormal mainly in cholestasis
◆ Alkaline phosphatase (ALP)
◆ γ-Glutamyl transferase (transpeptidase) (GGT)

Alkaline Phosphatase

Levels of alkaline phosphatase increase in cholestasis, mainly because of increased synthesis of the enzyme. An increased activity of serum alkaline phosphatase is sometimes the only abnormal finding when liver function tests are estimated. It may then be important to establish if the enzyme is of hepatic origin or from another organ, such as bone, by estimating alkaline phosphatase isoenzymes or the activity of another biliary enzyme, usually γ-glutamyl tranferase (GGT) (see chapter 12).

γ-Glutamyl Transferase

Increased serum activities of GGT are found in both hepatocellular and cholestatic disease. Higher activities are found in cholestasis, when levels greater than 50 times the upper limit of normal are not uncommon. Increased synthesis of GGT is induced by excessive ethanol intake.

KEY POINTS

HEPATIC ENZYMES

- Transaminase (ALT and AST) levels are raised mainly in hepatocellular disease

- Alkaline phosphatase level is raised mainly in obstructive disease

- Increases in serum GGT levels are modest in hepatocellular disease and marked in obstructive disease

---

Plasma Proteins in Liver Disease

Albumin has a half-life in serum of about 20 days and levels fall slowly if no synthesis occurs. Thus, serum albumin is usually normal in fulminant hepatic failure. However, in chronic liver diseases such as cirrhosis, impaired synthesis may lead to low serum levels. Serum globulins are often increased in cirrhosis, although electrophoresis of serum proteins is of limited value in

liver disease, because patterns of abnormalities lack specificity.

Serum protein levels are sometimes of value when investigating specific diseases. α_1-Antitrypsin (α_1-antiprotease) deficiency causes neonatal jaundice and cirrhosis in children and young adults. α-Fetoprotein is produced by the fetus but disappears from the circulation a few weeks after birth. Modest levels are found when hepatic regeneration occurs, e.g. during acute viral hepatitis, while very high values occur in hepatocellular carcinoma. Caeruloplasmin is low in most cases of Wilson's disease.

LIVER DISEASES

Different patterns of liver function test results (**Table 11.5**) are suggestive of groups of causes of different types of jaundice. Such classification is useful although only a general guide, as considerable overlap in test results occurs. Findings may not fit characteristic patterns, as hepatocellular disease often has cholestatic elements and hepatocellular failure occurs in advanced cholestasis.

Neonatal Jaundice

Neonatal jaundice is considered in chapter 18.

Congenital Defects in Bilirubin Transport

Gilbert's Disease (Syndrome)

Gilbert's disease is a common congenital disorder of bilirubin transport affecting approximately 2% of the population – males more than females. The pathogenesis of the condition is complex. The activity of UDP-glucuronyl transferase is reduced and defects in the uptake of bilirubin by hepatocytes also occur. Gilbert's disease characteristically causes mild, fluctuating

Table 11.5 Liver function tests in the differential diagnosis of jaundice

Test	Prehepatic	Hepatic	Cholestatic
Serum bilirubin	Unconjugated	Mixed	Conjugated
Urine bilirubin	Absent	Present	Present
Urine urobilinogen	Increased	Increased	Decreased
Alanine or aspartate aminotransferase (ALT, AST)	Normal	Marked increase	Slight increase
Alkaline phosphatase (ALP)	Normal	Slight increase	Marked increase

jaundice, serum bilirubin concentrations usually being 20–85 μmol l^{-1}. Haemolysis is absent, other liver function tests are normal and there are no histological changes in the liver. Gilbert's disease is a benign condition and life expectancy is normal. It often presents in young adults and must be differentiated from other conditions affecting this age group which can cause isolated unconjugated hyperbilirubinaemia, such as haemolysis or hepatitis. In Gilbert's disease, bilirubin concentrations increase with a 400 kcal diet and fall following phenobarbitone administration.

Other Congenital Transport Syndromes

Congenital transport disorders of bilirubin metabolism other than Gilbert's disease are rare. A severe congenital deficiency in UDP-glucuronyl transferase occurs in Crigler–Najjar syndrome, most patients dying in infancy from kernicterus. Transport of conjugated bilirubin from the hepatocyte is abnormal in the Rotor and Dubin–Johnson syndromes. These are chronic benign conditions in which conjugated hyperbilirubinaemia occurs. A blackish-brown pigment is found in the liver in the Dubin–Johnson but not in the Rotor syndrome.

Acute Viral Hepatitis

Hepatitis occurs as a complication of many viral infections although the term viral hepatitis usually refers to three types of infection (A, B and C). Hepatitis A is transmitted by the oro-faecal route while hepatitis B and C are transmitted by blood products or other body fluids. Attacks vary in severity and may be asymptomatic with only a transient rise in transaminases. The basic pathology of these infections is similar, and acute inflammation and hepatic necrosis occurs. Symptoms are often non-specific at presentation, including malaise, anorexia and nausea. Patients are anicteric at this stage although serum transaminases may be elevated significantly, sometimes exceeding 20 times the upper limit of normal. Serum transaminase activities usually peak before the onset of jaundice which occurs typically 3–4 days following the onset of symptoms, the urine often becoming dark and the faeces pale. Impaired excretion of bilirubin from hepatocytes is often the major cause of hyperbilirubinaemia which is therefore mainly conjugated. Urinary urobilinogen increases before the onset of jaundice owing to impaired hepatic uptake. Bilirubinuria is common. Modest increases in alkaline phosphatase may be seen but these are rarely greater than three times the upper limit of normal. In uncomplicated cases jaundice resolves after a few weeks.

Chronic Hepatitis

Chronic persistent hepatitis may follow acute viral hepatitis or be found by chance. Jaundice is unusual, transaminase activities often being the only abnormal biochemical finding, with levels rarely exceeding five times the upper limit of normal. Although these abnormalities may persist the clinical course is usually benign, cirrhosis being a rare complication. Chronic active hepatitis may result from persisting hepatitis B infection, other viral infections, autoimmune lupoid hepatitis, drug reactions or, unusually α_1-antitrypsin deficiency or alcohol abuse. Jaundice with very high serum transaminase activities is common; immunoglobulin levels are often high. Serum albumin concentrations may fall as the disease progresses.

Hepatic Cirrhosis

Cirrhosis is a diffuse process in which fibrosis and nodule formation follows hepatocellular necrosis. There are many causes (**Table 11.6**) cryptogenic cirrhosis being diagnosed when other causes have been excluded. The normal architecture of the liver is disrupted in cirrhosis, with changes in the blood supply resulting in portal hypertension and shunting of blood from the portal vein directly into the hepatic vein. However, biochemical function is often relatively normal. Slight increases in transa-

minases, particularly AST and GGT, are the commonest abnormalities, presumably reflecting continuing cell destruction, mild cholestasis, or enzyme induction. If progression occurs, hepatic function can become decompensated with a hepatocellular pattern of abnormalities. Jaundice is accompanied by increased urobilinogen and bilirubin excretion in urine. The synthesis of albumin may be impaired, with hypoalbuminaemia developing. Increases in serum immunoglobulins may occur, due to antigens that have been absorbed from the gut bypassing the filtering mechanisms in the hepatic sinusoids. Patients with cirrhosis are at increased risk of developing hepatocellular carcinoma, this sometimes being indicated by high α-fetoprotein concentrations in serum.

Hepatocellular and Acute (Fulminant) Hepatic Failure

Hepatocellular failure may result from almost all causes of liver disease including viral hepatitis, decompensated cirrhosis, drug overdoses, e.g. paracetamol, and prolonged cholestasis. Jaundice is often progressive and transaminases are usually raised, although they may fall terminally. Changes in nitrogen metabolism occur, including reduced urea synthesis and impaired deamination of amino acids, leading to increased concentrations of aromatic amino acids: tyrosine, phenylalanine, and methionine in plasma, with overflow aminoaciduria. The concentration of branched-chain amino acids, valine, leucine and isoleucine is reduced. The conversion of ammonia to urea is often impaired and blood levels of ammonia may rise. These correlate with the degree of hepatic encephalopathy, although ammonia is probably not the cause. Hypoglycaemia may occur owing to impaired gluconeogenesis. Endocrine changes may be found, at least in part due to reduced metabolism of hormones.

Table 11.6   Causes of hepatic cirrhosis

Chronic alcohol abuse
Viral hepatitis
Inherited metabolic disorders
◆ Haemochromatosis
◆ Wilson's disease
◆ Galactosaemia
◆ α_1-Antitrypsin deficiency
◆ Tyrosinaemia
◆ Type IV glycogen storage disease
Prolonged cholestasis
Hepatic venous outflow obstruction
◆ Heart failure
◆ Budd–Chiari syndrome
Lupoid hepatitis
Toxins, drugs
Cryptogenic cirrhosis

Table 11.7 Toxins and drugs causing liver damage

Hepatic changes	Type of injury	Drug
Hepatocellular damage	Dose-related	Carbon tetrachloride
		Alcohol
		Paracetamol
		Methotrexate
	Idiosyncratic	Halothane
		Antituberculous drugs
		Tricyclic antidepressants
		Valproate
Cirrhosis	Dose-related	Alcohol
		Methotrexate
Intrahepatic cholestasis	Dose-related	Anabolic steroids
		Azathioprine
	Idiosyncratic	Carbimazole
		Phenothiazines
		Sulphonylureas
Gallstones		Fibric acid analogues
		Oestrogens

Abnormalities in oestrogen and androgen metabolism occur and a degree of feminization is common in male patients. Testicular atrophy is common, with reduced testosterone levels, particularly in alcoholic patients. Plasma oestrogens are increased although not enough to explain feminization. Hyponatraemia is common, particularly in patients with ascites; water retention is probably the most important factor causing this.

Fulminant hepatic failure is caused by sudden massive necrosis or severe impairment of liver function. The most common causes are viral hepatitis or a drug reaction. Plasma albumin concentrations are initially normal and falling concentrations are associated with a poor prognosis, as are serum bilirubin levels greater than 400 μmol l^{-1}. Increasing serum α-fetoprotein levels may reflect hepatic regeneration.

Hepatic Malignancy

The liver is a common site for secondary carcinoma, multiple deposits often occurring. Increases in serum alkaline phosphatase and GGT due to tumours causing cholestasis in parts of the liver are common abnormalities of liver function tests.

Toxic Liver Damage

Liver injury may follow exposure to a number of pharmacological or chemical agents. With some, toxic effects are predictable and dose-related, while idiosyncratic reactions are responsible for others (**Table 11.7**). Idiosyncratic reactions may be caused by immunologically-mediated reactions or due to drug metabolites.

GALLSTONES

Most gallstones, unlike renal stones, do not contain calcium and are radiotranslucent. The main constituent of gallstones in Western countries is cholesterol. Several factors are thought to favour cholesterol gallstone formation, including supersaturation of the bile with cholesterol, and decreased biliary content of bile acids. The cholesterol content of bile increases with age. Oestrogens and treatment with fibric acid analogues reduce bile acid secretion, resulting in more lithogenic bile. In addition to the oestrogen effect the higher incidence of cholelithiasis in women, particularly multiparous women, may be explained by incomplete gall bladder emptying which occurs in late pregnancy, favouring cholesterol nucleation.

Gallstones, which contain little cholesterol, are composed largely of bilirubin and its calcium salts. They are usually small multiple-faceted stones which accompany chronic haemolysis and are often found in cirrhosis.

INVESTIGATION OF LIVER DISEASE

Biochemical liver function tests are an essential part of assessment of liver disease. However, most liver function tests are relatively insensitive as the liver has considerable functional reserve and tests must be interpreted with knowledge of the clinical details of the patient and the results of other investigations. These often include ultrasound examination, radiological procedures, clotting studies and liver biopsy. Biochemical liver function tests are undertaken to detect and follow the progress of liver disease, to check for effects such as drug toxicity and to establish patterns of liver disease.

FURTHER READING

Johnson PJ. Role of the standard 'liver function tests' in current clinical practice. *Annals of Clinical Biochemistry* 1989; **26**: 463–71

Laker MF. Liver function tests. *British Medical Journal* 1990; **301**: 250–1

Rustgi VK. Hepatic disease. *Medical Clinics of North America* 1989; **73**: 753–1053

Sherlock S, Dooley J. *Diseases of the Liver and Biliary System* (9th edn). Oxford: Blackwell, 1993

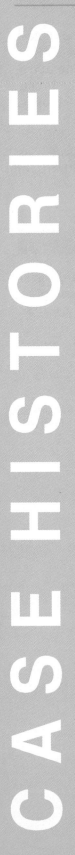

CASE 11:1

A 24-year-old-man who was otherwise well was thought to be mildly jaundiced and liver function tests were carried out:

bilirubin	39 μmol l^{-1}
ALT	35 U l^{-1}
alkaline phosphatase	85 U l^{-1}

What diagnoses must be considered?

CASE 11.2

The following liver function tests were obtained from a 72-year-old woman who was found to be jaundiced at a routine outpatient appointment 2 years after undergoing colectomy for a carcinoma of the colon.

bilirubin	75 μmol l^{-1}
ALT	40 U l^{-1}
alkaline phosphatase	950 U l^{-1}

What pattern of liver function abnormality is present and what is the most likely cause?

CASE 11.3

A 54-year-old man was seen in a lipid clinic because he had hypercholesterolaemia (total cholesterol 7.4 mmol l^{-1}) and two other risk factors for coronary heart disease were also present (poor family history and hypertension). He admitted to consuming 21 units of alcohol per week and the following liver function test results were received.

bilirubin	14 μmol l^{-1}
ALT	65 U l^{-1}
alkaline phosphatase	75 U l^{-1}

In view of the borderline abnormality in the ALT activity can further laboratory tests help to establish whether he is abusing alcohol?

ENZYMES IN BODY FLUIDS

INTRODUCTION

Enzymes are protein catalysts which are found in small amounts, mainly within cells although some, such as clotting factors and digestive enzymes, function naturally after secretion. However, most enzymes with diagnostic applications function within the cells in which they are synthesized and since they have a large molecular mass, they do not cross cell membranes readily. Thus, normally only small quantities of intracellular enzymes leak from cells into blood or other body fluids. The amounts are too low for enzyme mass to be measured, although their activities can be monitored. Enzyme activities in body fluids are often altered by pathological processes and measurement of body fluid enzymes is used to investigate disease. Most clinical enzyme measurements are made using serum, although occasionally other fluids, such as urine and gut secretions, are investigated. In general, increased rather than decreased activities of enzymes are of diagnostic interest in body fluids, although cellular enzymes are often deficient and measured in the investigation of inherited metabolic diseases (see chapter 18).

FACTORS AFFECTING SERUM ENZYME ACTIVITIES

The activity of an enzyme in the circulation depends on a balance between the rate of release from tissues, the presence of inhibitors, and the rate of removal (**Figure 12.1**).

Rate of Entry of Enzymes into Blood

The main factors affecting the rate of entry of enzymes into blood are the rate of synthesis, the mass of enzyme producing cells, and cell damage.

Enzyme Synthesis

The rate of enzyme synthesis is increased particularly in conditions affecting the liver. Biliary obstruction causes increased synthesis of enzymes located in the lining of the hepatobiliary tree. Some agents induce increased synthesis of enzymes by hepatocytes, examples including anticonvulsant drugs, particularly phenobarbitone and phenytoin. If a constant proportion of the enzymes produced leaks into the circulation, increased serum enzyme activities will result.

Mass of Enzyme Producing Cells

Serum alkaline phosphatase originating from bone reflects osteoblastic activity. This is increased, leading to high serum alkaline phosphatase activity in children who are actively growing, or where bone disease is present in which increased osteoblastic activity occurs, e.g. Paget's disease. The placenta produces alkaline phosphatase, causing increased levels in the third trimester. Metastatic carcinoma of the prostate produces increased acid phosphatase levels.

Cell Damage

Increased amounts may leak from tissues that are inflamed, necrotic, or metabolically abnormal, leading to increased serum levels. Examples include raised transaminase levels in hepatitis, creatine kinase (CK) following myocardial infarction and lactate dehydrogenase (LDH) in stored blood.

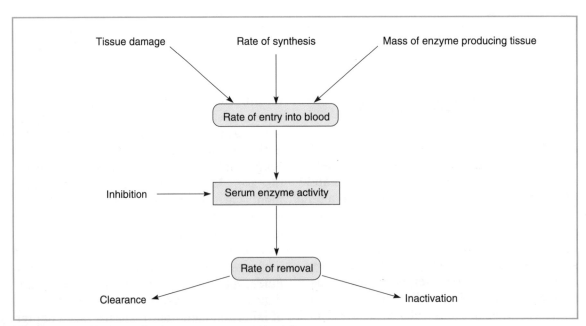

Figure 12.1 Factors affecting serum enzyme activity.

Table 12.1   Serum enzymes of diagnostic interest

Enzyme	Origin	Main applications
Acid phosphatase	Prostate, erythrocytes	Metastatic carcinoma of prostate
Alanine aminotransferase (ALT, SGPT)	Hepatocytes	Hepatocellular disease
Alkaline phosphatase (ALP)	Hepatobiliary tree	Cholestatic disease
	Bone	Bone disease
	GI tract, placenta, kidney	
Amylase	Pancreas	Acute pancreatitis
	Salivary glands	
Aspartate aminotransferase)	Hepatocytes	Hepatocellular disease
(AST, SGOT[2]	Cardiac muscle	Myocardial infarction
	Skeletal muscle	Muscle disease
Cholinesterase	Liver	Suxamethonium sensitivity, organophosphorus poisoning
Creatine kinase (CK)	Skeletal muscle	Muscle disease
	Heart muscle	Myocardial infarction
	Brain	
γ-Glutamyl transferase (GGT)	Liver	Cholestasis
	Pancreas	Alcohol abuse
Lactate dehydrogenase (LDH)	Cardiac muscle	Myocardial infarction
	Skeletal muscle	
	Erythrocytes, liver	

SGOT, serum glutamate-oxaloacetate transaminase; SGPT, serum glutamate-pyruvate transaminase.

Enzyme Inhibitors

The presence of circulating inhibitors of enzyme activity appears to have little effect on values determined in the laboratory. An exception is organophosphate poisoning which irreversibly inhibits cholinesterase.

Clearance of Enzymes

Serum enzyme activity is also affected by the rate of removal of enzymes from the circulation, although understanding of these mechanisms is incomplete. Possibilities include breakdown by proteases and removal by the reticuloendothelial system. Renal excretion appears unimportant, except for amylase which is small enough to be cleared by the kidney. Modest increases in serum amylase occur in chronic renal failure.

SPECIFICITY OF SERUM ENZYME MEASUREMENTS

Many enzymes which are used diagnostically originate from more than one tissue (**Table 12.1**), which potentially limits their specificity. Thus, increased serum CK could be due to myocardial infarction or skeletal muscle disease, and increased LDH occurs through multiple causes. This would limit the usefulness of enzyme measurements if their specificity was not increased. Greater specificity is achieved in three ways: interpreting investigations in the light of clinical features, test pattern recognition, and isoenzyme determination.

Test Results and Clinical Features

Serum aspartate aminotransferase (AST) activity may be raised due to myocardial infarction or because of diseases affecting hepatocytes, such as viral hepatitis. In practice, results rarely cause diagnostic confusion as the presenting features of the two conditions are very different. Occasionally, increased AST may originate from the liver because of complications of myocardial infarction, such as congestive cardiac failure.

Test Pattern Recognition

Investigations are rarely done in isolation and recognition of test patterns may aid differential diagnosis. Thus, alkaline phosphatase is raised in cholestasis and bone disease. In cholestasis, there are often increases in bilirubin and transaminase levels, while these do not occur in bone disease. If an isolated increase in alkaline phosphatase occurs, the estimation of γ-glutamyl tranferase may be helpful, as high serum activities of this enzyme occur in cholestasis while levels are normal in bone disease.

Isoenzymes

Multiple forms of enzymes (isoenzymes) occur which have similar catalytic activities but different structures. Different isoenzymes are often organ-specific and their determination may thus improve the specificity of enzyme tests. The heterogeneity of some isoenzymes is due to different protein subunits which are coded for by separate genes. Lactate dehydrogenase has four subunits of two different types (H and M); thus, five isoenzymes occur, H4 originating from the heart and M4 from the liver. Creatine kinase has two subunits, M and B; three isoenzymes occur, BB from brain, MM from skeletal muscle and MB from the heart. Other mechanisms are also responsible for heterogeneity, isoenzymes of alkaline phosphatase differing in their content of carbohydrate (sialic acid) residues attached to the protein chain.

Isoenzymes may be differentiated because of different physicochemical properties (by techniques such as electrophoresis), immunochemical properties (immunoassay) or chemical properties (differential activity for some substrates or susceptibility to inhibitors).

MAJOR ENZYMES OF DIAGNOSTIC INTEREST
Phosphatases

Acid Phosphatase
The richest source of acid phosphatase is the prostate, although significant amounts are also found in erythrocytes, liver spleen and platelets. Diagnostically, acid phosphatase measurements are used for monitoring metastatic carcinoma of the prostate, serum levels being raised in approximately 20% of cases where the tumour is confined to the gland, and 80% where there is spread of the tumour. Increased serum acid phosphatase may also occur occasionally in other prostatic conditions, particularly prostatitis and benign prostatic hypertrophy. Some acid phosphatase is released into the circulation when the prostate is examined *per rectum* and thus blood should be taken for estimation before this examination is undertaken. Serum acid phosphatase may also be increased through nonprostatic causes. These include haemolysis, bone disease, particularly Paget's disease and metastatic carcinoma of the breast and Gaucher's disease. Prostatic may be differentiated from nonprostatic acid phosphatase by the effect of enzyme inhibitors. Tartrate inhibits the prostatic enzyme while formaldehyde inhibits acid phosphatase from other sources.

Prostate-Specific Antigen
Prostate-specific antigen (PSA) is an enzyme which occurs in prostatic tissue and is raised in serum in a higher proportion of cases of metastatic carcinoma than acid

phosphatase. It is, however, less specific, as serum activities are also increased in many patients with benign prostatic hypertrophy.

ACID PHOSPHATASE

- The main sources of serum acid phosphatase are prostatic tissue and erythrocytes

- Serum acid phosphatase activity is raised in up to 80% of patients with metastatic carcinoma of the prostate

- Prostate-specific antigen is a more sensitive but less specific indicator of metastatic prostatic carcinoma

Alkaline Phosphatase

Alkaline phosphatase is found in high concentrations in the liver, bone, intestine, placenta and kidney although, except in pregnant women, the main sources of serum enzyme are the hepatobiliary tree and osteoblasts. Causes of increased serum activity of alkaline phosphatase are outlined in **Table 12.2**. Physiologically increased levels are seen during periods of active bone growth, particularly in infants and at puberty. Values increase during the second and third trimesters of pregnancy to about twice those normally seen in adults. Pathological increases in serum alkaline phosphatase occur mainly in hepatobiliary disease and bone disease. Rarely, serum alkaline phosphatase is elevated in patients with malignancy which does not affect liver or bone. This particular isoenzyme, named 'Regan' after a patient in whom it was described, resembles placental alkaline phosphatase and usually originates from carcinoma of the bronchus.

Serum alkaline phosphatase may be elevated in the absence of other biochemical abnormalities or clinical features to suggest the source. Under such circumstances the enzyme is usually derived from liver or bone and it is important to identify the tissue of origin. This can usually be done

Table 12.2 Causes of increased serum alkaline phosphatase activity

Physiological
- Infancy
- Puberty
- Pregnancy
- Intestinal isoenzyme

Bone disease
- Hyperparathyroidism
- Osteomalacia, rickets
- Paget's disease of the bone
- Osteomyelitis

Hepatobiliary disease
- Cholestasis
- Cirrhosis
- Hepatitis

Other
- Carcinoma of the bronchus

either by determining alkaline phosphatase isoenzymes or by estimating the activity of another enzyme, usually γ-glutamyl transferase, which rises in parallel with biliary alkaline phosphatase. Occasionally, isolated increases in serum alkaline phosphatase are due to the presence of an intestinal isoenzyme. This form of the enzyme is under genetic control and is usually found in subjects who secrete H blood group antigens into saliva and other body fluids.

Alkaline phosphatase activity in serum is usually estimated to detect increased levels. However, markedly reduced levels are found in the inherited condition hypophosphatasia, which is caused by defective bone calcification.

ALKALINE PHOSPHATASE

- The main sources of serum alkaline phosphatase are the hepatobiliary tree and bone

- Increased serum alkaline phosphatase activity from bone is associated with increased osteoblastic activity

- Increased serum alkaline phosphatase activity in liver disease is mainly due to cholestasis

Transaminases

Aspartate Aminotransferase

Aspartate aminotranferase (AST) is widely distributed, the heart, liver, skeletal muscle and kidney being rich sources. Smaller amounts are found in erythrocytes and slight increases can occur in haemolysis. Causes of increased serum sctivity of AST are outlined in **Table 12.3**. The major diagnostic applications are in the investigation of myocardial infarction, liver disease and muscle disease. Different isoenzymes of AST occur in the cytosol and mitochondria of the liver but differentiation of these and organ-specific forms of AST is not undertaken in clinical practice.

Alanine Aminotransferase

Alanine aminotransferase (ALT) is also widely distributed although the largest amounts occur in liver. Smaller amounts occur in the heart and ALT usually remains normal following myocardial infarction unless congestive cardiac failure occurs, causing release from the liver. Thus, ALT is more specific for liver disease than AST.

Table 12.3 Causes of increased serum aspartate aminotransferase activity

Physiological
◆ Neonates
Liver disease
◆ Hepatitis
◆ Hepatic necrosis
◆ Cholestasis
Cardiac disease
◆ Myocardial infarction
Diseases of skeletal muscle
◆ Crush injury
◆ Trauma
◆ Myopathy
From erythrocytes
◆ Haemolysis (intra- and extra-vascular)

γ-Glutamyl Transferase

γ-Glutamyl transferase (γ-glutamyl transpeptidase, GGT) is found in several tissues, the kidney being the richest source. Significant amounts are present in the liver and pancreas, the major diagnostic application of GGT measurements being in the investigation of hepatobiliary disease. γ-Glutyamyl tranferase is a microsomal enzyme, its synthesis being induced by ethanol and certain drugs, e.g. anticonvulsants. Modest elevations in serum levels may be seen in the absence of hepatocellular disease in 70–80% of patients who abuse alcohol, with more marked elevations occurring in the presence of alcoholic liver disease. γ-Glutamyl transferase is a less sensitive indicator of hepatocellular disease than transaminases but high serum levels occur in cholestasis, when increases may be seen before elevations of alkaline phosphatase are apparent.

Serum GGT activity sometimes increases following myocardial infarction and in congestive cardiac failure. This is probably due to hepatic congestion.

Amylase

Amylase is produced by the pancreas and salivary glands and its main diagnostic application is in the investigation of acute abdominal pain, the highest values being seen in acute pancreatitis (see chapter 10). Values greater than five times but less than 10 times the upper limit of normal may be seen in other causes of acute abdominal pain, particularly perforated peptic ulcer but also occasionally in intestinal obstruction. Abdominal pain and hyperamylasaemia are not uncommon in diabetic ketoacidosis, these features being related to the acidosis. Interestingly, such hyperamylasaemia usually results from increases in the salivary rather than the pancreatic isoenzyme.

Values greater than five times the upper limit of normal may be seen in acute renal failure with more modest increases (2–3 times the upper limit of normal) being found in chronic renal failure. These increases are explained by decreased urinary clearance of the enzyme. Reduced renal clearance is also the explanation for macroamylasaemia, a benign condition in which circulating amylase is either in a polymeric form or complexed with an immunoglobulin. In either form the enzyme is too large to be cleared by the glomerulus and serum activities are raised, usually 3–5 times the upper limit of normal.

> **KEY POINTS**
>
> ## AMYLASE
>
> - The main source of serum amylase in normal subjects is the salivary glands
>
> - The main source of elevated serum amylase activity is the pancreas
>
> - Serum amylase activities greater than 10 times the upper limit of normal are virtually diagnostic of acute pancreatitis

Cholinesterase

Two types of cholinesterase are found in man, acetylcholinesterase (or 'true' cholinesterase) and cholinesterase (pseudocholinesterase). Erythrocytes and nervous tissue are particularly rich in acetylcholinesterase while cholinesterase is synthesized mainly in the liver, significant amounts being released into serum. Acetylcholinesterase breaks down acetylcholine while cholinesterase has a broader spectrum of activity, hydrolysing both choline and non-choline esters.

Suxamethonium Sensitivity (Scoline Apnoea)

Suxamethonium (scoline) is a muscle relaxant with a short duration of action (3–4 minutes in most subjects) which is often used for procedures such as endotracheal intubation. Suxamethonium causes prolonged depolarization of motor end-plates and prevents a response to acetylcholine. Normally, suxamethonium is rapidly broken down by cholinesterase. However, occasionally, the drug is active for much longer periods, causing apnoea which lasts for several hours. This is sometimes due to electrolyte imbalance and dehydration but also occurs if a genetically determined atypical cholinesterase variant is present. Several variants have been described which are characterized by low activity and resistance to enzyme inhibitors, particularly dibucaine and fluoride. Patients with suxamethonium sensitivity are either homozygous for a single abnormal variant or have pairs of different variants with reduced activity. Heterozygotes can be identified by the response of their enzyme to inhibitors, and family studies are important to identify affected relatives who may be at risk when undergoing surgery.

Cholinesterase Deficiency

Cholinesterase is synthesized in the liver and serum levels are often low in hepatic disease. Organophosphorus insecticides, which are used in sheep dips, inhibit both cholinesterases and serum cholinesterase can be used to screen for poisoning.

Creatine Kinase

CK catalyses the phosphorylation of creatine. The richest source of the enzyme is skeletal muscle while cardiac muscle and brain also contain appreciable amounts. The main diagnostic application of CK is in the investigation of muscle disease, when the major circulating isoenzyme is CK-MM, and myocardial infarction, in which CK-MB predominates.

Lactate Dehydrogenase

Most tissues contain LDH and therefore measurements of the enzyme have low specificity. This may be improved by determining isoenzymes; five forms occur, the proportions of which vary between tissues. Isoenzymes can be determined by electrophoresis which separates different forms on the basis of their electrical charge, heart having a high proportion of fast-moving enzyme, while the least mobile form predominates in liver. The main diagnostic application of LDH measurements is in the investigation of myocardial infarction (see below) when the cardiac-specific form of the enzyme is of interest. Because electrophoresis is a manual technique which is not readily automated, an alternative approach to determining LDH is usually adopted – estimating the enzyme activity with a substrate specific to the isoenzyme type. LDH catalyses the reversi-ble oxidation of L-lactate to pyruvate but also has activity against other hydroxy- and keto-acids, including hydroxybutyrate (2-oxobutyrate). The cardiac isoenzyme has a high affinity for this substrate, while liver LDH reacts with it very slowly; therefore, the cardiac isoenzyme may be determined by measuring hydroxybutyrate dehydrogenase (HBD) activity.

SERUM ENZYMES IN DISEASE
Myocardial Infarction

Serum enzyme tests are used extensively in the investigation of suspected myocardial infarction. Necrosis of the myocardium, but not angina pectoris, leads to the release into the circulation of tissue enzymes, particularly CK, AST and LDH (HBD). These are released from the heart and cleared from the circulation at different rates (**Figure 12.2**). The first to rise is CK, activities being

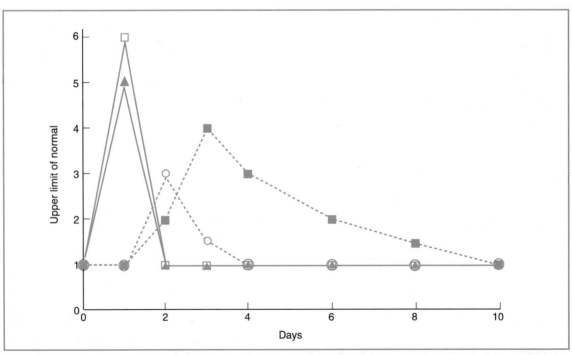

Figure 12.2 Pattern of increase of serum enzymes following myocardial infarction. ○ Aspartate aminotransferase; □ creatine kinase; ▲ creatine kinase muscle isoenzyme; ■ hydroxybutyrate dehydrogenase.

raised within 6 h of myocardial infarction. Total CK reaches a peak at 24–36 h, slightly later than the maximum activity of CK-MB. In uncomplicated cases, CK returns to normal in 3 days. Serum AST rises more slowly, reaching a maximum activity at about 48 h and returning to normal in 4–5 days. No significant elevations in HBD are seen for the first 24 h; values reach a maximum at about 3 days and remain elevated for up to 8 days. Thus, it is important to consider the timing of samples when interpreting test results. Thrombolytic therapy alters the pattern of enzymes, peak values being greater and occurring earlier.

CK and HBD are useful as early and late indicators of myocardial infarction, respectively, and are more specific than AST. However, CK from skeletal muscle may be raised following an intramuscular injection, chest compression for resuscitation or electrical defibrillation. The specificity of CK is increased by the measurement of CK-MB, although small amounts of this isoenzyme also occur in muscle, the proportion increasing in trained athletes and in patients with necrotizing muscle diseases. Subtypes of CK-MB have been described recently and the measurement of these may improve specificity. The activity of HBD may also be increased due to noncardiac factors, haemolysis being an important artefactual cause since erythrocyte LDH has similar properties to the cardiac isoenzyme.

Cardiac enzyme measurements are very sensitive indicators of myocardial infarction, being raised in over 95% of cases. However, they add little to diagnosis and management where the clinical features and ECG changes are characteristic. They are of particular value under the following circumstances.

1. When the clinical presentation is atypical, particularly if the characteristic chest pain is absent.
2. If the patient presents some time after a suspected event.
3. If there is difficulty in interpreting the electrocardiogram (ECG). The presence

of an arrhythmia or a previous myocardial infarction often leads to equivocal patterns.
4. If further infarction is suspected within a few days of a previous event.

The value of the magnitude of serum enzyme changes as a prognostic indicator of myocardial infarction is controversial. Some studies suggest the the degree of elevation is related to the size of the infarct, while small ante-mortem changes may occur in patients who die of massive infarction. The site rather than the size of infarction also affects prognosis.

Muscle Disease

Skeletal muscle is a rich source of several enzymes including CK, AST, ALT, aldolase and LDH. The measurement of total CK activity is the most widely used enzyme in the investigation of muscle damage, this being increased most frequently and showing the highest activities in diseases in which there is muscle fibre necrosis, particularly muscular dystrophies, polymyositis and rhabdomyolysis. Serum enzymes are usually normal in peripheral neuropathies and neuromuscular junction disorders but may be slightly elevated in motor neurone diseases.

Muscular Dystrophy

The muscular dystrophies are a group of genetically determined degenerative disorders of muscle, each type having distinct features. Duchenne (pseudohypertrophic) muscular dystrophy is an X-linked recessive disorder caused by an abnormal dystrophin gene and characterized by progressive weakness of muscles from the age of 5 years. Raised serum CK activities occur before the onset of clinical symptoms and values greater than 10 times the upper limit of normal are often seen, although these decline in the later stages of the disease. Serum CK is also elevated in approximately 75% of female carriers of the condition.

Becker's muscular dystrophy is a more benign form of pseudohypertrophic muscular dystrophy with a later age of onset, affected males sometimes reaching reproductive age. The pattern of elevations in serum CK is similar to that seen in Duchenne muscular dystrophy. Smaller elevations are usually seen in other forms of muscular dystrophy and in some, e.g. myotonic dystrophy, serum CK may be normal.

Toxic Myopathies

Many drugs and chemicals may produce local or generalized muscle damage. Intramuscular injections may cause muscle damage by two mechanisms, trauma and effect of the agent being injected. The latter may be caused by narcotic analgesics, a possible cause of elevated CK activity which should be considered in cases of suspected myocardial infarction. Various agents may cause a generalized myopathy, including alcohol, D-penicillamine and lipid-lowering agents such as fibric acid analogues and hydroxymethyl glutaryl coenzyme A (HMG-CoA) reductase inhibitors. Very rarely, rhabdomyolysis may result from treatment with HMG-CoA reductase inhibitors and CK is often monitored in patients receiving these drugs to identify susceptible individuals.

Malignant Hyperpyrexia

Malignant hyperpyrexia is a serious toxic myopathy, fortunately rare, in which rapid increases in body temperature, shock, and convulsions occur in susceptible individuals. This usually follows general anaesthesia although some cases have been described after the administration of muscle relaxants. High serum CK activities are seen during attacks and modest increases may persist after recovery, although this is not inevitable. Susceptibility appears to be determined genetically and elevated enzymes are sometimes found in affected relatives. Preoperative CK should be measured in patients with a family history of malignant hyperpyrexia or operative deaths.

Because the condition is rare and CK is an insensitive indicator of those at risk, generalized preoperative screening is unwarranted.

Traumatic Myopathies

Causes of trauma to muscles which may result in release of enzymes include surgery, intramuscular injections and postexercise changes. High serum CK values are found after operation and if myocardial infarction is suspected, CK-MB should be measured. Serum CK values usually return to normal within 48 h of a single intramuscular injection, although occasionally activities may remain elevated for up to a week. Vigorous exercise of short duration and prolonged moderate exercise may produce elevations in serum CK, particularly in untrained athletes.

Liver Disease

Enzyme measurements in the context of liver disease are discussed in chapter 11. Measurement of serum enzyme activities is useful in the differential diagnosis of jaundice and monitoring drug toxicity. One of the transaminases is used as an indicator of hepatocellular damage, ALT being more specific for this purpose than AST. Hepatocellular disease has only a modest effect on alkaline phosphatase and GGT (up to three times the upper limit of normal), unless an obstructive element also occurs. Typically, much higher values are seen in cholestasis, which causes increased synthesis of alkaline phosphatase and GGT in biliary canalicular cells, with solubilization of enzymes and release into the circulation. This occurs whether the obstruction is intra- or extra-hepatic, values often being 5–10 times the upper limit of normal.

Bone Disease

Serum alkaline phosphatase is usually normal in osteoporosis as osteoblastic activity is not increased, while modest increases are typical in osteomalacia and rickets. Transient increases occur due to healing fractures. Patients with primary or secondary hyperparathyroidism may show increased serum alkaline phosphatase activity if bony involvement occurs. Levels may be very high in Paget's disease of the bone (greater than 10 times the upper limit of normal), depending on the activity of the pathological process. Both primary and secondary bone tumours can cause increases in alkaline phosphatase, typically up to five times the upper limit of normal although higher levels are seen occasionally, particularly in osteogenic sarcoma.

Enzymes in Urine

Enzymes appear in urine from two sources, by filtration of plasma and by leaking from cells lining the urinary tract. Amylase is normally detected in urine, while other serum enzymes are too large to cross the glomerulus (see chapter 8). Several enzymes derived from renal tubular cells have been investigated as indicators of tubular damage, particularly when caused by renal transplant rejection, the most commonly used being alkaline phosphatase and *N*-acetyl-β-glucosaminidase (NAG). However, results have been found to be inconsistent and elevations of urinary enzymes lack specificity.

Haematological Disorders

Red cell enzymes activities may be abnormal because of an inherited deficiency or due to acquired disease. Many inherited defects have been described which result in haemolytic disease, spherocytosis or methaemoglobinaemia. Many genetic variants of glucose-6-phosphate dehydrogenase (G6PD) occur causing defective enzyme activity. These are relatively common in black and Mediterranean populations and cause haemolysis after exposure to oxidant drugs, such as primaquine, or fava beans. Synthesis of G6PD is controlled by an X-linked gene and therefore males predominantly are affected. Haemolytic anaemia may also be caused by other enzyme defects including those affecting pyruvate kinase, glutathione synthetase, hexokinase and enzymes of the glycolytic pathway. A detailed consideration of these is beyond the scope of the present book.

Red cell enzymes are sometimes measured in the diagnosis of vitamin deficiencies, e.g. transketolase in thiamine deficiency (see chapter 3). Elevated serum LDH activities (owing to increases in HBD) are found in various acquired haematological disorders including megaloblastic anaemias and leukaemias.

Tissue Enzymes

The estimation of tissue enzymes is usually undertaken in the investigation of inherited metabolic diseases, often being done on biopsy specimens from specific tissues. Most estimations are undertaken in specialized centres.

FURTHER READING

Hamm CW. New serum markers for acute myocardial infarction. *New England Journal of Medicine* 1994; **331**: 607–8

Moss DW. *Isoenzymes*. London: Chapman & Hall, 1982

Sherman KE. Alanine aminotransferase in clinical practice. *Archives of Internal Medicine* 1991; **151**: 260–5

Wilkinson JH (ed). *The Principles and Practice of Diagnostic Enzymology*. London: Edward Arnold, 1976

CASE 12.1

A 54-year-old man with a past history of myocardial infarction was admitted following the onset of acute central chest pain 3 h previously. The results of his ECG were equivocal. The following serum enzyme results were obtained.

Time	CK (U l^{-1})	AST (U l^{-1})
On admission	1150	85
After 24 h	560	40
After 48 h	200	25

Do these results suggest that the patient had suffered a myocardial infarction?

CASE 12.2

A 54-year-old woman presented to the accident room with acute abdominal pain of 4 h duration. The pain was epigastric and radiated through to the back. On examination the patient was distressed and hypotensive, and there was epigastric tenderness. Investigation showed that the serum amylase was 6500 U l^{-1}. What is the most probable diagnosis?

CASE 12.3

A 79-year-old man was investigated for abdominal discomfort and constipation. Investigations were unremarkable except for an abnormal alkaline phosphatase result which was detected in the liver function tests. These showed

bilirubin	17 μmol l^{-1}
ALT	42 U l^{-1}
alkaline phosphatase	550 U l^{-1}

What are the possible explanations for these findings?

13

THE PITUITARY AND HYPOTHALAMUS

INTRODUCTION

The pituitary gland is situated within the sella turcica in the sphenoid bone at the base of the skull and consists of two parts which have separate functions and secrete different hormones. The anterior part of the gland is of ectodermal origin, arising as an evagination from the roof of the pharynx, while the posterior pituitary is formed by a downgrowth from the floor of the third ventricle of the brain. After development, the posterior pituitary remains connected to the hypothalamus by the pituitary stalk through which runs the hypothalamo-hypophyseal tract. In contrast, there are no neural connections between the anterior pituitary and hypothalamus. The hypothalamus receives its blood supply from arteries which supply the base of the brain and capillaries from the median eminence of the hypothalamus drain through the connecting stalk to supply the anterior pituitary, which thus receives a portal blood supply.

THE HYPOTHALAMUS

The hypothalamus secretes several regulatory factors into blood supplying the anterior pituitary where they control the secretion of hormones, mostly by stimulation of hormone release although some regulatory factors inhibit secretion (**Table 13.1**). Anterior pituitary hormones are trophic, controlling the secretion of hormones by target glands – the thyroid, breast, adrenal glands, and gonads. The secretion of hypothalamic-releasing hormones is regulated as a result of negative feedback control by hormones produced by end organs, although there is also some feedback at the level of the pituitary (**Figure 13.1**). Higher centres of the brain affect

Table 13.1 Anterior pituitary hormones, their cell types and hypothalamic regulatory factors

Hormone	Cell type	Hypothalamic regulatory factor
Growth hormone	Acidophil	Growth hormone-releasing hormone (GH-RH) (stimulatory)
		Growth hormone release-inhibiting factor (somatostatin) (inhibitory)
Prolactin	Acidophil	Prolactin release-inhibiting hormone
Thyroid-stimulating hormone (TSH)	Basophil	Thyrotropin-releasing hormone (TRH)
Adrenocorticotrophic hormone (ACTH)	Basophil	Corticotrophin (CRF)
Luteinizing hormone (LH)	Basophil	Gonadotrophin-releasing hormone (Gn-RH)
Follicle-stimulating hormone (FSH)	Basophil	Gonadotrophin-releasing hormone (Gn-RH)

secretion of hypothalamic-releasing hormones and thus pituitary secretion. Hypothalamic-releasing factors are present in minute amounts in the brain; structurally they appear to be low molecular weight polypeptides. It is becoming clear that hypothalamic regulating factors have effects other than the regulation of pituitary secretion, with several additional actions being recognized for growth hormone release-inhibiting hormone (somatostatin). These include neurotransmission, inhibition of thyroid-stimulating hormone (TSH) release, and inhibition of the local release of hormones and exocrine secretions in the gastrointestinal tract.

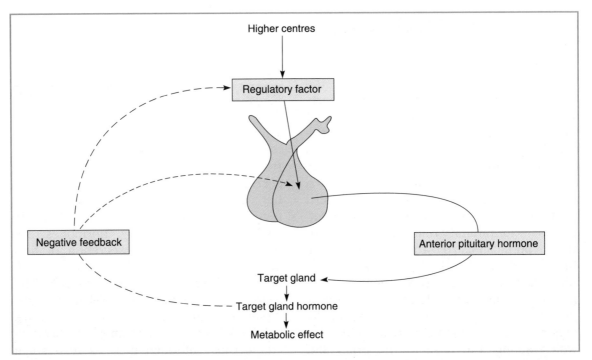

Figure 13.1 Negative feedback control of target organ hormones (dashed lines) on the secretion of hypothalamic-releasing hormones and pituitary trophic hormones.

THE HYPOTHALAMUS AND PITUITARY

- There are neural connections between the hypothalamus and posterior pituitary but not the anterior pituitary

- Blood from the hypothalamus supplies the anterior pituitary

- The secretion of anterior pituitary hormones is regulated by hypothalamic-releasing factors

THE ANTERIOR PITUITARY

The anterior pituitary contains several different cell types. Three are identified by conventional haematoxylin and eosin stains: chromophobe cells which contain little hormone, acidophil cells which synthesize growth hormone and prolactin, and basophils which contain gonadotrophins (luteinizing hormone (LH) and follicle-stimulating hormone (FSH)) and TSH (**Table 13.1**). Specific cell types for the production of each of the pituitary hormones are recognized by using immunochemical stains.

Anterior Pituitary Hormones

Growth Hormone

Growth hormone (GH)-secreting cells comprise approximately 50% of the anterior pituitary gland. Growth hormone is a single-chain peptide which contains 191 amino acids, the sequence of which is species specific. Secretion is regulated by two hypothalamic factors, growth hormone-releasing hormone (GH-RH) and growth hormone release-inhibiting hormone (somatostatin). Secretion occurs in short bursts, mainly at night during deep sleep. Levels rise in response to stress, during exercise, and in response to hypoglycaemia and certain amino acids, particularly arginine. Glucose infusion suppresses GH release.

Although GH is necessary for normal growth it does not appear to control this directly, but acts by stimulating the production of other hormones, somatomedins. The most important of these is somatomedin C (insulin-like growth factor 1, IGF-1) which is produced mainly in the liver. IGF-1 is structurally similar to insulin and circulating levels are relatively constant, in contrast to those of GH. Growth hormone has additional metabolic effects that antagonize many of the actions of insulin. Thus, it increases lipolysis and fatty acid release from adipose tissue and also stimulates hepatic glucose production. However, like insulin, it stimulates tissue uptake of amino acids.

GROWTH HORMONE

- GH secretion is regulated by two hypothalamic regulatory factors, GH-RH stimulating and somatostatin inhibiting secretion

- GH promotes growth through the action of somatomedins

- Growth hormone antagonizes the action of insulin on adipose tissue and carbohydrate metabolism

Thyroid Stimulating Hormone

TSH is a glycoprotein which, like the gonadotrophins and placental human chorionic gonadotrophin, contains α and β subunits. In each of these hormones the α subunits are very similar in structure, their biological properties depending on differences in the β subunits. Secretion of TSH is stimulated by thyrotropin-releasing hormone (TRH) and is inhibited by thyroid hormones, predominantly tri-iodothyronine (T3), somatostatin, dopamine and catecholamines. TSH stimulates the cellular processes leading to the synthesis and secretion of T3 and thyroxine (T4).

Adrenocorticotrophic Hormone

Adrenocorticotrophic hormone (ACTH) is a single-chain polypeptide which contains 39 amino acids. It is produced from a precursor protein, pro-opiomelanocortin, from which β-endorphin, a peptide with opiate properties, and β-lipotrophin are also produced. Pro-opiomelanocortin also contains the amino acid sequence of melanocyte-stimulating hormone, although this is not normally released into the blood in man. Release of ACTH is stimulated by corticotrophin-releasing hormone (CRH), and vasopressin also has a weak stimulatory effect. CRH secretion is regulated through negative feedback by circulating corticosteroids and also by other centres in the brain, secretion increasing in response to stress, hypoglycaemia and fever. ACTH secretion shows diurnal variation, the highest levels occurring in the early morning and lowest levels in the late evening.

Lipotrophins

Lipotrophins were so named because they were thought to have fat-mobilizing properties. This is no longer appears to be the case and their function is unknown.

Opiate Peptides

The enkephalins and endorphins are peptides with opiate effects which occur because they bind to opioid receptors, even though their structure is unrelated to that of morphine. While β-endorphin is derived from pro-opiomelanocortin, enkephalins are derived from different precursors and are synthesized largely in the adrenal medulla and autonomic ganglia. Opiate peptides occur widely throughout the central nervous system and appear to be neurotransmitters. They may also play a role in memory and in the response to stress and pain. Various addictions are thought to be related to abnormalities of these pep-

tides and acupuncture-mediated analgesia may be a result of their action.

Gonadotrophins

The gonadotrophins LH and FSH are, like TSH, glycoproteins, the specificity of their action depending on differences in β-subunits. The secretion of both LH and FSH is controlled by gonadotrophin-releasing hormone (Gn-RH, LH-RH) and puberty does not occur if Gn-RH is absent. Circulating levels of gonadotrophins are low in childhood and rise during puberty, after which they are secreted in a pulsatile manner. LH induces ovulation in females and initiates formation of the corpus luteum. It also stimulates oestrogen production indirectly through stimulating the synthesis of precursors by thecal cells, while FSH stimulates the granulosa cells of the ovarian follicle to produce oestradiol. In males LH stimulates testicular Leydig cells to produce androgens, while both LH and FSH are required for spermatogenesis in the seminiferous tubules. In women, there is both positive and negative feedback control of gonadotrophin secretion; in men, testosterone exerts negative feedback on LH secretion while FSH secretion appears to be regulated by inhibin, a peptide secreted by the seminiferous tubules.

Prolactin

Prolactin is a 198-amino-acid peptide which is similar in structure to growth hormone, its main function being to initiate and maintain lactation. Normally, prolactin secretion is inhibited, probably by the catecholamine dopamine. Like other anterior pituitary hormones, prolactin is secreted in a pulsatile manner. Circulating levels are higher at night than during the day and secretion increases as a result of stress, including the discomfort of venepuncture. Prolactin-secreting cells increase in number during pregnancy as a result of stimulation by oestrogens. The secretion of prolactin also increases and this, together with the action of oestrogens, leads to the development of breast tissue. Circulating prolactin levels are increased tenfold during lactation; further increases occur through a reflex resulting from nipple stimulation, which stimulates the flow of milk. Other hormones are also required for normal lactation including oestrogens, progesterone, thyroxine and oxytocin.

THE POSTERIOR PITUITARY

The posterior pituitary hormones vasopressin and oxytocin are synthesized in the supraoptic and paraventricular nuclei of the hypothalamus, and pass in neural tracts to the posterior pituitary, where they are stored in granules. They differ from anterior pituitary hormones in that secretion is not regulated by hypothalamic hormones.

Posterior Pituitary Hormones

Vasopressin

Vasopressin (antidiuretic hormone, ADH) is a cyclical peptide which contains 9 amino acids, these being very similar to those found in oxytocin. A precursor is synthesized in the hypothalamus, the active hormone being formed as vasopressin is transported to the posterior pituitary. The main function of vasopressin is the fine control of water balance through actions on the distal convoluted tubule and collecting duct. Vasopressin conserves water by increasing the permeability of the tubule, which allows water to flow down the osmotic gradient between the interstitial fluid of the kidney and the tubular lumen (see chapter 8).

The major physiological factor controlling vasopressin release is the osmotic gradient between extracellular and intracellular fluid (ECF, ICF), secretion increasing when ECF osmolality increases. Other factors regulating vasopressin secretion include decreased plasma volume, through effects on stretch

receptors in the left atrium, and baroreceptors which are found in the aorta and carotid arteries. Reduced blood pressure is a potent stimulus of vasopressin secretion, and the hormone has a pressor effect, helping to compensate for reductions in blood pressure. Other factors stimulating vasopressin secretion include stress, pain and various drugs including nicotine, chlorpropamide, tricyclic antidepressants and anticonvulsants.

KEY POINTS

VASOPRESSIN

- Vasopressin is synthesized in hypothalamic nuclei and stored in the posterior pituitary gland

- The main factor controlling vasopressin secretion is extracellular fluid osmolality

- Vasopressin regulates the fine control of water balance through actions in the kidney

---

Oxytocin

The structure of oxytocin is similar to that of vasopressin, there being differences in two amino acids. Oxytocin release from the posterior pituitary is stimulated by nerve impulses from the hypothalamus, the stimulus for which is breast suckling. Oxytocin leads to contraction of myoepithelial cells in the breast, causing milk to flow. A role for oxytocin in the induction of labour has been suggested, although this has not been confirmed.

DISORDERS OF THE PITUITARY

Hypopituitarism

Causes

Hypopituitarism is a deficiency of one or more pituitary hormones which may result from many conditions (**Table 13.2**). The

Table 13.2   Causes of hypopituitarism

Tumours
◆ Pituitary adenomas
◆ Hypothalamic tumours
  Craniopharyngiomas
  Neural tumours
◆ Secondary tumours
Infectious disease
◆ Tuberculosis
◆ Syphilis
◆ Encephalitis
Granulomatous disease
◆ Sarcoidosis
◆ Histiocytosis
Vascular
◆ Sheehan's postpartum necrosis
◆ Severe hypotension
◆ Pituitary apoplexy
Trauma
◆ Head injury
Iatrogenic
◆ Hypophysectomy
◆ Irradiation
Isolated defects
◆ Deficiency of releasing hormone
◆ Suppression by prolonged administration of
  target organ hormone

most common cause is a pituitary or hypothalamic tumour which destroys anterior pituitary secretory cells. This is most often a chromophobe adenoma in adults or a craniopharyngioma in children. Other important causes include destruction of the pituitary by surgery or radiation, and necrosis of the pituitary in the postpartum period. The anterior pituitary is susceptible to hypotension because its arterial blood supply is at a low pressure and this susceptibility is increased in pregnancy because of enlargement of the gland. However, pituitary necrosis is now very rare as a result of modern obstetric practice.

Clinical Features

The clinical features depend on which pituitary hormones are deficient and the pathological process causing the disease. Tumours of the pituitary may lead to visual disturbances as a result of pressure on the optic chiasma. Destruction of secretory cells will lead to deficiencies of hormones, partial hypopituitarism occurring more frequently than complete failure of hormone production. Growth hormone and gonadotrophin secretion usually fail first in progressive disease, with ACTH and TSH deficiency occurring later; vasopressin secretion is often maintained unless very advanced disease is present. Defective GH secretion leads to growth retardation in children and an increased tendency to hypoglycaemia in adults. Gonadotrophin deficiency leads to menstrual disturbances and infertility in women, decreased libido and loss of body hair in men, and delayed puberty in children. Loss of adrenal and thyroid secretions due to lack of trophic hormones may mimic primary failure of these organs. Panhypopituitarism may cause coma, hypoglycaemia, sodium depletion and hypothyroidism being possible contributory metabolic factors.

Isolated deficiencies of pituitary hormones can occur owing to defects in the secretion of hypothalamic-releasing hormones. Congenital GH deficiency leads to short stature in children which can be treated by hormone replacement. However, human growth hormone must be used because of species specificity. Originally this was prepared from human pituitary glands removed at autopsy, although this has been discontinued because of the development of Creutzfeld–Jacob disease in a small number of recipients. Growth hormone for therapeutic use is now produced using recombinant DNA technology.

Isolated gonadotrophin deficiency may occur in association with a defective sense of smell (Kallman's syndrome).

Investigation

Imaging techniques are important for assessing the pituitary, these including plain X-rays, computerized tomography (CT) scanning and magnetic resonance imaging. Basal levels of pituitary and target organ hor-

Table 13.3 Insulin tolerance test for the investigation of hypopituitarism

---

- ◆ The test is contraindicated in patients with myocardial ischaemia, epilepsy, unequivocal hypocortisolism. Medical supervision of the test is required.
- ◆ The patients is fasted from midnight although water is allowed.
- ◆ An intravenous cannula is inserted at 08.30 hours.
- ◆ After 30 min blood is taken for glucose, cortisol and growth hormone estimation.
- ◆ Insulin (0.1 unit kg^{-1}) is infused*.
- ◆ Blood is withdrawn at 30, 45, 60 and 90 min after injection for glucose, cortisol and growth hormone analysis.
- ◆ The test is terminated with administration of a glucose drink, the patient remaining on the ward for a further 2 h.

---

*0.10 units kg^{-1} if hypopituitarism is strongly suspected and in children; 0.15 units kg^{-1} in normal subjects; 0.3 units kg^{-1} in acromegaly or Cushing's disease

mones should be measured and may be low. However, fluctuations of these due to diurnal variations complicates interpretation and concentrations may be normal in the presence of disease, since there is considerable functional reserve. Impairment of functional reserve may be investigated by dynamic tests which stimulate or inhibit secretion.

Insulin Sensitivity (Tolerance) Test The insulin sensitivity test, outlined in **Table 13.3**, assesses growth hormone and ACTH reserve, the secretion of these normally increasing in response to hypoglycaemia. The dose of insulin required to produce hypoglycaemia depends on the clinical state of the patient, those with hypopituitarism being more sensitive to insulin than normal subjects. Patients with Cushing's disease and acromegaly are less sensitive to hypoglycaemia, as these conditions result from increased concentrations of counter-regula-

tory hormones. The dose of insulin is usually determined by the condition which is suspected, but hypoglycaemia may not develop if the patient is insulin resistant and the test will need to be repeated with a higher dose of insulin. The test is positive if adequate hypoglycaemia (<2.2 mmol l^{-1}) develops and growth hormone and cortisol levels do not rise. Growth hormone levels should exceed 40 mU l^{-1}, while levels between 20 and 40 mU l^{-1} are equivocal. Cortisol concentrations should increase by at least 170 nmol l^{-1}: the levels fail to rise in pituitary disease and primary adrenal failure. With the introduction of powerful imaging techniques the insulin sensitivity test is being used less often in the initial diagnosis of hypopituitarism, although it is useful in assessment of pituitary reserve when a pituitary tumour has been removed.

Other Dynamic Tests Pituitary reserve may also be investigated following the injection of TRH or Gn-RH, to assess the secretion of TSH or LH and FSH. In addition, TRH and Gn-RH may injected together with insulin in a combined pituitary function test, the combined sampling protocols including the time points of the individual tests. The TRH and Gn-RH tests are considered in the chapters dealing with the appropriate target organs – Chapter 14 for the TRH test and chapter 16 for the Gn-RH test.

Other Investigations Glucagon injection can be used to assess pituitary reserve when the insulin tolerance test is contraindicated; this stimulates both growth hormone and ACTH secretion, although it is not as reliable a stimulus as insulin. Arginine infusion can be undertaken to assess growth hormone reserves. Gonadotrophin reserve can be assessed by giving clomiphene which competes with gonadal steroids for hypothalamic receptors, the normal effect being secretion of LH and FSH.

HYPOPITUITARISM

- Hypopituitarism is caused most commonly by a pituitary or hypothalamic tumour

- Partial hypopituitarism is more common than a complete failure of hormone production

- Dynamic function tests have a greater utility in detecting impaired pituitary function than measuring basal hormone concentrations

Excess Growth Hormone Secretion

Excess growth hormone secretion causes gigantism if it occurs before fusion of the epiphyses and acromegaly after fusion. Acromegaly is almost always due to a pituitary adenoma, although increased production of GH-RH can occur very rarely, either as a result of a tumour in the hypothalamus or because GH-RH is produced ectopically by a bronchial carcinoid or a pancreatic islet cell tumour. Skeletal and soft tissue overgrowth occurs in acromegaly which leads to increased hand and foot size, enlargement of the tongue, prognathism and coarsening of facial features. These may be obvious in some cases but in others comparison with earlier photographs may be helpful. Hypertension, arthritis and muscle symptoms are common. Headaches occur and local effects of the tumour include destruction of other pituitary cells leading to hypopituitarism or diabetes insipidus. Menstrual disturbances are common and men often complain of a loss of libido and potency. Metabolic effects include diabetes mellitus, growth hormone being an insulin antagonist.

Investigation

Growth hormone levels rise in response to stress and in some patients the discomfort of venepuncture is sufficient to elevate serum concentrations; thus, random levels may be misleading. A glucose tolerance test in which glucose and growth hormone levels are measured simultaneously may be helpful. Normally, growth hormone levels are suppressed by increased serum glucose concentrations, but this fails to occur in acromegaly.

Hyperprolactinaemia

The causes of hyperprolactinaemia are outlined in **Table 13.4**. There are several physiological causes and prolactin is often synthesized by functioning pituitary tumours. Diseases of the hypothalamic–pituitary stalk lead to hyperprolactinaemia by preventing dopamine, which inhibits prolactin secretion, from reaching the pituitary. Most drugs which cause hyperprolactinaemia interfere with the action of dopamine. Clinical features of hyperprolactinaemia include gonadal dysfunction and galactorrhoea. Amenorrhoea or anovulatory cycles

Table 13.4 Causes of hyperprolactinaemia

Physiological
◆ Stress, sleep, coitus, pregnancy, suckling
Pituitary tumours
◆ Prolactinomas
◆ Mixed adenomas (prolactin and growth hormone or adrenocorticotrophic hormone (ACTH) secretion)
Pituitary stalk or hypothalamic disorder
◆ Pituitary stalk section (surgery, head injury)
◆ Tumours (craniopharyngioma, glioma)
◆ Granulomas (sarcoid, tuberculosis, Hand–Schuller–Christian disease)
Drugs
◆ Dopamine blockers (phenothiazines, metoclopramide, haliperidol)
◆ Dopamine depleting agents (reserpine, methyldopa)
◆ Others (oestrogens, thyroid-stimulating hormone (TSH))
Hypothyroidism
Chronic renal failure
Ectopic secretion

are common in women while impotence occurs in men.

Investigation

Serum prolactin levels should be measured in patients who have symptoms suggestive of hypogonadism or galactorrhoea. Samples should be taken from unstressed patients; venous cannulation allows the stress of venepuncture to pass before blood samples are drawn. Impaired response to TRH injection occurs in patients with prolactinomas although the response is too variable for this to form the basis of a diagnostic test. Imaging techniques are important, contrast-enhanced CT scanning often being used, although functioning tumours may be too small to be visualized (microadenomas).

Management

Bromocriptine is a long-acting dopamine agonist which inhibits prolactin secretion – up to 80% of prolactinomas shrink with this treatment. Pituitary irradiation or surgery is required in some patients, particularly when suprasellar extension of the tumour has occurred.

ACTH-Secreting Tumours

Tumours which secrete ACTH cause Cushing's disease. This is considered in chapter 14.

Diabetes Insipidus

Diabetes insipidus is caused by deficient production of vasopressin or occurs as a result of a failure of the renal tubules to respond to vasopressin (**Table 13.5**). Impaired vasopressin action leads to polyuria, owing to reduced water conservation by the kidney.

Cranial Diabetes Insipidus

Removal of the pituitary gland does not lead to permanent diabetes insipidus even

Table 13.5 Causes of diabetes insipidus

Cranial
◆ Tumours
Craniopharyngiomas
Pituitary tumours
Secondary tumours
◆ Granulomas
Sarcoidosis
Tuberculosis
Hand–Schuller–Christian disease
◆ Trauma
◆ Vascular
Nephrogenic
◆ Inherited
◆ Metabolic
Hypokalaemia
Hypercalcaemia
◆ Drugs
Lithium
Demeclocycline
◆ Renal disease
Pyelonephritis
Polycystic disease
Obstructive uropathy

though vasopressin is secreted by the posterior lobe. This is because the hypothalamus is unaffected and vasopressin is still synthesized. However, temporary diabetes insipidus may follow pituitary removal, head injury, or pituitary stalk section. Similarly, pituitary tumours do not cause diabetes insipidus unless suprasellar extension occurs. Craniopharyngioma is the commonest primary neoplasm while secondary tumours can cause vasopressin deficiency, the primary sites most commonly being the breast and lung. Other space-occupying hypothalamic lesions include granulomatous diseases. Associated deficiencies of anterior pituitary hormones may occur as a result of space-occupying lesions. In approximately 30% of cases of diabetes insipidus the cause is unknown.

Nephrogenic Diabetes Insipidus

Nephrogenic diabetes insipidus may be inherited, the congenital condition being a rare sex-linked disorder. Several acquired diseases cause polyuria which is resistant to the administration of vasopressin (**Table 13.5**).

Clinical Features

The main features are polyuria, polydipsia and thirst. The urine volume is usually moderately increased (up to 6 l day^{-1}) but occasionally massive volumes are passed – over 20 l per day. Loss of large volumes of urine causes the serum osmolality to rise, which stimulates the thirst mechanism; fluid loss and replacement are normally balanced and dehydration does not occur. However, dehydration can occur rapidly if fluid is restricted.

Investigation

Many causes of polyuria, such as diabetes mellitus, hypokalaemia, hypercalcaemia and chronic renal failure can be investigated by appropriate biochemical methods. The diagnosis of diabetes insipidus may be obvious from the clinical features but sometimes the condition must be differentiated from other causes of polyuria, particularly psychogenic polydipsia. Vasopressin is not measured routinely in blood but diabetes insipidus and psychogenic polydipsia can usually be differentiated by the water deprivation test (**Table 13.6**). The kidney responds in psychogenic polydipsia by increasing urinary concentration, while no such effect is seen in diabetes insipidus.

Water Deprivation Test The kidney will concentrate urine if:

1. Vasopressin secretion and action are normal.
2. There is not an excessive amount of solute being excreted.
3. Fluid intake is not excessive.
4. The rate of urea synthesis is normal.

Causes of polyuria such as diabetes mellitus should be excluded before the test is undertaken and the test should not be

Table 13.6 The water deprivation test

- The test must be closely supervised.
- A light breakfast is allowed and the test is started at 8.30 am.
- Subjects are deprived of fluids for 8 h; smoking is not allowed.
- The patient is weighed before the test and after 4, 6, 7 and 8 h.
- Urine is collected hourly, the volumes recorded and samples saved for the determination of osmolality.
- Blood is taken for osmolality measurements at the midpoint of each urine collection.
- If the patient's weight falls by more than 3% during the test, plasma osmolality is checked. Consider stopping the test.
- After 8 h water is allowed and desmopressin 2 μg is given intramuscularly.
- Urine is collected half-hourly for 2 h.

carried out in patients with hypothyroidism or Addisons's disease. In addition to a fall in urine volume, the osmolality of urine from normal subjects will increase to >600 mmol kg^{-1}, while their plasma osmolality will not increase above 300 mmol kg^{-1}. In diabetes insipidus, the volume of urine remains high and it is dilute. Plasma osmolality increases to >300 mmol kg^{-1} while urine osmolality is less than that of plasma. Failure to concentrate urine during the test confirms the diagnosis of diabetes insipidus. Concentration of urine after administration of vasopressin indicates cranial diabetes insipidus while failure to do so suggests nephrogenic

KEY POINTS

DIABETES INSIPIDUS

- Cranial diabetes insipidus results from a lack of production of vasopressin

- Nephrogenic diabetes insipidus is caused by failure of the kidneys to respond to vasopressin

- Diabetes insipidus may be differentiated from psychogenic polydipsia by the water deprivation test

diabetes insipidus. The plasma osmolality is often low at the start of the test in psychogenic polydipsia and does not increase to more than 300 mmol kg^{-1}. Occasionally, such patients have a minor degree of impairment in urinary concentration but this is not as severe as in patients with diabetes insipidus.

FURTHER READING

Bierich JR. Aetiology and pathogenesis of growth hormone deficiency. *Baillière's Clinical Endocrinology and Metabolism* 1992; **6**: 491–511

Gaillard RC. Pituitary gland emergencies. *Baillière's Clinical Endocrinology and Metabolism* 1992; **6**: 57–75

Hall R, Besser M. *Fundamentals of Clinical Endocrinology* (4th edn). Edinburgh: Churchill Livingstone, 1989

Ho KY, Evans WS, Thorner MO. Disorders of prolactin and growth hormone secretion. *Clinics in Endocrinology and Metabolism* 1985; **14**: 821–43

Robinson AG. Disorders of antidiuretic hormone secretion. *Clinics in Endocrinology and Metabolism* 1985; **14**: 55–89

Vance ML. Hypopituitarism. *New England Journal of Medicine* 1994; **330**: 1651–62

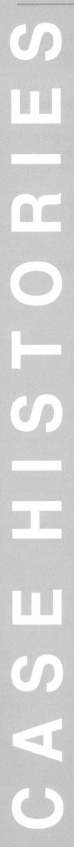

CASE 13.1

A 50-year-old woman with familial hypercholesterolaemia was evaluated in a lipid clinic. There was nothing of note in her past history, except for a premature menopause at the age of 38 years and previous investigations for coronary heart disease (CHD); these included a coronary angiogram, which was normal. On examination there was scant axillary hair. In addition to hypercholesterolaemia, investigations showed the following:

serum LH	<1 U l^{-1}
serum FSH	1.3 U l^{-1}
serum TSH	1.2 U l^{-1}

Explain these results.

CASE 13.2

A 32-year-old woman consulted her general practitioner because of galactorrhoea which persisted after she had finished breast feeding her second child 18 months previously. Menstruation was normal. Some investigations were carried out by her general practitioner including the following:

serum growth hormone	21 mU l^{-1}
serum prolactin	450 mU l^{-1}

Do these results explain her galactorrhoea?

CASE 13.3

A 42-year-old man had developed coarsening of his facial features and acromegaly was suspected. An oral glucose tolerance test was performed, during which growth hormone measurements were undertaken.

Time (min)	Glucose (mmol l^{-1})	Growth hormone (mU l^{-1})
0	6.2	48
30	7.4	56
60	8.5	52
90	9.2	65
120	8.7	53
150	7.6	48
180	6.8	49

Do these results support the diagnosis of acromegaly?

CASE 13.4

A 24-year-old man complained of thirst and increasing urine output which had been increasing over the course of several months. No glycosuria was present and blood glucose levels taken fasting and 2 h postprandially were normal. He was admitted for investigations which included a water deprivation test. After 7 h the test was stopped and vasopressin administered because of the following test results:

Time (h)	Weight (kg)	Serum osmolality (mmol kg^{-1})	Urine osmolality (mmol kg^{-1})
0	74	287	110
6	71	310	190

What do these results indicate?

THE THYROID GLAND

INTRODUCTION

The thyroid is the largest endocrine gland in the body and is located in the neck, although it originates from the floor of the pharynx. Remnants of thyroid tissue may therefore be found anywhere between the base of the tongue and the normal gland position, which is anterior and lateral to the trachea. The normal gland weighs approximately 20 g, consists of two lobes connected by a narrow isthmus and is composed of numerous functional units, follicles. Each follicle is spherical and lined with epithelial cells which surround a central space containing colloid. Follicular cells concentrate iodine and synthesize two major hormones, thyroxine (T4) and tri-iodothyronine (T3), which are stored prior to secretion in colloid. Follicles are separated by connective tissue in which are scattered C cells. These synthesize calcitonin, a hormone of uncertain function in man (see chapter 9).

HORMONE SYNTHESIS AND SECRETION

Concentration of iodine within follicular cells is required for the synthesis of thyroid hormones; this occurs by an active transport process. Iodine is oxidized by a peroxidase enzyme system and linked with tyrosine to form mono- and di-iodotyrosine within thyroglobulin. These are coupled together to form T4 and T3 (**Figure 14.1**).

Secretion of thyroid hormones is preceded by reabsorption of colloid droplets

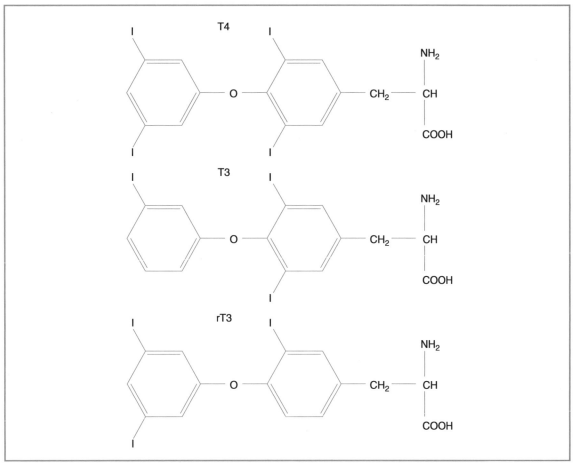

Figure 14.1 Structures of thyroid hormones. Thyroxine (T4) is the main hormone produced by the thyroid gland, while biological activity is due mostly to tri-iodothyronine (T3), which is produced largely in peripheral tissues from T4. Reverse T3 (rT3) is also produced from thyroxine by deiodination in peripheral tissues.

into follicular cells by pinocytosis (**Figure 14.2**). Within the cells, the colloid droplets fuse with lysosomes which contain proteolytic enzymes. These hydrolyse thyroglobulin, thus releasing thyroid hormones which are secreted into the circulation. Small amounts of thyroglobulin taken up by follicular cells escape hydrolysis and drain into the lymphatic system and thus enter the blood stream.

Thyroid Hormones in Blood

The concentration of T4 in blood is approximately 70 times greater than that of T3. T4 and T3 are rapidly bound to proteins in plasma following release from the gland, a very small proportion of each, less than 1%, circulating as free hormones. The metabolic activity of the hormones is determined by this free fraction, T3 being approximately four times more active than T4. Three plasma proteins bind thyroid hormones, thyroid-binding globulin (TBG), thyroid-binding prealbumin (TBPA), and albumin. Over 70% of thyroid hormones are bound to TBG, approximately 20% to albumin and the remainder to TBPA. The thyroid-binding proteins provide a readily accessible buffer of hormones to tissues and also limit losses of the low molecular weight hormones through the kidney. However, an inherited deficiency of TBG has been described where

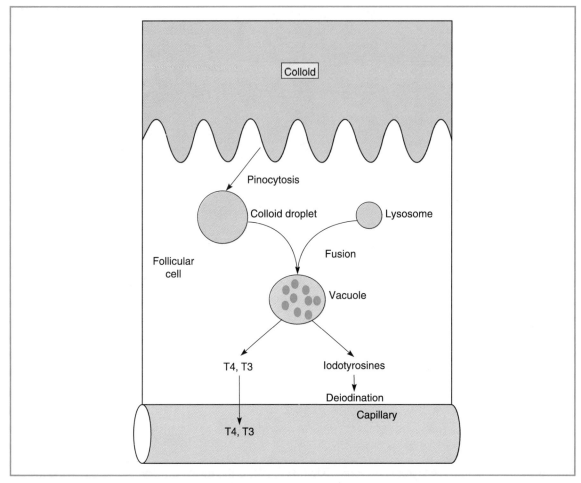

Figure 14.2 The process of thyroid hormone secretion. Colloid enters follicular cells by pinocytosis through microvilli and then fuses with lysosomes which contain proteolytic enzymes. These break down thyroglobulin, liberating thyroid hormones and iodotyrosines which have not been coupled. Thyroid hormones are released, while iodotyrosines are reutilized. T3, tri-iodothyronine; T4, thyroxine.

the subjects suffer no ill effects; thus, the protein is not essential. Causes of altered TBG levels are outlined in **Table 14.1**.

Control of Thyroid Secretion

Synthesis and release of thyroid hormones is controlled by thyroid-stimulating hormone (TSH) produced by the pituitary, the secretion of which is in turn regulated by thyrotrophin-releasing hormone (TRH) synthesized in the hypothalamus (**Figure 14.3**). There is negative feedback by the thyroid hormones mainly on TSH and also on TRH secretion. It is unclear to what extent higher centres affect TRH release.

TSH is a glycoprotein with α and β subunits, the α subunit having a similar structure to the α subunits of luteinizing hormone (LH), follicle-stimulating hormone (FSH) and human chorionic gonadotrophin (hCG), while the biological and immunological characteristics of TSH depend on the β subunits. In addition to regulation by TRH, TSH synthesis is inhibited by dopamine and somatostatin. TSH acts by binding to specific receptors on follicular cells, leading

Table 14.1 Causes of altered thyroid-binding globulin concentrations

Increased
- ◆ Genetic
- ◆ Neonatal
- ◆ Pregnancy
- ◆ Drug therapy
  Oestrogens and oral contraceptives
  Phenothiazines

Decreased
- ◆ Genetic
- ◆ Protein-losing states
- ◆ Endocrine disease
  Acromegaly
  Cushing's disease
- ◆ Drug therapy
  Anabolic steroids, androgens
  Phenytoin
  Glucocorticoids

LABORATORY ASSESSMENT OF THYROID FUNCTION

Total Thyroxine and Free Thyroxine Index

to activation of intracellular adenylate cyclase and protein kinases.

Biological Effects of Thyroid Hormones

Some di-iodotyrosine is released from the thyroid gland although biological activity is due to T4 and T3. Free hormones enter cells in peripheral tissues where the effect of T4 appears to result from its conversion to T3. Some T4 is converted to reverse T3 (rT3) although this is inactive. The conversion to rT3 increases under some circumstances, particularly in severe nonthyroidal illness (see below). Receptors for thyroid hormones are found in nuclei, the binding of T3 leading to transcription of messenger RNA coding for proteins which regulate cellular metabolism.

Thyroid hormones are essential for normal growth and development, dwarfism being a feature of congenital thyroid deficiency, cretinism. They increase the turnover of carbohydrates, lipids and proteins, and the rate of oxygen consumption.

The concentrations of T4 found in the serum of normal adults are 54–142 nmol l^{-1}; higher values are found in neonates. The concentration of total T4 in blood generally discriminates well between euthyroid patients and those with abnormal thyroid function. However, discrepancies between measured T4 and thyroid status may occur as a result of changes in the concentrations of binding proteins (**Table 14.1**). Increases or decreases in these cause corresponding changes in the serum total T4 concentration without any variation occurring in the level of free, physiologically active hormone. Thus, serum total T4 levels may be misleading and concentrations of the free hormone are more useful.

One approach to this is to calculate a free thyroxine index (FTI) which reflects free T4 (fT4). This involves a second measurement which estimates the unoccupied T4 binding sites present in the patient's serum, the test being based on the principle that the number of TBG binding sites occupied by T4 is proportional to the amount of fT4 present. This procedure corrects T4 for changes in TBG, although misleading results can still occur and the FTI is less

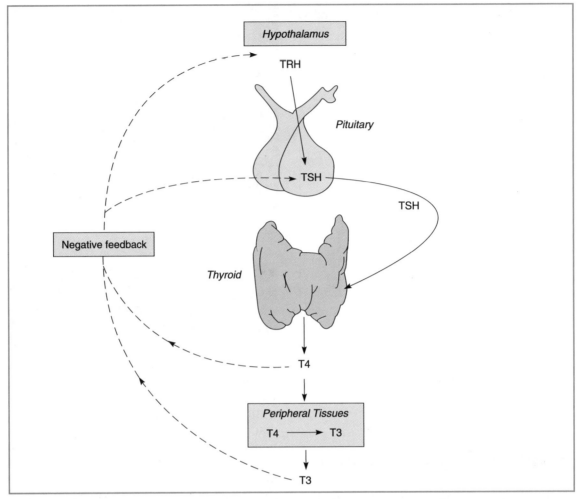

Figure 14.3 The control of thyroid hormone secretion. Thyrotrophin-releasing hormone (TRH) secreted by the hypothalamus stimulates thyroid-stimulating hormone (TSH) production by the pituitary which, in turn, stimulates the synthesis and secretion of thyroxine (T4) by the thyroid. The main active thyroid hormone, tri-iodothyronine (T3), is produced mostly by deiodination of T4 in peripheral tissues. Both T4 and T3 control the release mainly of TSH by negative feedback (dashed arrows).

sensitive than free hormone measurements. Early techniques for free hormone measurement were indirect and rather cumbersome but direct, extremely sensitive immunoassays have since been introduced.

Free Thyroxine

Measurements of fT4 are not affected by variations in TBG and therefore discriminate more reliably than total T4 between normal and abnormal thyroid function when there are abnormalities of TBG. Some fT4 methods

give low results in patients with hypoalbuminaemia or severe nonthyroidal illnesses such as liver disease or cardiac failure, although newer methods are less susceptible to these problems. The levels of fT4 found in healthy subjects are 12–28 pmol l^{-1}.

Tri-iodothyronine

Free and total T3 measurements discriminate well between hyperthyroid and euthyroid patients in patients who are otherwise healthy, although free T3 concentrations are affected by low serum albumin levels. Both T4 and T3 levels are raised in most patients with overt hyperthyroidism although occasional thyrotoxic patients have a normal T4 while the T3 is elevated (T3 toxicosis). The investigation is of little value in the diagnosis of hypothyroidism. The reference range is 3–9 pmol l^{-1}.

Thyroid-Stimulating Hormone

The diurnal variation of TSH secretion is small, in contrast to some pituitary hormones, and therefore the time of blood sampling for analysis is not critical. Serum TSH measurement is a sensitive indicator of primary thyroid failure, as reduced synthesis of thyroid hormones decreases negative feedback on the pituitary gland, thus increasing TSH levels. These are sufficient to increase synthesis of thyroid hormones in compensated hypothyroidism and the clinical features of hypothyroidism do not occur. Secretion of TSH is suppressed in hyperthyroidism but early measurement techniques used in clinical practice were not sensitive enough to detect these low levels, and so additional dynamic tests of thyroid function, such as the TRH test, were used. However, extremely sensitive methods for TSH estimation are now available which can quantify the very low levels that occur in hyperthyroidism and discriminate these from the concentrations found in normal subjects. As serum TSH can differentiate between most subjects with hypothyroidism, hyperthyroidism and normal subjects many laboratories now use serum TSH as the first line of investigation in the assessment of thyroid dysfunction. However, values may be abnormal in conditions other than hyper- and hypo-thyroidism (**Table 14.2**) and thus the finding of altered TSH concentrations may require further investigation. Free T4 is helpful in differentiating the causes of abnormal TSH levels (**Figure 14.4**). The reference range for serum TSH is 0.15–3.0 mU l^{-1}.

Table 14.2 Causes of changes in serum thyroid-stimulating hormone (TSH) concentrations

Increased
◆ Hypothyroidism
◆ Drugs (amiodorone, lithium)

Decreased
◆ Hyperthyroidism
◆ Pituitary failure
◆ Nonthyroidal illness
◆ Treated hyperthyroidism
◆ Early pregnancy

Neonates are screened for cretinism in some countries by measuring TSH using blood spots collected by heelprick and dried onto filter paper; these are collected in screening programmes for phenylketonuria. Values are usually very high in cretinism and fewer false-positive results occur than with thyroxine measurement.

Thyrotrophin-Releasing Hormone Test

This test involves collecting blood for TSH analysis, following which 200 mg TRH is injected intravenously and further blood samples are taken for TSH 20 min and 60 min following injection. Some patients experience nausea, dizziness and flushing following the injection but this passes rapidly. In normal subjects the serum TSH value increases by >2 mU l^{-1}, a rise of <1 mU l^{-1} is an absent response and an increase >20 mU l^{-1} is an exaggerated response. In a delayed response the 60-min value is greater than the 20-min value.

Previously, this investigation has been used widely in the diagnosis of thyrotoxicosis when other tests of thyroid function gave equivocal results. However, sensitive TSH measurements have now replaced widespread use of the TRH test in this way, and it is now used mostly for the investigation of hypothalamic or pituitary

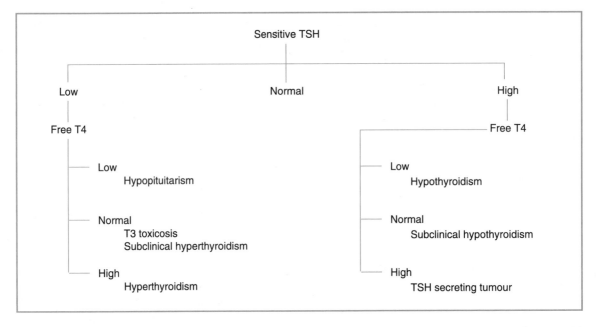

Sensitive TSH

Low — Normal — High

Low — Free T4

Low
Hypopituitarism

Normal
T3 toxicosis
Subclinical hyperthyroidism

High
Hyperthyroidism

High — Free T4

Low
Hypothyroidism

Normal
Subclinical hypothyroidism

High
TSH secreting tumour

Figure 14.4 Suggested scheme for the interpretation of biochemical thyroid function tests. TSH, thyroid-stimulating hormone; T3, tri-iodothyronine; T4, thyroxine.

disease. In pituitary disease causing hypothyroidism there is usually little TSH secretion in response to TRH administration, while in hypothalamic disease there may be a delayed response. The TRH test can be administered together with insulin and gonadotrophin-releasing hormone (Gn-RH) in the combined test of pituitary function.

Other Investigations

Isotope Uptake
Scanning of the thyroid following administration of an isotope taken up by the gland, most often technetium-99m pertechnetate (^{99m}Tc) given by intravenous injection, will differentiate areas that are active from those that are nonfunctioning. Areas that do not take up isotope may be malignant, contain a cyst or may be suppressed by autonomous nodules. Patchy uptake occurs in a multinodular gland while diffuse uptake occurs in Graves' disease. Scanning can also identify ectopic thyroid tissue.

Thyroid Autoantibodies
Antimicrosomal and antithyroglobulin antibodies are present in high titres in most patients with Hashimoto's disease, although low titres of these antibodies occur in some apparently normal individuals. The antibodies are directed against thyroid cell components. Thyroid-stimulating immunoglobulins (antibodies) which are directed against the TSH receptor or closely related sites occur in many patients with Graves' disease. Interaction of antibodies with these sites often leads to cell stimulation.

KEY POINTS

THYROID FUNCTION TESTS

- Concentrations of total serum thyroid hormones may be changed by altered levels of binding proteins

- The first line investigation of thyroid function is serum TSH concentration

- Serum fT4 levels are useful in interpreting abnormal TSH concentrations

DISORDERS OF THYROID FUNCTION

Hypothyroidism

Causes

Hypothyroidism from birth leads to cretinism and developmental abnormalities, while severe hypothyroidism in adults causes myxoedema. The major causes of hypothyroidism are shown in **Table 14.3**. Over 95% of cases are caused by primary thyroid disease, while less than 5% are suprathyroid in origin. The commonest cause in Western countries is autoimmune thyroiditis (Hashimoto's disease) in which progressive destruction of hormone-secreting tissue occurs. Antithyroid therapy, either with drugs or surgery, and neonatal hypothyroidism are also relatively common causes. Goitre predominates in areas where iodine deficiency is endemic.

Clinical Features

Hypothyroidism is more common in women than men and most patients present between the ages of 30 and 60 years. The clinical presentation is variable, gross hormone deficiency sometimes being associated with minor clinical features. In overt hypothyroidism there is weight gain, hoarseness of the voice and slow speech, lack of energy, thickening of facial features as a result of accumulation of mucopolysaccharides in the dermis, sensitivity to the cold and dryness of the skin and hair. Prolongation of the relaxation phase of deep tendon reflexes may be found. Depressive disorders or paranoid or agitated states may occur. Very rarely coma complicates myxoedema. Patients often complain of symptoms due to carpal tunnel syndrome and muscle cramps. The heart size may be increased, hypertrophy, pericardial effusions and dilatation being contributory causes. Menstrual disturbances and infertility are common in women. Laboratory investigations often show hypercholesterolaemia, increased serum creatine kinase activities and macrocytic anaemia. Mild or nonspecific features often occur in patients with mild hypothyroidism, particularly cold intolerance, lack of energy and puffiness around the eyes. Clinical features are seen rarely in hypothyroidism secondary to hypopituitarism.

Investigation

The serum TSH concentration is elevated in primary thyroid disease, including subclinical hypothyroidism, and reduced in hypothyroidism secondary to hypothalamic or pituitary disease. Thyroid failure is excluded if the level is normal. Serum fT4 is reduced in overt hypothyroidism and is normal in subclinical hypothyroidism; it may be normal in mild hypothyroidism. Thyroid autoantibodies may indicate the cause, high titres occurring in autoimmune thyroiditis.

Management

Thyroid deficiency is usually treated by giving thyroxine, small doses being administered initially (50 μg daily), these being increased after several weeks if necessary. The mean replacement dose is 150 μg daily. Effective treatment suppresses elevations of serum TSH to within the normal reference range, while excessive replacement reduces TSH levels to below normal.

Table 14.3 Causes of hypothyroidism

Primary hypothyroidism
◆ Developmental and inherited abnormalities
◆ Autoimmune thyroiditis (Hashimoto's disease)
◆ Postsurgery
◆ Antithyroid drugs
◆ Endemic goitre
Secondary hypothyroidism
◆ Pituitary disease
◆ Hypothalamic disease

HYPOTHYROIDISM

- Hypothyroidism leads to cretinism in infants and myxoedema in adults

- The commonest cause of hypothyroidism in adults is Hashimoto's disease

- Serum TSH concentrations are elevated in primary hypothyroidism

Thyroid Function in Nonthyroidal Illness

Severe illness, stress, or trauma may cause changes in thyroid hormone metabolism. Conditions producing such changes include myocardial infarction, liver disease, diabetes mellitus, surgery, and fever. Serum levels of total T4 are usually reduced largely, but not entirely, due to reductions in concentrations of binding proteins. Reduced peripheral conversion of T4 to T3 also occurs, deiodination of T4 leading to increased synthesis of inactive rT3. Serum levels of TSH may be reduced. It is important to be aware that many conditions may cause abnormalities in thyroid function tests and to restrict such investigations in the presence of severe illness.

Hyperthyroidism

Causes

The term thyrotoxicosis refers to the clinical and biochemical features which result from excessive thyroid hormone production. The main causes of hyperthyroidism are outlined in **Table 14.4**. The most frequent cause in Western countries is Graves' disease. This is caused by antibodies to TSH receptors in the thyroid which mimic the effect of TSH, leading to stimulation of the gland, hyperplasia, hypertrophy and thus diffuse thyroid enlargement. Excessive amounts of thyroid

Table 14.4 Causes of hyperthyroidism

Graves' disease
Toxic multinodular goitre
Toxic adenoma
Thyroiditis

hormones are secreted, producing the clinical features of hyperthyroidism.

Clinical Features

Graves' disease affects women more frequently than men, the peak incidence being in the third and fourth decades. Clinical features include weight loss, increased appetite, tiredness, irritability, insomnia, heat intolerance, tachycardia and palpitations, atrial fibrillation in the elderly, and muscle weakness. Many of these features are due directly to increased thyroid hormone levels, while others appear to result from increased sympathetic activity, symptomatic improvement occurring with the use of β-adrenergic blocking drugs such as propanolol. Changes may occur in the eye, including lid retraction and exophthalmos. The pathogenesis of these changes is unclear although one possibility is the production of antibodies directed against antigens in the extraocular muscles.

Investigation

Serum levels of TSH are suppressed and these can be differentiated from normal values using sensitive assays. Very rarely, thyrotoxicosis may be due to a TSH-secreting tumour. The serum fT4 concentration is usually raised although this is normal in approximately 5% of cases, the T3 level being increased (T3 toxicosis). The TRH test shows a lack of response of serum TSH to TRH injection. Thyroid antibodies are useful in investigating the cause of hyperthyroidism.

Management

Thyrotoxicosis is treated by antithyroid drugs, partial thyroidectomy or radioactive iodine. Carbimazole inhibits the synthesis of hormones within the gland, while propylthiouracil also reduces the peripheral conversion of T4 to T3. The serum fT4 levels fall rapidly with successful treatment, although serum levels of TSH often remain suppressed for several months. Relapses are common in patients with Graves' disease treated with antithyroid drugs, while the risk of hypothyroidism is high with radioactive iodine treatment. Long-term follow-up is essential to detect relapses or hypothyroidism regardless of form of therapy used; biochemical monitoring includes fT4 and TSH measurements.

KEY POINTS

HYPERTHYROIDISM

■ The commonest cause of hyperthyroidism is Graves' disease

■ Serum TSH concentrations are suppressed

■ The fT4 levels are raised in 95% of cases while increases in fT3 concentrations only occur in 5%

Goitre

A goitre is an enlargement of the thyroid gland. Some cases are caused by inadequate thyroid hormone secretion which leads to increased TSH production, resulting in thyroid enlargement. This compensates for hormone deficiency in some but not all cases. Thyroiditis may also lead to gland enlargement and can also cause thyrotoxicosis. Goitre also results from thyroid tumours and can occur for no obvious cause and with no functional abnormality (nontoxic goitre). Thus patients with goitre may be hypothyroid, euthyroid or hyperthyroid.

FURTHER READING

Brent GA. The molecular basis of thyroid hormone action. *New England Journal of Medicine* 1994; **331**: 847–53

Hall R, Besser M. Chapter 5. *Fundamentals of Clinical Endocrinology*. Edinburgh: Churchill Livingstone, 1989

John R. Screening for congenital hypothyroidism. *Annals of Clinical Biochemistry* 1987; **24**: 1–13

Nicoloff JT, Spencer CA. The use and misuse of sensitive thyrotropin assays. *Journal of Clinical Endocrinology and Metabolism* 1990; **71**: 553–8

Toft AD. Thyroxine therapy. *New England Journal of Medicine* 1994; **331**: 174–80

Toft AD (ed.). Hyperthyroidism. *Clinics in Endocrinology and Metabolism* 1985; **14**: 299–511

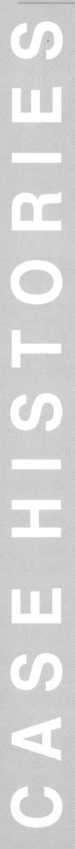

CASE 14.1

A 54-year-old woman was referred to a lipid clinic because of hypercholesterolaemia which persisted at levels between 8.2 and 9.5 mmol l^{-1}, despite following appropriate dietary advice. Among investigations to establish whether there was a secondary cause for hypercholesterolaemia thyroid function tests were undertaken.

serum TSH   17.4 mU l^{-1}
serum free T4   13 pmol l^{-1}

Comment on her thyroid function.

CASE 14.2

A 48-year-old woman complained to her general practitioner of palpitations. Upon questioning she admitted that she was also intolerant of heat and thyrotoxicosis was suspected. However, T4 concentration was normal and she was therefore referred to an endocrine clinic for further evaluation. The following were her thyroid function test results.

serum TSH   <0.1 mU l^{-1}
serum free T4   17 pmol l^{-1}

Has thyrotoxicosis been eliminated?

CASE 14.3

A 56-year-old woman receiving treatment with thyroxine for hypothyroidism was seen on four occasions at follow up with the following thyroid function test results. The dose of thyroxine had not been changed during these visits.

Visit	TSH (mU l^{-1})	Free T4 (pmol l^{-1})
1	13	21
2	8	14
3	4	17
4	12	21

Can you explain these results?

15

THE ADRENAL CORTEX

INTRODUCTION

The adrenal glands are situated retroperitoneally at the upper pole of each kidney. The adrenals consist of two distinct areas, an outer cortex, which is derived from mesoderm and synthesizes steroid hormones, and the inner medulla, which is derived from ectoderm and synthesizes catecholamines. This chapter considers disorders of the adrenal cortex, the medulla being considered in chapter 17. The adrenal cortex consists of three zones, an outer zona glomerulosa, the zona fasciculata and the inner zona reticularis. Glucocorticoids and adrenal androgens are synthesized in the two inner layers while the zona glomerulosa produces aldosterone.

ADRENOCORTICAL HORMONES

Biosynthesis

A large number of different steroid hormones have been isolated from the adrenal cortex, some in very small amounts. The principal glucocorticoid is cortisol, although significant amounts of corticosterone are also synthesized. Aldosterone is the major mineralocorticoid while the most important androgens are dehydroepiandrosterone, androstenedione and testosterone. Small amounts of oestrogens and progestagens are also produced. All are synthesized from cholesterol, a 27-carbon steroid, by removal of carbon side-chains; progestagens, glucocorticoids and mineralocorticoids have 21 carbon atoms, androgens 19 carbon atoms

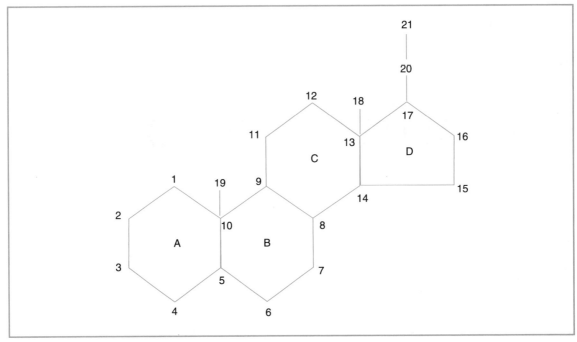

Figure 15.1 The nomenclature for numbering adrenal steroids. Each ring of the steroid nucleus is designated by a letter and each carbon atom by a number. Adrenal steroid have 21 carbon atoms (cortisol, aldosterone) or 19 carbon atoms (androgens). The side chain on the D ring is removed in the synthesis of androgens.

and oestrogens 18 carbon atoms. The nomenclature for numbering adrenal steroids is outlined in **Figure 15.1** and an overview of the biosynthetic pathways leading to adrenal steroid synthesis is shown in **Figure 15.2**.

Transport

There are two cortisol-binding proteins in plasma, a specific binding protein, transcortin (cortisol-binding globulin), and albumin. Transcortin has a high affinity but low capacity for binding cortisol, while albumin has a lower affinity. Over 95% of cortisol in blood is protein-bound under normal circumstances, the physiologically active fraction being the free hormone. The binding capacity of transcortin in normal subjects is approximately 700 nmol l^{-1} cortisol and when this concentration is exceeded part of the excess is bound to albumin and a greater proportion circulates as the free hormone. The concentration of transcortin increases in pregnancy and with oestrogen therapy, including the contraceptive pill; levels decrease in chronic liver disease. Circulating aldosterone is not bound to cortisol-binding globulin; however, approximately 60% is bound to albumin. Like other sex hormones adrenal androgens and oestrogens are transported bound mainly to sex hormone-binding globulin, with a small amount being albumin bound.

KEY POINTS

ADRENAL STEROIDS

- Cortisol is the principal glucocorticoid hormone produced by the adrenal while aldosterone is the principal mineralocorticoid hormone

- Androgens, oestrogens and progestogens are produced by the adrenal

- Adrenal steroids are predominantly protein bound in plasma, either to specific globulins or albumin

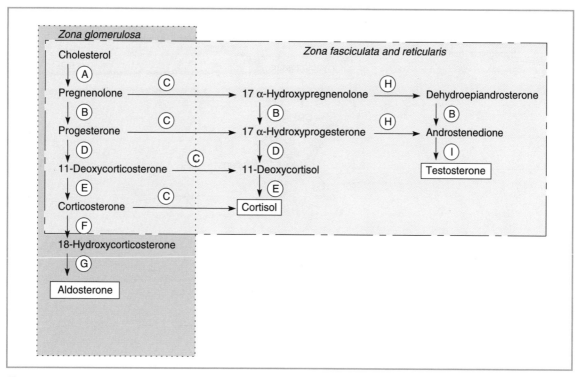

Figure 15.2 Outline of the biosynthesis of adrenal steroids. Enzymes involved in the process are designated by letters (A, cholesterol desmolase; B, 3β-hydroxysteroid dehydrogenase; C, 17α-hydroxylase; D, 21-hydroxylase; E, 11β-hydroxylase; F, 18-hydroxylase; G, 18-dehydrogenase; H, 17,20 desmolase; I, 17β-hydroxysteroid dehydrogenase). The details of oestrogen synthesis have been omitted; they are produced from androgens. The conversions which take place in the zona glomerulosa are outlined in the dotted box while the dashed box includes the conversions which occur in the zona fasciculata and the zona reticularis.

Control of Secretion

Cortisol Secretion

The control of cortisol secretion is outlined in **Figure 15.3**. Cortisol production is controlled mainly by adrenocorticotrophic hormone (ACTH) which is produced in basophil cells in the anterior pituitary. The major control on ACTH secretion is exerted by corticotrophin-releasing factor (CRF), which is produced in the hypothalamus. Cortisol exerts negative feedback inhibition on both ACTH and CRF secretion. There is marked circadian variation in the secretion of CRF, ACTH and cortisol, levels being greatest about the time of waking and lowest in the late evening. If a different sleeping pattern is adopted, as in night workers, the pattern of

hormone secretion changes accordingly. Stressful stimuli increase cortisol secretion through the release of CRF, these including pyrogens, surgery, hypoglycaemia, trauma, anxiety and exercise. The effect of stress overrides the normal circadian rhythm.

Aldosterone Secretion

The major controlling mechanism of aldosterone secretion is the renin–angiotensin system (**Figure 15.4**). Renin is secreted by the juxtaglomerular apparatus in the kidney which is sensitive to changes in both blood pressure and sodium concentration; hypotension and sodium loss stimulate secretion. Renin is a proteolytic enzyme and acts on angiotensinogen, which is produced in the liver, to produce angiotensin I. This is

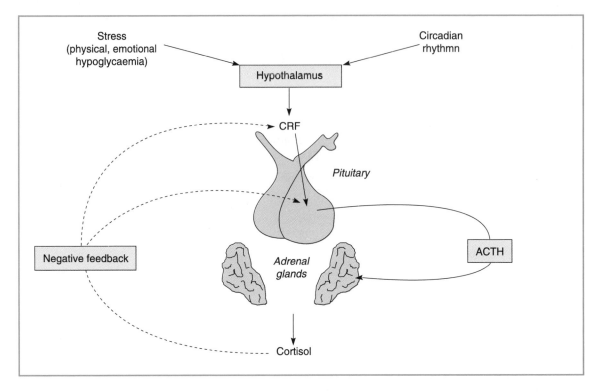

Figure 15.3 The hypothalamic–pituitary–adrenal axis and its role in the regulation of cortisol secretion. Positive stimulation is shown by solid arrows and negative feedback inhibition by dashed arrows. The release of adrenocorticotrophic hormone (ACTH), which stimulates cortisol secretion, is controlled by corticotrophin-releasing hormone (CRF). The secretion of CRF by the hypothalamus is regulated by negative feedback from cortisol and also by higher centres.

converted to angiotensin II by angiotensin-converting enzyme which is synthesized mainly in the lungs and also in vascular endothelium. Angiotensin II is a powerful vasocontrictor and also acts on the zona glomerulosa of the adrenal to produce aldosterone. Other factors controlling renin secretion include the sympathetic nervous system and potassium. The sympathetic nervous system increases renin secretion when the upright posture is adopted and high plasma potassium levels inhibit secretion. Aldosterone secretion is stimulated, to some extent, by ACTH, although this is an acute effect and not sustained for more than a few hours.

Androgen Secretion

The secretion of adrenal androgens is controlled by ACTH, not gonadotrophins.

KEY POINTS

CONTROL OF ADRENAL STEROID SECRETION

- The synthesis of cortisol is regulated by the hypothalamic–pituitary–adrenal axis

- The regulation of aldosterone synthesis is controlled mainly by the renin–angiotensin system

- Renal gonadal steroid synthesis is regulated by ACTH, not gonadotrophins

Biological Effects of Adrenal Steroids

Adrenal steroids enter cells by diffusion and bind to cytoplasmic receptors, forming

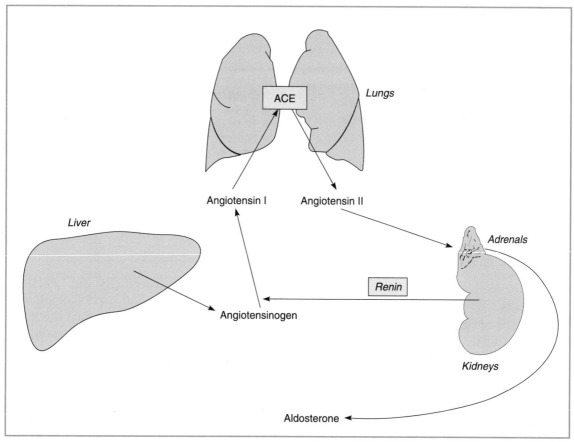

Figure 15.4 The control of aldosterone secretion. Angiotensinogen is synthesized by the liver and is converted to angiotensin I by renin, the secretion of which is stimulated by hypotension and sodium depletion. Angiotensin I is converted to angiotensin II by angiotensin-converting enzyme which is found mainly in the lungs. Angiotensin II has a direct pressor effect and also stimulates the secretion of aldosterone which promotes sodium retention.

complexes which are transferred to the nucleus where they induce synthesis of ribonucleic acid (RNA) and thus regulatory proteins.

Cortisol

Cortisol has significant effects on energy metabolism. It antagonizes the effect of insulin, enhancing gluconeogenesis, promotes the deposition of fat with a central distribution, and increases catabolism of proteins. Other actions include anti-inflammatory properties and increasing the number of circulating polymorphonuclear leukocytes, although lymphocyte levels are decreased. Glucocorticoids have weak

mineralocorticoid properties, increasing renal tubular sodium reabsorption and increasing potassium excretion. They antagonize the effect of vasopressin on the renal tubule, enhancing water excretion.

Aldosterone

Aldosterone increases sodium reabsorption in the distal convoluted tubule of the kidney by an exchange mechanism in which potassium and hydrogen ions are excreted. This is not a direct exchange mechanism but rather one in which sodium transport affects transmembrane potential, thus enhancing the flow into the lumen of positively charged ions which are present in high concentrations within the tubular cell. Aldosterone also stimulates sodium transport in the salivary glands, sweat glands and in the gastrointestinal tract. It is the principal mineralocorticoid in healthy subjects, although there are small contributions to this activity from cortisol and corticosterone.

Androgens

Adrenal androgens have very little virilizing effect when secreted in normal amounts, although they have a masculinizing effect when secreted in excess in women, and produce precocious development of secondary sexual characteristics in prepubertal boys.

Oestrogens

The amount of oestrogens produced by the normal adrenals is too small to have a biological effect, although oestrogen-secreting adrenal tumours may occur rarely and produce pathological effects by excess secretion. Patients with oestrogen-dependent breast carcinomas may improve after adrenalectomy or with suppression of ACTH secretion.

KEY POINTS

ADRENAL STEROID ACTION

- Cortisol is an insulin antagonist and promotes the central deposition of fat

- Cortisol has a weak mineralocorticoid action

- Aldosterone stimulates transmembrane transport of sodium in the salivary glands, skin, and gut, in addition to the kidney

---

ASSESSMENT OF ADRENAL FUNCTION

Serum Cortisol

Serum cortisol is usually measured by radioimmunoassay using antibodies with a

Table 15.1 Causes of elevated serum cortisol concentrations

Increased cortisol secretion
◆ Cushing's syndrome
◆ Exercise
◆ Meals
◆ Stress
◆ Anxiety, depression
◆ Obesity
◆ Alcohol abuse
◆ Chronic renal failure
Increased cortisol binding globulin
◆ Congenital
◆ Oestrogen therapy
◆ Pregnancy

high degree of specificity for cortisol, although prednisone and prednisolone may interfere with the assay. Standard times for specimen collection have been adopted because of circadian variation in secretion, 08.00–09.00 hours being the period of maximum, and 22.00–24.00 hours being the period of minimum secretion. Stress during specimen collection may increase levels and the use of an indwelling cannula is sometimes necessary to avoid this. The concentration of serum cortisol is reduced in hypoadrenalism and the causes of elevated serum cortisol concentrations are outlined in **Table 15.1**. The pattern of cortisol secretion is important in addition to the amount secreted, the normal circadian pattern often being lost in Cushing's syndrome.

Urinary Cortisol

Cortisol is metabolized mainly in the liver; products including 17-hydroxysteroids are formed which retain some glucocorticoid activity and are excreted in the urine. A small amount of cortisol is excreted unchanged, this being related to concentration of free cortisol in serum and to the rate of adrenal secretion. The measurement of cortisol in a 24-h urine collection is a sensitive test of excess cortisol secretion, although the test discriminates poorly between normal and reduced secretion.

Plasma ACTH

Plasma ACTH concentration is an important investigation in the assessment of adrenal function. Elevated levels are seen in Addison's disease as a result of a failure of the normal negative feedback effect of adrenal hormones, while levels are low in adrenal insufficiency due to hypothalamic or pituitary disease. Levels are suppressed in Cushing's syndrome if caused by an adrenal tumour or exogenous steroid administration, while levels are modestly elevated by ACTH-producing pituitary tumours. Concentrations are usually markedly elevated in ectopic ACTH secretion.

Aldosterone

Aldosterone measurements are undertaken most often in the investigation of primary hyperaldosteronism. Since aldosterone secretion is affected by posture, levels are usually measured in the morning after overnight recumbency, and also after adopting the upright posture. Specimens must be collected under carefully controlled conditions: diuretic and antihypertensive therapy should be withdrawn 4–6 weeks before investigation, and adequate sodium intake is necessary. Renin concentration is usually measured simultaneously as plasma renin activity, this being the amount of angiotensin I generated by plasma.

Adrenal Androgens

Methods are available for the measurement of several adrenal androgens including dehydroepiandrosterone (DHEA), dehydroepiandrosterone sulphate (DHEA-S) and androstenedione. These are of value in the investigation of congenital adrenal hyperplasia and hirsuitism in women.

Urinary Steroid Profiles

Chromatographic techniques, particularly gas–liquid and high-performance liquid chromatography, allow the simultaneous estimation of many steroids, together with their metabolites. Using these, it is possible to obtain a profile of steroid excretion which may be valuable in the investigation of inherited defects of adrenal steroid synthesis, particularly congenital adrenal hyperplasia.

Dynamic Function Tests

Although measurements of hormone levels are essential in investigating suspected adrenocortical disease their sensitivity is limited because they may not detect minor degrees of dysfunction and are affected by factors such as stress. To overcome these difficulties dynamic function tests are often used, these having the additional advantage that they often give some indication of the cause of dysfunction. Some are suitable for outpatients while others are performed best on inpatients.

Dexamethasone Suppression Tests

Dexamethasone is a potent synthetic steroid which, by negative feedback, suppresses secretion of CRF and thus ACTH and cortisol. Dexamethasone does not interfere with cortisol measurement.

Overnight Suppression Test An overnight suppression test is often used as an outpatient screening test. Dexamethasone (1 mg) is given at bedtime and the patient attends for a blood test the following morning at 09.00 hours, the serum cortisol concentration normally being less than 100 nmol l^{-1}. The value is usually greater than this in Cushing's syndrome, although false-positive results can occur. The serum cortisol level fails to suppress in approximately 15% of patients with obesity and also in a number of other conditions including alcohol abuse, recent acute illness, anxiety and depression.

Two-Day Low-Dose Dexamethasone Suppression Test Dexamethasone (0.5 mg) is taken 6-hourly for 2 days, and serum cortisol is then measured. The criterion for a positive result is the same as for the overnight test, the number of false-positive results in obesity being lower.

High-Dose Dexamethasone Suppression Test The procedure is similar to the 2-day low dose test except that 2 mg of the drug is given 6-hourly. The test is used in the differential diagnosis of Cushing's syndrome, suppression of serum cortisol by >50% being characteristic of pituitary-dependent Cushing's syndrome, while suppression does not occur in adrenal tumours or ectopic ACTH production.

Insulin Tolerance Test

The insulin tolerance test is outlined in chapter 13. A normal response indicates an intact hypothalamic–pituitary–adrenal axis and rules out adrenal insufficiency or impaired pituitary reserve. Because of the risk of hypoglycaemia and the greater inconvenience of the procedure, many endocrinologists now use the short synacthen test for the initial investigation of the hypothalamic–pituitary–adrenal axis.

ACTH Stimulation Tests

The administration of ACTH allows the assessment of adrenocortical reserve. Synacthen is a synthetic analogue of ACTH which is as potent as the native hormone but causes fewer allergic reactions.

Short ACTH Stimulation (Synacthen) Test This investigation, which does not require fasting and can be carried out at any time, is performed by injecting 250 μg synacthen intramuscularly. Serum cortisol is measured before and at 30 and 60 min after injection. The basal level should be >150 nmol l^{-1}, stimulated levels should exceed 550 nmol l^{-1}

and the increment should be >200 nmol l^{-1}. An impaired response is occasionally found in normal subjects although a normal response excludes Addison's disease. The test does not differentiate between Addison's disease, secondary adrenocortical insufficiency or suppression of the adrenal by exogenous steroids.

Prolonged ACTH Stimulation Test This investigation is carried out in patients who have failed to respond to the short synacthen test and is also used to differentiate between primary and secondary adrenocortical insufficiency. Serum cortisol concentration is measured before and after the intramuscular injection of a depot preparation of synacthen (1 mg), values rising during the test in secondary adrenocortical insufficiency owing to the response of the adrenal to stimulation. No such response is seen in Addison's disease. This investigation is performed infrequently, as plasma ACTH levels usually differentiate between primary and secondary adrenal failure.

CRF Stimulation Test

Increased secretion of ACTH and cortisol following the injection of CRF is seen in pituitary-dependent Cushing's syndrome, while there is little or no response in patients with ectopic ACTH production or an adrenal tumour.

DISORDERS OF ADRENAL FUNCTION
Adrenocortical Insufficiency

Adrenocortical insufficiency may result from a primary disease of the adrenals (Addison's disease) or secondary to a failure of ACTH production.

Addison's Disease

Causes Addison's disease results from destruction of the adrenal cortex (**Table 15.2**) and deficiency of both glucocorticoids and mineralocorticoids occurs. Addison's

Table 15.2 Causes of Addison's disease

Autoimmune disease
Infections
◆ Tuberculosis
◆ Viral (AIDS)
◆ Meningococcus
Bilateral secondary carcinoma
Congenital adrenal hyperplasia

AIDS, acquired immune deficiency syndrome.

disease is caused most commonly by auto-immune disease which sometimes occurs in association with autoimmune disease affecting other organs, particularly the thyroid; the incidence of diabetes mellitus, pernicious anaemia and ovarian failure also increases.

Clinical Features The onset of disease is usually insidious with tiredness, weakness, anorexia, nausea, apathy and ill-defined abdominal pain. Hyperpigmentation is a characteristic but not inevitable finding, this being caused by increased pituitary secretion of ACTH and β-lipotrophin. Increased production of pituitary hormones occurs because of reduced negative feedback of cortisol, ACTH and β-lipotrophin being derived from the same precursor molecule (see chapter 13). Hypoglycaemia occurs frequently due to a reduction in the antagonistic effect of cortisol on insulin action. Postural hypotension is often found, this being due to sodium and fluid depletion as a result of mineralocorticoid deficiency. Acute adrenocortical insufficiency may occur as the initial presentation of Addison's disease or in patients with chronic features who suffer an acute stress. Volume depletion, anorexia, nausea and vomiting may be severe and patients may be shocked; abdominal pain is frequent. Hyperpigmentation may be absent if the disease is of acute onset.

Secondary Adrenal Insufficiency

Hyperpigmentation does not occur in adrenocortical insufficiency secondary to loss of pituitary secretions. Although an acute clinical presentation is sometimes seen, chronic features are more common. Aldosterone secretion is preserved as this is not dependent on ACTH and therefore the electrolyte abnormalities seen in Addison's disease are absent (see below).

Investigation of Adrenocortical Insufficiency

The plasma sodium concentration is typically reduced, together with the serum total CO_2, while plasma potassium levels are elevated; these findings result from reduced mineralocorticoid action. Plasma urea concentrations are often elevated. In severe cases the morning cortisol levels are often reduced; in milder cases they may fall within the normal range, although serum cortisol concentrations do not increase in response to ACTH stimulation (short synacthen test). Primary and secondary causes of adrenocortical insufficiency may be differentiated using the prolonged ACTH stimulation test or plasma ACTH levels, these being elevated in Addison's disease and reduced in pituitary or hypothalamic disease.

Management of Adrenocortical Insufficiency

Patients with Addison's disease require permanent replacement therapy with glucocorticoids and mineralocorticoids, the requirements for these increasing during intercurrent illnesses and stresses such as trauma or operation.

KEY POINTS

ADRENOCORTICAL INSUFFICIENCY

■ Addison's disease (primary adrenocortical insufficiency) is caused most commonly by autoimmune destruction of the adrenal glands

■ The secretion of both cortisol and aldosterone is impaired in Addison's disease

■ Aldosterone secretion is maintained in secondary adrenocortical insufficiency

Table 15.3 Causes of Cushing's syndrome

Pituitary-dependent (Cushing's disease)
Ectopic ACTH production
Adrenal adenoma
Adrenal carcinoma
Exogenous administration
◆ Steroids
◆ ACTH

ACTH, adrenocorticotrophic hormone

Hyperfunction of the Adrenal Cortex

Excess cortisol secretion causes Cushing's syndrome, excess aldosterone secretion hyperaldosteronism and excess adrenal androgen production causes virilism. The clinical features of these conditions may overlap.

Cushing's Syndrome

Causes

Cushing's syndrome, which is due to excess production of glucocorticoids, has several causes (**Table 15.3**). These include excess ACTH secretion, either from the pituitary (Cushing's disease), as a result of ectopic production by tumours of nonpituitary origin, due to the administration of exogenous ACTH. The precise cause of hypersecretion by the pituitary of ACTH is not clear in all cases; some have a basophil adenoma while in others the defect appears to be hypersecretion of CRF. The majority of cases of nonendocrine secretion of ACTH are due to small-cell carcinomas of the bronchus, although the syndrome can result occasionally from benign tumours. Non-ACTH dependent causes include tumours of the adrenal gland or exogenous steroid administration.

Clinical Features

Clinical features include an increase in adipose tissue in characteristic sites, parti-

cularly the face, producing 'moon' facies, the interscapular area leading to the formation of a 'buffalo' hump, and within the abdomen, resulting in truncal obesity. The face is usually plethoric. Cortisol mobilizes protein from peripheral tissues and loss of muscle mass occurs, leading to thin limbs and muscular weakness. Purple striae occur on the abdomen and the skin is thin and abnormally fragile. Impaired glucose tolerance is common, cortisol being a gluconeogenic hormone. Severe osteoporosis may occur, leading to pathological fractures. Hypertension is common and psychiatric disturbances occur, including depression and psychosis. In women, increased adrenal androgen secretion can lead to hirsuitism, acne, oligomenorrhoea and amenorrhoea.

Investigation

The utility of biochemical investigations in the differential diagnosis of Cushing's syndrome is outlined in **Table 15.4**. Basal serum cortisol measurements are rarely helpful as these are normal in many patients with Cushing's syndrome. Determination of the circadian rhythm of cortisol secretion is rarely useful in outpatients because of the stress of the procedure. Investigations can be performed usefully on outpatients include 24-h urinary cortisol secretion and the low-dose dexamethasone suppression test. If both these tests are normal Cushing's syndrome is extremely unlikely. False positive results do occur in depressed patients, obesity, alcohol abuse and intercurrent illness and therefore further inpatient investigations are required to confirm the diagnosis. These include determination of circadian rhythm of cortisol secretion after the patient has settled into the ward environment so that any stress resulting from this is minimized. The normal circadian pattern of cortisol secretion is lost in Cushing's disease but retained in obesity. The insulin tolerance test is sometimes used to discriminate between Cushing's syndrome and conditions giving false positive results in other investigations – serum

Table 15.4 Biochemical investigations in the differential diagnosis of Cushing's syndrome

Test	Pituitary-dependent	Ectopic ACTH production	Adrenal tumour
Plasma cortisol	Loss of circadian rhythm	Very high	Loss of circadian rhythm
Urinary cortisol	Raised	Very high	Raised
Dexamethasone suppression			
Low dose	No suppression	No suppression	No suppression
High dose	Suppression	No suppression	No suppression
Plasma ACTH	Modestly raised	Raised	Low

ACTH, adrenocorticotrophic hormone

cortisol levels fail to suppress in Cushing's syndrome, despite adequate hypoglycaemia. It is important to note that greater amounts of insulin are required to produce hypoglycaemia in Cushing's syndrome than normal because of insulin resistance.

The high-dose dexamethasone suppression test is used in the differential diagnosis of Cushing's syndrome, suppression of serum cortisol levels usually occurring in pituitary-dependent disease. Suppression is unusual in ectopic ACTH production and adrenal tumours. Plasma ACTH is very low in adrenal tumours, normal to high in pituitary-dependent disease and usually very high in ectopic ACTH production. Patients with Cushing's disease often have hypokalaemia and metabolic alkalosis, these sometimes being very profound, particularly in patients with ectopic ACTH production.

KEY POINTS

CUSHING'S SYNDROME

- The commonest cause of Cushing's syndrome is pituitary-dependent bilateral adrenal hyperplasia

- Clinical features of Cushing's syndrome include central obesity and loss of muscle mass

- Increased adrenal androgen secretion may occur in Cushing's syndrome

Hyperaldosteronism

Hyperaldosteronism may either be primary, when the cause lies within the adrenal gland, or secondary, when hypersecretion is caused by stimuli external to the gland.

Primary Hyperaldosteronism (Conn's Syndrome)

Primary hyperaldosteronism leads to sodium retention, hypokalaemia and hypertension. Excessive hormone secretion causes increased sodium reabsorption and potassium loss from the kidney, sodium retention leading to an expansion in extracellular volume and hypertension. However, oedema is rare as patients escape the mineralocorticoid effects of aldosterone. The causes of primary hyperaldosteronism include adenoma, hyperplasia and carcinoma of the adrenal.

Investigation Patients should not be receiving drug therapy when investigations are carried out and sodium balance should also be controlled, as sodium depletion from diuretic therapy or low intake can decrease potassium excretion and mask hypokalaemia. If these precautions are followed, persistent hypokalaemia associated with inappropriately high urinary losses is characteristic of primary hyperaldosteronism. Metabolic alkalosis also occurs, owing to increased distal tubular secretion of H^+

ions. Plasma aldosterone concentrations are elevated in primary hyperaldosteronism while plasma renin activity is suppressed.

Secondary Hyperaldosteronism

Secondary hyperaldosteronism occurs when aldosterone secretion is stimulated by excessive activation of the renin–angiotensin system. Increased aldosterone secretion occurs physiologically during pregnancy – oestrogens increase plasma renin activity. Secretion of renin occurs very commonly postoperatively as a physiological response to hypotension induced by anaesthesia. Severe hypertension stimulates renin secretion by causing renal vasoconstriction. Renin-secreting juxtaglomerular tumours occur but are extremely rare. Secondary hyperaldosteronism develops in several conditions associated with oedema or ascites formation including cirrhosis, nephrotic syndrome and congestive cardiac failure, due to reduced effective intravascular volume. Juxtaglomerular hyperplasia

occurs in Bartter's syndrome leading to severe secondary hyperaldosteronism. The characteristic findings in secondary hyperaldosteronism are elevated plasma renin activity, sodium retention and increased urinary potassium excretion.

Congenital Adrenal Hyperplasia

Causes

Congenital adrenal hyperplasia is caused by a group of inherited defects of enzymes which control the biosynthesis of adrenocortical steroids (**Figure 15.2**). Deficiencies are due to autosomal recessive mutations which usually present in childhood, although partial defects may be expressed in adults. The most common defect, which is found in over 90% of cases, is C-21 hydroxylase deficiency in which the formation of 11-deoxycortisol, the precursor of cortisol, is reduced. This leads to ineffective negative feedback inhibition of cortisol on ACTH

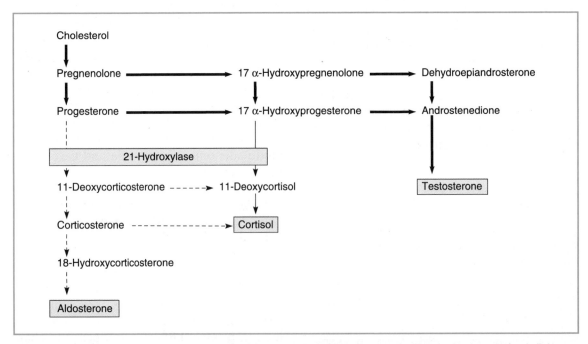

Figure 15.5 The pathogenesis of congenital adrenal hyperplasia caused by 21-hydroxylase deficiency. As a result of the defective enzyme the synthesis of aldosterone and cortisol is reduced leading to reduced negative feedback inhibition. The synthesis of intermediates and hormones proximal to the block is increased.

secretion, which in turn is increased. This stimulates the synthesis of steroid intermediates proximal to the block in the pathway, causing increased androgen production (**Figure 15.5**). 21-Hydroxylase is also required for aldosterone production and thus the synthesis of this may also be reduced.

Clinical Features

Increased androgen secretion in 21-hydroxylase deficiency causes ambiguous genitalia in females at birth, while accelerated somatic growth, penile enlargement and pubic hair development may occur in boys. Adrenal androgen and gonadal steroid production is reduced in C-17 hydroxylase deficiency, leading to ambiguous genitalia in males and delayed puberty and primary amenorrhoea in females. Salt loss, vomiting and dehydration occur in approximately 60% of patients. A hypertensive form of congenital adrenal hyperplasia occurs with C-11 hydroxylase deficiency owing to the accumulation of 11-deoxycorticosterone, a potent mineralocorticoid. Increased synthesis of mineralocorticoids leads to hypokalaemic alkalosis, hypertension and suppressed plasma renin activity. Marked elevations of corticosterone and deoxycorticosterone levels occur.

Investigation

Investigations include measuring electrolytes and precursor concentrations in blood and their metabolites in urine. Plasma sodium concentrations are usually low while potassium levels are elevated. Serum 17-hydroxyprogesterone levels are often raised while pregnanetriol, a metabolite of this intermediate, is excreted in increased amounts.

FURTHER READING

Hall R, Besser M. Chapters 6 and 8. *Fundamentals of Clinical Endocrinology*. Edinburgh: Churchill Livingstone, 1989, pp. 153–184 and pp. 197–204

Stewart PM, Corrie J, Seckl JR, Edwards CRW, Padfield PL. A rational approach for assessing the hypothalamo-pituitary-adrenal axis. *Lancet* 1988; **i**; 1208–10

White PC. Disorders of aldosterone biosynthesis and action. *New England Journal of Medicine* 1994; **331**: 250-8

White PC, New MI, Dupont B. Congenital adrenal hyperplasia. *New England Journal of Medicine* 1987; **316**: 1519–24, 1580-6

CASE HISTORIES

CASE 15.1

A 24-year-old woman had felt generally unwell for about a month, with vomiting for the past 4 days. She had felt weak for 2 days and had collapsed on the day of her admission to hospital. She was unconscious when seen in the accident and emergency room and the following investigations were carried out:

sodium	114 mmol l^{-1}
potassium	5.7 mmol l^{-1}
chloride	96 mmol l^{-1}
total CO_2	17 mmol l^{-1}
urea	29.5 mmol l^{-1}
creatinine	175 μmol l^{-1}
urinary glucose	Negative
urinary ketones	Negative

What do you think is going on?

CASE 15.2

A 3-month-old baby was investigated for failure to thrive and the following results were obtained:

sodium	121 mmol l^{-1}
potassium	5.9 mmol l^{-1}
chloride	96 mmol l^{-1}
total CO_2	15 mmol l^{-1}
urea	15.6 mmol l^{-1}
creatinine	72 μmol l^{-1}

What is the most probable diagnosis?

CASE 15.3

A 53-year-old man was referred to outpatients because of muscle weakness and weight loss. He was unwell and therefore admitted to hospital. The following investigations were carried out:

pH	7.58
P_{O_2}	7.2 kPa
P_{CO_2}	6.7 kPa
sodium	144 mmol l^{-1}
potassium	2.1 mmol l^{-1}
chloride	86 mmol l^{-1}
total CO_2	43 mmol l^{-1}
urea	6.9 mmol l^{-1}
creatinine	92 μmol l^{-1}
blood glucose	17.5 mmol l^{-1}

Explain these abnormalities.

GONADAL FUNCTION AND PREGNANCY

MALE GONADAL FUNCTION

Introduction

The main function of the gonads is to produce gametes for reproduction and to regulate sexual characteristics. Chromoso-mal sex is established at fertilization and this determines the development of the gonads during intrauterine life. Development is identical in male and female fetuses for approximately 6 weeks after fertilization, the primitive gonads then developing into either testes or ovaries (gonadal sex). The differentiation into testes is controlled by genes on the short arm of the Y chromosome. By 8 weeks spermatogenic cords have developed, and Leydig cells and Sertoli cells have differentiated. The Sertoli cells secrete a glycoprotein which inhibits the development of the Müllerian duct system and testosterone is secreted by Leydig cells, promoting development of the Wolffian duct system into the vas deferens, epididymis, seminal vesicles and ejaculatory ducts. Masculinization of the external genitalia occurs under the influence of androgens, development of the penis being complete by 14 weeks (phenotypic sex). In the absence of a Y chromosome the primitive gonads develop into ovaries.

NORMAL MALE GONADAL FUNCTION
The Testis

The testis consists of two components, the seminiferous tubules which produce sperm and Leydig cells which produce androgenic hormones.

Testicular Hormones
The biosynthesis of testosterone from cholesterol in the Leydig cells follows a similar pathway to testosterone synthesis in the adrenal (see **Figure 15.2**). Over 95% of testosterone is protein bound after secretion into the circulation. Testosterone is the main androgenic hormone and promotes the development of secondary sexual characteristics, although conversion to 5α-dihydrotestosterone in target organs is required for this function. Testosterone is also an anabolic hormone, promoting growth and protein synthesis. Androgens are essential for the early stages of spermatogenesis, testosterone diffusing into the seminiferous tubules from adjacent Leydig cells. Spermatogenesis also depends on follicle-stimulating hormone (FSH) which increases the activity of Sertoli cells. Some peripheral conversion of testosterone to oestradiol (aromatization) occurs, particularly in adi-

pose tissue, the amount formed increasing with adiposity. Testosterone is inactivated, mainly in the liver, to form 17-oxosteroids which are excreted in urine as sulphates and glucuronides. The testis also secretes inhibin, a peptide hormone which inhibits FSH secretion.

Hypothalamic–Pituitary Control of Testicular Function

Gonatrophin-releasing hormone (Gn-RH) is secreted in a pulsatile fashion by hypothalamic neurones into the hypothalamic-hypophyseal portal blood system. It stimulates the release of both luteinizing hormone (LH) and FSH. Testosterone exerts negative feedback control at the level of both the hypothalamus and the pituitary, where it inhibits the secretion of LH. Secretion of FSH is regulated by feedback of inhibin (**Figure 16.1**). Suppression of testicular function occurs in hyperprolactinaemia.

KEY POINTS

MALE GONADAL FUNCTION
- Testosterone is secreted by Leydig cells in the testis
- Testosterone exerts negative feedback on LH secretion
- FSH secretion is regulated by inhibin, a peptide hormone secreted by the testis

ASSESSMENT OF MALE GONADAL FUNCTION

Clinical Features

Inadequate androgen action during embryogenesis causes hypospadias, microphallus and cryptorchidism, while failure of Leydig cell function before puberty causes delayed puberty and impaired beard growth, libido and sexual function. Leydig cell failure after puberty may be more difficult to detect from

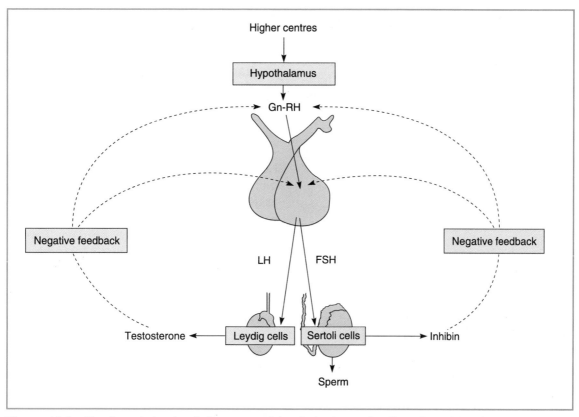

Figure 16.1   The hypothalamic–pituitary–gonadal axis in the male. Gonadotrophin-releasing hormone (Gn-RH) is produced in the hypothalamus and stimulates the secretion of both luteinizing hormone (LH) and follicle-stimulating hormone (FSH). LH promotes the synthesis of testosterone by Leydig cells, testosterone exerting negative feedback inhibition at the level of the hypothalamus and pituitary. FSH stimulates spermatogenesis by Sertoli cells, which also produces inhibin, this exerting negative feedback inhibition. Positive stimulation, solid arrows; negative feedback, dashed arrows.

clinical features since, once established, beard growth is usually maintained.

Serum Testosterone

The secretion of testosterone is pulsatile with peaks every 60–90 min. The range of levels in normal adults is 9–28 nmol l^{-1}, the majority of serum testosterone being bound to protein in normal subjects. Approximately 65% is bound to sex-hormone-binding globulin (SHBG), 30% is albumin-bound and approximately 2% is free, this being the physiologically active fraction. Serum total testosterone levels are affected by the concentrations of SHBG and the levels of testosterone can be corrected for this;

normal free hormone concentrations are 250–750 pmol l^{-1}.

Serum Gonadotrophins

The pulsatile variations in serum LH are greater than those of FSH and samples are usually collected at a standard time, around 09.00 hours, to minimize this effect. Serum testosterone levels are also required for correct interpretation, low values of both hormones imply hypothalamic–pituitary disease while high LH with low testosterone concentrations occur in primary testicular failure. Isolated increases in serum FSH usually indicates disease of the germinal epithelium.

Serum Prolactin

The measurement of serum prolactin levels is important in disordered testicular function as hyperprolactinaemia leads to impaired spermatogenesis.

Serum Oestrogens

Serum oestradiol is usually <200 pmol l^{-1} in men; oestrone levels are rather higher, up to 300 pmol l^{-1}. Elevated levels may be due to increased synthesis (adrenal disease or testicular tumours), decreased metabolism of oestrogens (liver disease), or increased aromatization of androgens (obesity).

Dynamic Function Tests

Three main dynamic function tests to assess hypothalamic–pituitary gonadal function have been described, although they are now used less frequently than in the past as the sensitivity of gonadotrophin and gonadal steroid assays have improved. Dynamic function tests are now used to assess borderline deficiencies in hormone secretion.

Clomiphene Stimulation Test

Clomiphene is an anti-oestrogen which interferes with negative feedback on the pituitary, leading to increased LH and FSH secretion. Clomiphene (3 mg kg^{-1} body weight) is given for 7 days and blood tested for LH and FSH levels before administration and on days 4, 7 and 10. A lack of response suggests that hypogonadism is due to hypothalamic or pituitary disease. This test is now rarely used

Gn-RH Stimulation Test

The rationale for this investigation is that administration of Gn-RH (100 μg) will differentiate between hypothalamic and pituitary causes of hypogonadism, increased gonadotrophin secretion occurring in hypothalamic but not pituitary disease. However, patients with hypothalamic disease often fail to respond unless the pituitary is primed by repeated low-dose Gn-RH administration followed by a single high dose.

Human Chorionic Gonadotrophin Stimulation Test

Human chorionic gonadotrophin (hCG) stimulates Leydig cells and can be used to assess testicular testosterone secretion. Human chorionic gonadotrophin (2000 iu) is injected intramuscularly on days 0 and 3 of the test, and serum testosterone is measured before each injection and 2 days after the second injection. No response is seen in primary testicular failure while levels increase in hypothalamic–pituitary disease.

Other Investigations

Sperm counts and testicular biopsies are often important for the evaluation of disordered testicular function.

DISORDERS OF MALE GONADAL FUNCTION
Sexual Precocity

Abnormally early sexual development, before 9 years of age, is caused by increased androgen production. It is usually characterized by virilization without spermatogenesis, although spermatogenesis can occur. Sexual precocity may be caused by gonadotrophin-independent conditions, in which the development of the hypothalamus and pituitary is appropriate for the age, or gonadotrophin-dependent, in which spermatogenesis can occur if there is premature hypothalamic–pituitary activation (**Table 16.1**). Rarely, sexual precocity may be characterized by feminization: this is considered in feminizing syndromes (see below).

Table 16.1 Causes of sexual precocity in boys

Gonadotrophin independent (virilizing) syndromes
◆ Leydig cell tumours or hyperplasia
◆ Congenital adrenal hyperplasia
◆ Adrenal tumours
◆ Androgen administration
Gonadotrophin-dependent syndromes
◆ Idiopathic
◆ Human chorionic gonadotrophin (hCG)-secreting tumours
◆ Central nervous system disorders
   Tumours
   Infections
   Injuries

Hypogonadism

The clinical features of hypogonadism are determined by the time of onset, ambiguous genitalia resulting from defects occurring during early intrauterine development, delayed puberty from conditions which affect later stages of development, and reduced libido, infertility and impotence resulting if the disease occurs postpuberty.

Delayed Puberty

Puberty is occasionally delayed until 16–18 years with somatic growth continuing until 20 years. Such delay is not necessarily associated with disease and may need to be differentiated from delayed puberty due to pathological disorders. These include chromosomal abnormalities such as Klinefelter's syndrome (XXY), although partial puberty usually occurs in this condition. Other causes include poor diet, chronic systemic disease such as renal failure or coeliac disease, and endocrine conditions such as hypopituitarism, hypothyroidism, abnormalities of testicular development, mild degrees of androgen resistance and isolated gonadotrophin deficiency (Kallman's syndrome). Kallman's syndrome is caused by a deficiency in Gn-RH secretion and is often associated with a defective sense of smell; FSH, LH and testosterone levels are low. Administration of Gn-RH can correct these hormonal abnormalities and initiate spermatogenesis.

In addition to full clinical examination investigations should include assessment of chromosome karyotype, pituitary function and bone age, together with measurement of serum testosterone, FSH, LH and prolactin concentrations. The differentiation of isolated gonadotrophin deficiency from delayed puberty can be difficult, although measuring the response of LH secretion to Gn-RH injection may be helpful, as this increases as puberty approaches.

Abnormal Testicular Function in Adults (Hypogonadism)

The causes of hypogonadism in adults are outlined in **Table 16.2**. Impaired function

Table 16.2 Causes of male hypogonadism

Primary
◆ Congenital disorders
   Chromosomal abnormalities (Klinefelter's syndrome)
   Inherited defects in androgen synthesis
   Androgen resistance
   Cryptorchidism
   Varicocoele
◆ Acquired testicular disorders
   Viral orchitis (mumps)
   Trauma
   Radiation
   Drugs (including cytotoxic drugs, alcohol, spironolactone)
◆ Systemic disease affecting testicular function
   Liver disease
   Renal disease
   Sickle cell disease
   Neurological disease (dystrophia myotonica, paraplegia)
Secondary
◆ Hypothalamic–pituitary disease
   Panhypopituitarism
   Gonadotrophin deficiency
   Hyperprolactinaemia
◆ Other endocrine diseases
   Cushing's syndrome

may affect both spermatogenesis and testosterone production, or these may be reduced selectively. Infertility and impotence are the main symptoms. Primary hypogonadism is due to testicular disease, while secondary hypogonadism results from hypothalamic–pituitary or systemic disease.

Primary Hypogonadism Chromosomal abnormalities which cause gonadal dysgenesis, including Klinefelter's syndrome (XXY), may present as hypogonadism rather than delayed puberty. Primary sexual differentiation is often normal and partial puberty usually occurs. The seminiferous tubules are hyalinized and nonfunctional although Leydig cells are well developed. Gonadotrophin production is unimpaired, levels usually being elevated after puberty. Several inherited defects of androgen synthesis have been described which cause phenotypic abnormalities varying from normal males with hypospadias to apparent females with absent Müllerian duct differentiation (male pseudohermaphroditism). Failure of androgen synthesis may also occur in congenital adrenal hyperplasia. Defects in androgen action vary in severity from partial insensitivity, in which sexual differentiation and maturation are almost normal, to testicular feminization, in which there is complete resistance to androgen action (see below).

Bilateral cryptorchidism (undescended testes) causes infertility, although testosterone secretion is impaired only rarely. Orchitis complicates various viral infections, including mumps. There may be no residual impairment of testicular function but atrophy of seminiferous tubules occurs in up to 25% of affected adults; testosterone production is unaffected. A varicocoele results from the retrograde flow of blood from the abdomen into the internal spermatic vein, leading to warming of the testis and impaired function of the seminiferous tubules. Radiation damage may affect both spermatogenesis and testosterone secretion. Drugs affect testicular function in

various ways; spironolactone blocks androgen synthesis, while cytotoxic drugs commonly interfere with spermatogenesis. Marihuana inhibits LH secretion, testosterone production and sperm motility. Chronic prolonged alcohol abuse may cause low testosterone synthesis independently of any effect on liver function.

Testicular function is often abnormal in systemic disease. Atrophy of the testes is common in cirrhosis of the liver, serum oestradiol being increased, testosterone decreased and sperm motility impaired. Renal failure causes impairment of both spermatogenesis and testosterone synthesis, increased testosterone levels occurring after dialysis. This is due to a defect at the level of the testis, serum gonadotrophin concentrations being increased. Impaired sexual maturation and testicular atrophy is common in sickle-cell disease and impaired testosterone production occurs in dystrophia myotonica.

Secondary Hypogonadism Hypothalamic–pituitary disorders cause hypogonadism owing to decreased gonadotrophin production. This occurs because of destruction of gonadotrophin-producing cells in panhypopituitarism. Kallman's syndrome usually presents as delayed puberty although less severely affected subjects have been described with partial defects in either LH or FSH production or both. Acquired gonadotrophin deficiency can occur in Cushing's syndrome, hypercortisolism suppressing LH production independently of the effect of a space-occupying pituitary lesion. Prolactinomas may destroy gonadotrophin-producing cells although hyperprolactinaemia also impairs Gn-RH secretion.

Feminizing Syndromes Feminization in males ranges from gynaecomastia, the most common manifestation, to male pseudohermaphroditism (**Table 16.3**). Gynaecomastia is induced by oestrogens and physiological breast enlargement sometimes occurs in the newborn, resulting from maternal or placen-

Table 16.3 Feminizing syndromes in males

Physiological
◆ Neonatal
◆ Pubertal
◆ Ageing
Defects in androgen production
◆ Inherited disorders of testosterone synthesis
◆ Defects in androgen action
   Complete – testicular feminization
   Partial – male pseudohermaphroditism
Increased oestrogen production
◆ Human chorionic gonadotrophin
   (hCG)-secreting tumours
◆ Testicular tumours
◆ Increased substrate availability
   Increased synthesis of androstenedione,
   e.g. adrenal disease
   Decreased metabolism of androstenedione,
   e.g. liver disease
Drugs
◆ Oestrogens
◆ Inhibitors of testosterone synthesis or action
   Cytotoxic drugs, spironolactone, cimetidine
◆ Mechanism uncertain
   Phenothiazines, tricyclic antidepressants,
   marihuana, heroin

FEMALE GONADAL FUNCTION

Introduction

Oestrogen synthesis occurs *in utero* from about 6 weeks although differentiation of primitive germ cells occurs later in females than males, ovarian follicles developing from 12 weeks gestation. As an inhibiting factor is not secreted, the Müllerian duct system differentiates to form fallopian tubes, the uterus and the upper third of the vagina. The external genitalia develop the female pattern in the absence of a Y chromosome. Phenotypic sex is well established at birth, and further development occurs at puberty when the secondary sexual characteristics are developed. This coincides with rapid increases in gonadal steroid secretion in the early teens as a result of increasing gonadotrophin secretion. At the same time, increased secretion of adrenal androgens occurs which promotes secondary sexual hair development.

tal oestrogens. Breast enlargement, which may be unilateral, is seen sometimes at puberty and gynaecomastia can occur in otherwise healthy elderly men, and is probably caused by increased conversion of androgens to oestrogens in peripheral tissues. Pathological gynaecomastia may occur because of defective testosterone secretion, increased oestrogen secretion, or due to drugs.

Inherited defects in testosterone synthesis can cause phenotypic abnormalities which range from hypospadias to female external genitalia with absent Müllerian duct structures (male pseudohermaphroditism). Testosterone secretion is normal in testicular feminization and the karyotype is XY, although testosterone receptors are absent and therefore target organs do not develop. As the testes produce oestrogens in addition to testosterone breast development occurs.

NORMAL FEMALE GONADAL FUNCTION

The Ovary

Like the testis, the ovary produces gametes for reproduction and also hormones which control sexual characteristics.

Ovarian Hormones

Ovarian steroid hormones are synthesized from cholesterol, different cell types in the ovary containing varying amounts of the enzymes controlling oestrogen biosynthesis (**Figure 16.2**).

Oestrogens Oestrone and oestradiol are both synthesized and are interconvertible, although oestradiol is the more potent hormone. Oestrogen synthesis occurs main-

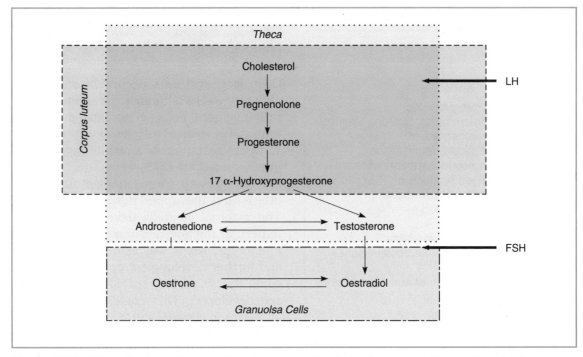

Figure 16.2 Biosynthetic pathways of oestrogen synthesis in the ovary. Conversions in the corpus luteum are enclosed within the dashed box, the theca in the dotted box, and the granulosa in the grey box. The main sites of action of luteinizing hormone (LH) and follicle-stimulating hormone (FSH) are indicated by the heavy arrows.

ly in the granulosa cells of the corpus luteum by aromatization of precursors produced by thecal cells. Circulating oestrogens in ovulating women are derived from two sources, approximately 60% being oestradiol synthesized by the ovaries. The remainder is mainly oestrone synthesized principally from androstenedione in peripheral tissues, particularly adipose tissue. Oestrogen production after the menopause is due to this latter mechanism. LH promotes the initial stages of steroidogenesis while FSH stimulates the final stage of oestrogen synthesis, aromatization. Oestrogens promote the development of secondary sexual characteristics, particularly uterine growth, thickening of the vaginal mucosa and breast development. The principal urinary oestrogen is oestriol which is produced from the metabolism of both oestradiol and oestrone.

Progesterone Progesterone is synthesized mainly in the corpus luteum and induces secretory activity and stromal changes in the endometrium, preparing the uterus for implantation should fertilization occur. Fertilization maintains progesterone secretion, which inhibits ovulation and leads to further development of the breast. Other effects of progesterone include increasing body temperature.

Peptide Hormones In addition to producing steroid hormones the ovary also synthesizes two peptide hormones, relaxin and inhibin. Relaxin is secreted during pregnancy and facilitates delivery of the fetus, loosening the ligaments of the symphysis pubis and softening the cervix. As in males, inhibin inhibits FSH secretion.

Androgens The ovary secretes several androgens including androstenedione, testosterone and dehydroepiandrosterone, these being produced mainly by the thecal cells (**Figure 16.2**). Androstenedione is secreted by the adrenals in addition to the ovaries and is metabolized in peripheral tissues, particularly adipose tissue, to form testosterone and oestrone. Some testosterone is also secreted directly by the adrenal cortex, which also secretes other weaker androgens, particularly dehydroepiandrosterone and dehydroepiandrosterone sulphate.

The Menstrual Cycle

The menarche is preceded by the development of cyclical secretion of gonadotrophins. Hypothalamic control of gonadotrophin secretion is mediated by the pulsatile secretion of gonadotrophin-releasing hormone (Gn-RH or LH-RH). Pulsatile gonadotrophin secretion is seen initially during sleep in the immediate prepubertal period. This pulsatile secretion of gonadotrophins, which has a periodicity of approximately 90 min, is maintained with the onset of menstruation, although further cyclical biochemical changes are superimposed. Before puberty, the hypothalamic–pituitary controlling mechanism is sensitive to negative feedback by the low levels of circulating sex steroids, but this sensitivity decreases in the prepubertal period. This leads to increased gonadotrophin secretion and thus to increased oestrogen secretion and the

physical changes of puberty.

The normal menstrual cycle is divided into follicular (proliferative) and luteal (secretory) phases. A dominant follicle develops during the follicular phase which migrates to the surface of the ovary. Oestradiol secretion increases, this being marked in days preceding ovulation. Oestradiol also has the effect of increasing the sensitivity of the pituitary to Gn-RH while at the same time decreasing the hypothalamic secretion of Gn-RH. Oestrogen secretion falls as the follicle becomes fully mature, progesterone secretion increasing. As a result of these changes, Gn-RH secretion increases significantly and a surge in LH secretion occurs (**Figure 16.3**). This induces ovulation, the follicle ruptures, and the ovum is released. The granulosa cells of the follicle form the corpus luteum which secretes large amounts of progesterone. This, together with oestradiol, stimulates proliferation of the endometrium. If pregnancy does not occur secretion by the corpus luteum falls, progesterone and oestradiol secretion decreases and menstrual bleeding occurs.

The Menopause

The ovaries become less responsive to gonadotrophins as the menopause approaches and the cycles become longer. This is due to exhaustion of follicles; as the development of these decreases the production of oestrogens falls. This in turn reduces the negative feedback control of gonadotrophin secretion. Thus, the serum levels of LH and FSH increase with the onset of the menopause. The hormonal changes lead to vasomotor instability (hot flushes), the precise cause of which is uncertain, although hormone replacement therapy usually alleviates these. Decreased breast size and atrophy of the urogenital epithelium result from the reduced oestrogen secretion. In addition, an increased risk of osteoporosis develops and changes occur in serum lipoproteins, particularly a fall in HDL-cholesterol.

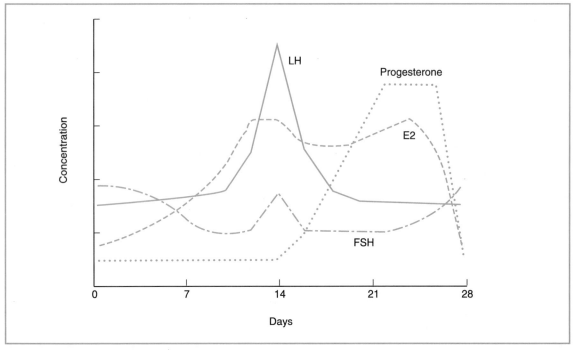

Figure 16.3 Typical pattern of serum gonadotrophin and gonadal steroid concentrations in the menstrual cycle. LH, luteinizing hormone; FSH, follicle-stimulating hormone; E2, E2-oestradiol.

ASSESSMENT OF FEMALE GONADAL FUNCTION

The assessment of ovarian function includes a careful history and examination, including a menstrual history and noting the development of secondary sexual characteristics. In addition, laboratory investigations are required in many cases to confirm a clinical diagnosis or to monitor hormone treatment.

Serum Gonadotrophins

Considerable variation in normal serum levels occurs, owing to the pulsatile nature of gonadotrophin secretion. The range of LH is 2–12 U l^{-1} and FSH 1–10 U l^{-1} in women with normal menstrual cycles, although levels 2–3 times higher than this occur near ovulation. Serum gonadotrophins are useful in the evaluation of amenorrhoea. Increased levels occur due to primary gonadal failure, either physiological (menopause) or pathological, while levels are low or undetectable in hypothalamic–pituitary disease. An elevated LH:FSH ratio is seen in the polycystic ovary syndrome (see below).

Oestrogens

The secretion of oestrogen is cyclical, the reference ranges for 17β-oestradiol being 70–370 pmol l^{-1} during the follicular phase, 280–1720 pmol l^{-1} at the ovulatory peak (usually days 11–15 of the menstrual cycle), and 90–870 pmol l^{-1} during the luteal phase. The estimation of 17β-oestradiol is less useful in investigating amenorrhoea than gonadotrophin levels, past oestrogen status being indicated by secondary sexual characteristics. Measurement of serum 17β-oestradiol is used to monitor anovulatory women during treatment to induce ovulation and in women undergoing *in vitro* fertilization.

Progestagen Withdrawal Test

Current oestrogen status can be assessed by a progestagen withdrawal test in which medroxyprogesterone acetate (10 mg per day for 5 days) is given orally. If menstrual bleeding occurs within 7–10 days of this then oestrogenization was adequate to produce withdrawal bleeding.

Progesterone

Pre-ovulation serum progesterone levels are <5 nmol l^{-1}, while levels increase to >20 nmol l^{-1} after ovulation. Progesterone measurements are used to demonstrate ovulation, although this can be assessed more simply by measuring body temperature. Progesterone is thermogenic and a rise in temperature in the luteal phase of the cycle suggests ovulation has occurred.

Androgens

Hirsutism or virilization implies excess androgen secretion owing to increased testosterone production by the adrenal or ovary, or as a result of increased peripheral production from androstenedione. Serum testosterone levels in women are normally <2.6 nmol l^{-1} while androstenedione levels are <13 nmol l^{-1}.

DISORDERS OF FEMALE GONADAL FUNCTION

Precocious Puberty

True precocious puberty is characterized by the early development of secondary sexual characteristics and ovulatory menstrual cycles, while menstrual cycles do not occur in precocious pseudopuberty. Most cases of precocious puberty are idiopathic while approximately 10% are caused by brain disorders, including tumours and infections. Ovarian cysts or tumours are the commonest cause of precocious pseudopuberty.

Amenorrhoea

Amenorrhoea is primary when menstruation has never occurred, or secondary if menstruation has ceased. Conditions leading to secondary amenorrhoea may also cause oligomenorrhoea – scanty and infrequent menstruation. Some disorders can cause primary or secondary amenorrhoea and therefore a classification based on the type of disorder is more useful than dividing causes according to whether menstruation has occurred or not. The causes of amenorrhoea are outlined in **Table 16.4**.

Amenorrhoea in the Absence of Secondary Sexual Characteristics

The menarche occurs by 15 years in over 95% of girls in the UK, while breast devel-

Table 16.4 Causes of amenorrhoea

Amenorrhoea in the absence of secondary sexual characteristics
- Gonadal agenesis
- Turner's syndrome
- Congenital adrenal hyperplasia
- Hypogonadotrophic hypogonadism (Kallman's syndrome)
- Central nervous system disorders (e.g. craniopharyngioma)

Amenorrhoea with normal secondary sexual characteristics
- Anatomical abnormalities
- Primary gonadal disorders
  Testicular feminization
  Premature ovarian failure
  Polycystic ovarian syndrome
  Ovarian tumours
- Hypothalamic–pituitary disorders
  Stress
  Anorexia nervosa
  Extreme physical training
  Systemic disease

opment starts a few years earlier. Causes of amenorrhoea in the absence of secondary sexual development include ovarian and hypothalamic–pituitary disorders. In the absence of development of the gonads (gonadal agenesis), the phenotype will be female but with no features of Turner's syndrome, whether the karyotype is 46XX or 46XY. In addition to lack of sexual maturation, features of Turner's syndrome (45XO) include short stature, webbed neck, and chest and elbow deformities. Ovarian failure can also occur in congenital adrenal hyperplasia, as some of the enzymes deficient in this syndrome are required for gonadal steroid synthesis. Lack of Gn-RH production (Kallman's syndrome) and central nervous system disorders such as craniopharyngioma are hypothalamic–pituitary causes of amenorrhoea with sexual immaturity.

Amenorrhoea with Normal Secondary Sexual Characteristics

Pregnancy must always be considered as a possible cause of amenorrhoea in patients with normal sexual development. If this is ruled out anatomical abnormalities of the reproductive tract, primary gonadal disorders and hypothalamic–pituitary disorders should be considered.

Anatomical Abnormalities Anatomical defects causing amenorrhoea include labial fusion, which may follow infection, and congenital abnormalities such as imperforate hymen, transverse vaginal septum and absence of Müllerian structures. In addition to congenital abnormalities, stenosis of the cervix may follow surgery and the endometrium may be destroyed following vigorous curettage.

Primary Gonadal Disorders Patients with testicular feminization have a female phenotype, a 46XY karyotype, an absent uterus and scanty sexual hair development (see above). Occasionally, premature ovarian failure occurs in women under the age of 40 years from a variety of causes including

infection (mumps orchitis), radiation injury, chemotherapy and autoimmune disease of the ovaries. This may be an isolated finding or occur in association with other autoimmune diseases such as hypothyroidism or systemic lupus erythematosus.

Amenorrhoea or oligomenorrhoea are features of the polycystic ovary syndrome, in which obesity and hirsutism are also common. The ovaries are usually abnormal with a thickened capsule, multiple small follicles and hyperplastic thecal cells. There appears to be excess androgen production from the adrenals and ovaries which leads to increased peripheral oestrogen synthesis in adipose tissue. This has a positive feedback of LH secretion and a negative feedback on FSH secretion, causing elevation in the LH:FSH ratio. This is consistent with the finding that ovulation is induced in many patients by the anti-oestrogen, clomiphene. Oestrogen-producing ovarian tumours often cause amenorrhoea or oligomenorrhoea.

Hypothalamic–Pituitary Disorders Stress in women may lead to amenorrhoea owing to impaired secretion of Gn-RH. Amenorrhoea occurs in anorexia nervosa, gonadotrophin levels being reduced although the mechanism responsible is not understood. Extreme physical training, systemic diseases such as renal failure, chronic liver disease and malabsorption, and endocrine disorders such as hypothyroidism and hyperthyroidism may lead to reduced gonadotrophin secretion. Pituitary necrosis or tumours may destroy gonadotrophin-producing cells while hyperprolactinaemia inhibits the normal pulsatile secretion of Gn-RH.

Investigation of Amenorrhoea

History and physical examination may suggest conditions such as Turner's syndrome, testicular feminization or congenital anatomical abnormalities. Hirsutism should be assessed and investigated if found (see below). Pregnancy should be considered and excluded before further investigation, however unlikely this appears. Chromosomal abnormalities, systemic diseases and extragonadal endocrine disorders should be considered. Serum gonadotrophin levels should be determined, these being high in primary gonadal failure but low in hypothalamic–pituitary disease. Levels of FSH are high in primary ovarian failure while LH levels are elevated more than FSH in polycystic ovary syndrome. If gonadotrophin levels are low it is essential to measure serum prolactin, imaging of the pituitary fossa being indicated if the serum prolactin level is elevated. Oestrogen status can be assessed by progestagen withdrawal (see above) – bleeding within 1 week of stopping progestagen administration indicates adequate oestrogenization, the cause often being polycystic ovary syndrome. If bleeding does not occur, a hypothalamic–pituitary disorder or an anatomical abnormality of the reproductive tract, such as destruction of the endometrium, are the most probable causes. If the findings are unclear these conditions can be differentiated by administering oral oestrogen for 3 weeks with medroxyprogesterone acetate being added for the last 7 days. Withdrawal bleeding occurs in hypothalamic–pituitary amenorrhoea but not with a uterine abnormality. Dynamic function tests, Gn-RH or clomiphene stimulation, often fail to distinguish hypothalamic from pituitary causes of amenorrhoea.

Hirsutism and Virilism

Hirsutism is an increase in body hair with a male pattern of distribution while virilization includes additional features of masculinization, such as deepening of the voice, temporal balding, clitoral hypertrophy and muscle development. Hair distribution is affected by genetic in addition to endocrine factors, there being considerable diversity between different ethnic groups. Secondary sexual hair development in the lower pubic triangle and axillae is dependent on adrenal androgens in women as well as men. Additional hair growth in the typically male pattern, including the upper pubic triangle, chest and beard, depends on higher levels of androgens produced normally by the testis. Polycystic ovary syndrome is a common cause of hirsutism (see above), some patients having normal menstrual cycles. Other causes include congenital adrenal hyperplasia, Cushing's syndrome and androgen-producing tumours. The last of these, which may arise in the ovary or adrenal, are uncommon and often associated with virilization.

Most women with hirsutism have increased androgen production, serum total testosterone being increased in approximately 40% of cases, while free testosterone is increased in many more owing to decreases in SHBG levels. Elevated serum LH levels suggest polycystic ovary syndrome, while increased 17-hydroxyprogesterone levels suggest congenital adrenal hyperplasia. Frank virilization with grossly elevated serum total testosterone levels or increased dehydroepiandrosterone sulphate concentrations suggest a neoplastic cause. Clinical features of Cushing's disease should be investigated appropriately.

Infertility

Infertility, often defined as a lack of conception after 1 year of unprotected intercourse, is due to factors affecting the male partner in approximately 40% of cases. Hypogonadism must be investigated but the commonest cause is idiopathic azospermia or oligospermia. In addition to amenorrhoea female causes of infertility include pelvic disease.

PREGNANCY

Major hormonal changes occur during pregnancy, these being detected soon after implantation of the conceptus. These endocrine changes are necessary for fetal development and result in metabolic adaptations that can lead to complications, such as gestational diabetes.

Human Chorionic Gonadotrophin

Following fertilization, the conceptus develops before implantation in the uterus, which occurs 6–7 days later. Within 24 h of implantation, the first measurable product of the placenta, hCG, is detected in the maternal plasma, the concentration doubling every 2 days in early pregnancy and reaching a peak approximately 8 weeks after conception. hCG can be detected in the urine within 2 days of implantation. The main physiological role of hCG is to maintain the corpus luteum and stimulate progesterone secretion.

hCG is a glycoprotein with two subunits, the α chain being almost identical in structure to the α subunit in LH, FSH and thyroid-stimulating hormone (TSH). Although similar in structure to LH, the β subunit has significant sequence differences which allow specific antibodies to be raised, these being used to measure hCG by immunochemical techniques. Detection in urine forms the basis of an early pregnancy test, this being positive before a menstrual period is missed. hCG is also produced by trophoblastic tumours (hydatidiform mole and chorioncarcinoma) and its concentrations are measured as a tumour marker in these conditions (see chapter 17).

Human Placental Lactogen

Human placental lactogen (hPL) is also a peptide hormone synthesized by the syncytiotrophoblast, and is detectable 20 days after the last menstrual period. Levels increase rapidly during the first trimester and more slowly during the remainder of pregnancy. The physiological function of hPL is unclear, although it has several properties including a weak growth hormone-like action, glucose-sparing effects and promotion of lipolysis.

Progesterone

Adequate progesterone secretion is required for implantation, and secretion increases throughout pregnancy, initially from the corpus luteum and later from the placenta, this becoming the most important source after 8 weeks. Progesterone stimulates uterine growth and inhibits uterine contractions. Together with oestrogens it stimulates breast development.

Oestrogens

Oestrogen secretion also increases throughout pregnancy, the initial source being the corpus luteum, the placenta becoming the major site of synthesis after 8 weeks. Oestrogens induce uterine and breast growth. The main urinary oestrogen of pregnancy is oestriol, synthesis of which occurs by a mechanism that involves fetal as well as placental metabolism (**Figure 16.4**). A precursor, pregnenolone, is synthesized in the placenta from cholesterol, pregnenolone being converted to dehydroepiandrosterone (DHEA) in the fetal adrenal cortex. This is conjugated to DHEA sulphate in the fetal liver and adrenal, increasing its solubility. Conversion of DHEA sulphate to oestriol occurs in the placenta.

Assessment of Feto-Placental Function

Because oestriol synthesis requires contributions from both the placenta and fetus, measurement of urinary oestriol has been used to assess feto-placental development. Low levels are often found in fetal death, and in at-risk pregnancies – falling levels have been found to correlate with fetal distress.

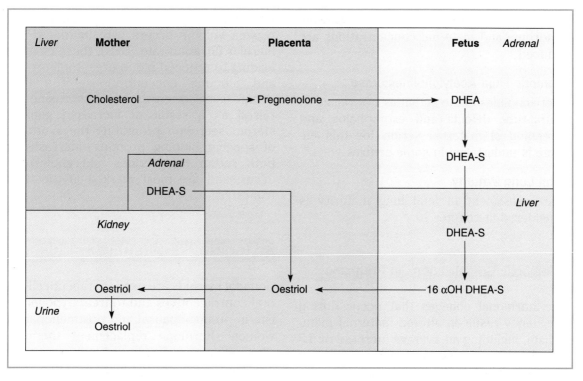

Figure 16.4 Outline of the biosynthesis of oestriol by the feto-placental unit. DHEA, dehydroepiandrostenedione; DHEA-S, dehydroepiandrostenedione sulphate; 16 αOH DHEA-S, 16 α-hydroxydehydroepiandrostenedione sulphate.

However, falling levels of oestriol do not always occur with impending fetal death and this investigation, together with other biochemical assessments of hormonal changes in pregnancy, have largely been replaced by assessment of fetal growth using ultrasound.

KEY POINTS

PREGNANCY

- Urinary hCG excretion increases within 7 days of fertilization

- Progesterone and oestrogen secretion is increased, initially from the corpus luteum, and later from the placenta

- Progesterone and oestrogens stimulate uterine growth and breast development and progesterone inhibits uterine contractions

Detection of Fetal Abnormalities

α-Fetoprotein

α-Fetoprotein is an oncofetal antigen which is synthesized early in fetal development by the yolk sac, and later by the liver. Hepatic synthesis of α-fetoprotein falls as term approaches, α-fetoprotein being replaced as the predominant protein in serum by albumin. α-Fetoprotein leaks across the placenta into the maternal circulation during pregnancy, the amount depending on the amount produced by the fetus. This is increased in the presence of neural-tube defects and measurement of maternal α-fetoprotein measurement is therefore undertaken to screen for this disorder. Raised maternal concentrations are not specific for neural-tube defects as increased placental transfer also occurs in multiple pregnancies and exomphalos.

α-Fetoprotein production is low in Down's syndrome and maternal concentrations are reduced.

Amniotic Fluid Acetylcholinesterase

Acetylcholinesterase activities are raised in neural-tube defects and exomphalos and screening of maternal serum for this enzyme is undertaken in some centres.

Fetal Lung Maturity

The assessment of fetal lung maturity is considered in chapter 19.

Metabolic Complications in Pregnancy

The hormonal changes that occur during pregnancy result in altered maternal metabolism, including an average increase of 3.5 kg in body weight, excluding the products of conception, this being most marked in the first two trimesters. Insulin secretion increases during pregnancy with insulin resistance occurring in the second half of pregnancy, as hPL, progesterone and increased cortisol secretion antagonize insulin action. This sometimes causes diabetes mellitus in women who were nondiabetic before pregnancy (gestational diabetes). Urinary glucose excretion should be monitored at antenatal clinic visits to check this possibility, although glycosuria may develop during pregnancy because of a reduced renal tubular reabsorptive capacity for glucose. Glycosuria should be investigated and, if necessary, a glucose tolerance test performed.

Pre-eclampsia is characterized by hypertension, proteinuria, oedema and high fetal mortality. Urinary protein should be checked routinely at antenatal clinic visits. Increased serum urate levels indicate a poor fetal prognosis.

Altered hormonal metabolism in pregnancy lead to changes in the values of many biochemical tests. Expansion of the plasma volume occurs with increased glomerular filtration rate (GFR), these changes leading to reduced blood urea, total protein and albumin concentrations. The total serum levels of cortisol and thyroxine are raised as a result of increased gonadal steroid secretion promoting the synthesis of specific binding proteins. Increases in both serum triglycerides and cholesterol occur, and are most marked in the third trimester.

EXOGENOUS GONADAL STEROIDS

Gonadal steroids are used therapeutically as oral contraceptives and to treat hypogonadism in premenopausal and postmenopausal women (hormone replacement therapy). Their effects on hormone-binding proteins are similar to those seen in pregnancy. Oestrogens increase high-density lipoprotein (HDL)-cholesterol and lower low-density lipoprotein (LDL)-cholesterol. Their effect on triglyceride levels depends on the route of administration, these increasing with oral but not transdermal oestrogens. Progestagens lower HDL-cholesterol.

FURTHER READING

Butt WR, Blunt SM. The role of the laboratory in the investigation of infertility. *Annals of Clinical Biochemistry* 1988; **25**: 601–9

Chang RJ (ed.). Hirsutism. *Clinical Obstetrics and Gynaecology* 1991; **34**: 794–882

Hall R, Besser M. Chapters 9–11. *Fundamentals of Clinical Endocrinology*. Edinburgh: Churchill Livingstone, 1989, pp. 205–75

Wang CA, Swerdloff RS. Evaluation of testicular function. *Baillière's Clinical Endocrinology and Metabolism* 1992; **6**: 405–34

CASE 16.1

A man of 32 years was investigated for infertility. He was found to have oligospermia and the following results were also obtained:

serum LH	21 U l^{-1}
serum FSH	24 U l^{-1}
serum testosterone	3.5 nmol l^{-1}

What is the probable diagnosis?

CASE 16.2

An 18-year-old boy was investigated for delayed puberty and the following investigations were carried out:

serum LH	<1 U l^{-1}
serum FSH	1 U l^{-1}
serum testosterone	4 nmol l^{-1}

What abnormality is present?

CASE 16.3

A woman of 28 years was investigated because of hirsutism and irregular periods. She was moderately overweight (body mass index, BMI, 32). The following endocrine investigations were carried out on day 5 of her menstrual cycle:

serum FSH	6 U l^{-1}
serum LH	19 U l^{-1}
serum testosterone	4.7 nmol l^{-1}
serum prolactin	350 mU l^{-1}

Are these results abnormal?

CASE HISTORIES

METABOLIC ASPECTS OF NEOPLASIA

INTRODUCTION

Some tumours secrete products such as peptides or proteins which, in addition to producing local consequences, cause generalized metabolic effects (paraneoplastic syndromes) while others secrete vasoactive products (catecholamines and 5-hydroxytryptamine). Tumour secretions are also important as indicators of the presence of a pathological process and can sometimes be used in the investigation of neoplastic disease (tumour markers). Neoplastic endocrine syndromes and tumour markers are considered in this chapter.

HORMONE-SECRETING NONENDOCRINE TUMOURS

Hormones and hormone precursors can be detected in small quantities, using very sensitive immunochemical techniques, in many organs which do not normally function as endocrine tissues. When tumours develop in these tissues increased amounts of hormones may be synthesized and secreted into the circulation, producing syndromes which are often said to be due to 'ectopic' hormone production; however, this term is not strictly accurate. These hormones are nearly always peptide or protein in nature and are usually, although not always, produced by malignant tumours. While hormones can be produced by a wide variety of tumours most cases of ectopic hormone production result from a relatively small number of causes (**Table 17.1**). The individual syndromes are considered in detail in the chapters in which the metabolic effects are considered.

The cellular basis of ectopic hormone production is unclear. It has been suggested that derepression of genes coding for hormone production occurs, although this

Table 17.1 Metabolic syndromes and ectopic hormone production

Syndrome	Hormone	Main site of origin
Hypercalcaemia	Parathyroid hormone (PTH)-related peptide	Bronchial carcinoma (squamous cell)
Syndrome of inappropriate antidiuretic hormone secretion (SIADH)	Vasopressin	Bronchial carcinoma (small cell)
Cushing's syndrome	Adrenocorticotrophic hormone (ACTH)	Bronchial carcinoma (small cell)
Hypoglycaemia	Insulin-like growth factor	Mesenchymal tumours
Precocious puberty in boys	Human chorionic gonadotrophin (hCG)	Hepatoblastoma

is unlikely to explain clear associations between tumour types and hormones. In addition, no increase in hormone mRNA has been found in such tumours. An alternative possibility is that tumours may result from growth of a particular cell type or clone. Hormone secretion could then be caused by growth of cells which produce small amounts of hormones normally, or growth of more primitive cells capable of expressing hormones which are synthesized by immature cells. The latter mechanism could also explain the production of fetal proteins such as α-fetoprotein. Alternative possibilities include dedifferentiation and arrested differentiation. In dedifferentiation, neoplastic cells revert to a more primitive level, producing products which were synthesized at an earlier developmental stage. In arrested differentiation, the development of cells only occurs to a stage in which secretion occurs.

CATECHOLAMINE-SECRETING TUMOURS

The highest density of catecholamine-secreting cells in the body is in the adrenal medulla, although these chromaffin cells, so called because of their affinity for chromium salts, are also found elsewhere in the sympathetic nervous system. Catecholamine-secreting tumours include phaeochromocytomas and neuroblastomas.

Biosynthesis of Catecholamines

The biosynthesis of catecholamines is outlined in **Figure 17.1**. The precursor of catecholamines is tyrosine which is hydroxylated to form DOPA (3,4-dihydroxyphenylalanine). DOPA is decarboxylated to form dopamine, which is further metabolized to form the other catecholamines, noradrenaline and adrenaline. Dopamine is found in high concentrations in the brain, where it is a neurotransmitter, and in noradrenergic neurones, where it is a precursor of noradrenaline. Noradrenaline is found in the adrenal medulla, central nervous system and sympathetic nerves, while adrenaline is synthesized mainly in the adrenal medulla.

Phaeochromocytoma

Phaeochromocytomas are catecholamine-secreting tumours which are found mainly in the adrenal medulla, although tumours also occur in sympathetic ganglia. Occasionally, phaeochromocytomas develop in patients with an autosomal dominant trait for

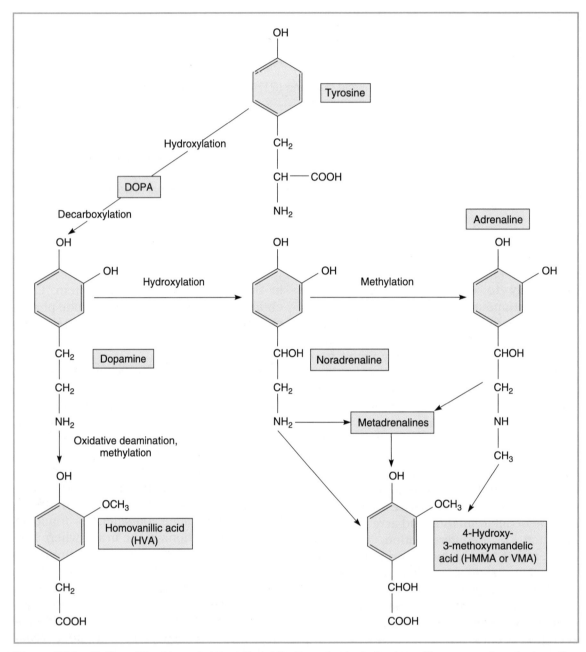

Figure 17.1 Outline of the biosynthesis and metabolism of catecholamines. The conversion of adrenaline and noradrenaline to 4-hydroxy-3-methoxymandelic acid (HMMA) involves two reactions, methylation (to form metadrenalines) and oxidative deamination, which can occur in either order.

developing the tumours in association with other abnormalities, such as neurofibromatosis (von Recklinhausen's disease) or medullary carcinoma of the thyroid and parathyroid hyperplasia (multiple endo-crine neoplasia type II). Most phaeochromocytomas secrete adrenaline and noradrenaline although some also secrete dopamine, which suggests malignancy. Most are benign and solitary although multiple tumours are found occasionally; approximately 10% of phaeochromocytomas are malignant.

Clinical Features

Although rare, phaeochromocytoma is an important cause of hypertension; it can be cured by successful surgical removal of the tumour. Hypertension, which results from the secretion of catecholamines, is sustained in approximately 60% of cases, while in 40% it is paroxysmal. Occasionally, hypotension is found when patients assume the upright posture (orthostatic hypotension). This is thought to result from decreased plasma volume caused by excess circulating catecholamines. Other clinical features resulting from catecholamine secretion include anxiety, palpitations and excessive sweating. Severe cardiac dysrhythmias and myocardial infarction can occur. Impaired glucose tolerance is seen in some patients, increased hepatic glucose production and inhibition of insulin secretion being contributory factors.

Investigation

The initial diagnosis of phaeochromocytoma is based on measurement of catecholamines or their metabolites in plasma or urine. It is important to be aware of potential interference as tests of catecholamine secretion, drugs and dietary constituents affect the results obtained with some techniques. Patients with persistently raised blood pressure usually have unequivocally elevated catecholamines while these may be raise intermittently in those with paroxysmal hypertension. In patients with persistent hypertension the diagnosis will be suggested by finding elevated urinary excretion of 4-hydroxy-3-methoxymandelic acid (HMMA or vanillylmandelic acid, VMA), metadrenalines or free catecholamines; it is usual to undertake three urine collections. Patients with episodic catecholamine excretion are more difficult to investigate effectively. Plasma catecholamine levels during an attack or a timed urine collection

immediately following an attack can be helpful. Considerable precautions are required in blood sampling and a venous cannula should be used to avoid the stress associated with venepuncture. Even with careful standardization of blood collection, plasma catecholamine levels may be slightly elevated in anxious patients and these may be difficult to distinguish from those seen as a result of a small tumour. In such cases a pentolinium suppression test may be helpful. Pentolinium blocks catecholamine secretion and plasma levels fall to normal following the intravenous injection of 2.5 mg in anxious subjects, while suppression does not occur in phaeochromocytoma. Once the diagnosis is established the tumour should be located by imaging techniques, either computerized tomography (CT) scanning or magnetic resonance imaging, prior to surgery.

KEY POINTS

PHAEOCHROMOCYTOMA

- Phaeochromocytoma is a catecholamine-producing tumour which occurs most commonly in the adrenal medulla

- Although phaeochromocytoma is a rare cause of hypertension it is important to diagnose as most cases are curable by surgery

- Excessive catecholamine production and hypertension may be intermittent

Neuroblastoma

Neuroblastoma is one of the most common malignant tumours of childhood and occurs in tissues of neural crest origin; it almost always presents in the first decade of life. The most common site is the adrenal medulla, although occasionally neuroblastomas occur in the sympathetic chain. The histology varies from relatively benign, well-differentiated to highly malignant, undifferentiated tumours. Because of their origin neuroblastomas can synthesize large quantities of catecholamines. The most common product is dopamine, which is not vasoactive. Urinary excretion of its metabolite, homovanillic acid, is measured to investigate the tumour. Rarely, noradrenaline is secreted and hypertensive crises can occur in these patients.

CARCINOID TUMOURS

Carcinoid tumours originate from chromaffin cells found in the small and large intestine, the bronchi, the pancreas, and very rarely in other organs. Approximately 90% occur in the gastrointestinal tract. They are characteristically slow-growing, although metastases occasionally occur. Some chromaffin cells synthesize 5-hydroxytryptamine (5-HT, serotonin) normally and the carcinoid syndrome results from excessive secretion of this. 5-HT is metabolized to 5-hydroxyindole acetic acid (5-HIAA) in the body, this metabolic end-product being excreted in urine (**Figure 17.2**). Clinical features include cutaneous flushing, diarrhoea, bronchial constriction, valvular cardiac disease and hypotension. 5-HT is normally metabolized in the liver and severe symptoms may indicate that hepatic metastases have occurred and 5-HT is being

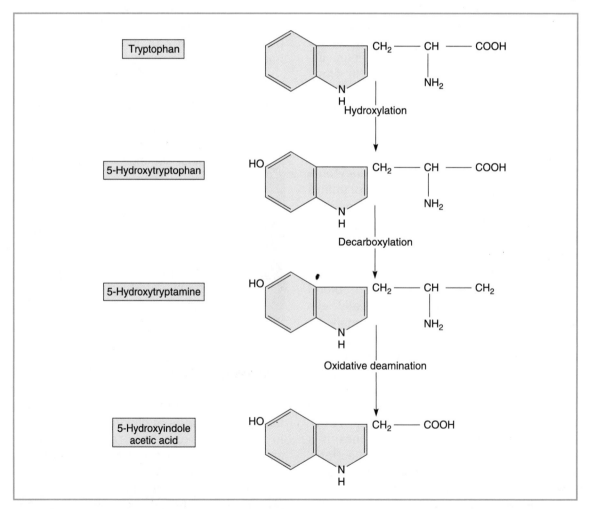

Figure 17.2 Outline of the synthesis and metabolism of 5-hydroxytryptamine.

secreted into the systemic circulation. Diagnosis is usually based on finding elevated urinary excretion of 5-HIAA. Some foods elevate levels and paracetamol may cause falsely elevated levels by interfering with some assays.

TUMOUR MARKERS

A tumour marker is a substance which is expressed by a neoplasm and can be monitored in diagnosis and management of the tumour. Such markers can be cellular, such as the Ph1 chromosome in chronic myeloid leukaemia, or expressed on cell surfaces, e.g. the presence of only κ or λ light chains on the surface of lymphocytes in myeloma. However, the term tumour marker is usually used in a more restricted sense to indicate a substance that is synthesized by a tumour in abnormal amounts and secreted into the circulation where it can be measured. Tumour markers have the following clinical applications:

1. To diagnose tumours, e.g. urinary 5-HIAA in carcinoid syndrome. However, in general, tumour markers are not specific enough for this purpose.
2. To screen high-risk individuals for the presence of tumours. Examples include measurement of calcitonin in families with multiple endocrine neoplasia type 1, calcitonin secretion being increased in medullary carcinoma of the thyroid. Patients with alcoholic cirrhosis are at increased risk of developing hepatocellular carcinoma and detection of α-fetoprotein in serum may indicate the development of a tumour.
3. To monitor the effectiveness of treatment, falling levels indicating that therapy has been successful.
4. To detect recurrence of tumours. If treatment of a tumour has been followed by falling levels of tumour markers, rising concentrations of these may well indicate that recurrence or metastasis has occurred.

Catecholamines and their metabolites in phaeochromocytoma and serotonin and its metabolites in carcinoid syndrome are measured for these purposes. Many other substances which can be thought of as tumour markers are considered elsewhere in this book, including paraproteins, parathyroid hormone (PTH)-related peptide, serum enzymes and faecal occult blood. Some of these are relatively specific, such as PTH-related peptide and elevated 5-HIAA excretion, while others, such as elevated serum enzyme activities, are nonspecific, since levels are often raised in the absence of tumour. Substances do not necessarily have to be specific to be useful tumour markers since the absolute concentration may be measured for monitoring response to treatment and recurrence. Tumour markers not considered elsewhere include α-fetoprotein, carcinoembryonic antigen and human chorionic gonadotrophin (hCG). The role of these as tumour markers is outlined below.

α-Fetoprotein

The use of α-fetoprotein in the investigation of fetal abnormalities is discussed in chapter 16. After birth, serum α-fetoprotein levels are very low but high concentrations can occur as a result of increased synthesis by hepatocellular carcinomas and some testicular and gastrointestinal tract malignancies. Serum α-fetoprotein levels can be raised in benign conditions, particularly hepatitis. Therefore high concentrations are not absolutely specific for tumours, although they are suggestive. Monitoring levels is useful in assessing the response to treatment.

Carcinoembryonic Antigen

Carcinoembryonic antigen is a group of glycoproteins, raised serum concentrations of which were thought to be specific for bowel cancer when they were first described. However, levels are high in a variety of nonmalignant conditions including inflammatory bowel disease, hepatitis, alcoholic cirrhosis and even cigarette smoking. Although elevated levels of carcinoembryonic antigen (CEA) are nonspecific, serial measurements are often undertaken in colorectal malignancies which produce CEA to monitor the response to treatment. Falling levels indicate successful treatment, while increasing concentrations following treatment suggest recurrence.

Human Chorionic Gonadotrophin

The role of this glycoprotein in pregnancy is considered in chapter 16. In addition to its production by the normal placenta hCG is secreted by trophoblastic tumours, particularly chorioncarcinoma, and germ-cell tumours of the testis and ovary. In trophoblastic tumours the levels of hCG reflect tumour mass and can be used to screen patients with a hydatidiform mole for the development of chorioncarcinoma. In germ-cell tumours its role is in monitoring response to treatment.

Prostatic Specific Antigen

Prostatic specific antigen is considered in chapter 12.

FURTHER READING

Beastall GH, Cook B, Rustin GJS, Jennings J. A review of the role of established tumour markers. *Annals of Clinical Biochemistry* 1991; **28**: 5–18.

Hall R, Besser M (eds). Chapters 7 and 19. *Fundamentals of Clinical Endocrinology*. Edinburgh: Churchill Livingstone, 1989, pp. 185–96 and pp. 420-42.

Odell WD, Appleton WS. Humoral manifestations of cancer. Chapter 34. In: Wilson JD, Foster DW (eds). *Williams Textbook of Endocrinology*. Philadelphia: WB Saunders, 1992, pp. 1599–618.

Roberts LJ II, Oates JA. Disorders of vasodilator hormones: the carcinoid syndrome and mastocytosis. Chapter 35. In: Wilson JD, Foster DW (eds). *Williams Textbook of Endocrinology*. Philadelphia: WB Saunders, 1992, pp. 1619–34.

CASE 17.1

A 43-year-old man complained to his general practitioner that he was suffering from frequent headaches. On direct questioning he indicated that these were often associated with sweating and on examination his blood pressure, when lying down, was 185/120 mmHg. What investigations must be performed?

CASE 17.2

A 35-year-old woman was referred to surgical outpatients because of intermittent diarrhoea for several months. The diarrhoea was not watery and she never passed blood. On direct questioning she reported breathlessness which had become apparent over the last few weeks. During the course of the consultation she was flushed and admitted that this occurred frequently when she felt stressed. What diagnosis must be considered?

CASE 17.3

A 5-year-old child was referred to a paediatric oncology unit with a mass in the abdomen. Urinary catecholamine metabolites were quantified and the following results obtained:

homovanillic acid	37 μmol 24 h^{-1}
(reference range for this age group	6–24 μmol 24 h^{-1})
4-hydroxy-3-methoxymandelic acid	13 μmol 24 h^{-1}
(reference range for this age group	4–13 μmol 24 h^{-1})

What is the cause of the abnormal results?

CASE HISTORIES

CLINICAL BIOCHEMISTRY AT THE EXTREMES OF AGE

THE ELDERLY

Introduction

The investigation of elderly patients requires special consideration for four main reasons.

1. The values for many biochemical tests in healthy elderly subjects are different from those seen in younger age groups.
2. Some diseases affecting elderly patients are seen rarely in younger age groups.
3. The clinical presentation of common diseases may be atypical compared with the features seen in younger age groups.
4. Test results are more likely to be affected by medical treatment than in younger patients.

Reference Ranges

Many biochemical investigations show changes with age in addition to differences between the sexes. The choice of a healthy aged population on which to base reference ranges poses some difficulties since the prevalence of clinically apparent or occult disease is high. In addition, surveys of the elderly living at home have shown that many receive medication that can affect test results. Reference ranges should ideally be performed on elderly subjects who are free from disease and are receiving no medication. In practice, this is rarely achieved, community-based data often being used which include subjects on medication, specific exclusions being made for those receiving relevant drugs, e.g. thyroid hormone replacement for reference ranges for thyroid function tests.

Renal Function

Renal function declines progressively with age, plasma urea concentrations rising (**Figure 18.1**) and creatinine clearance falling. Although plasma creatinine levels also increase with age, this is often less marked as lean body mass tends to fall in the elderly. The mean glomerular filtration rate (GFR) corrected to a body surface area of 1.73 m^2 is 140 ml min^{-1} at the age of 30 and this declines to 97 ml min^{-1} at the age of 80 years. The number of functioning nephrons in each kidney decreases with age, the decline being greatest after the fifth decade; the reason for this is not fully understood. The upper limit of the reference range for plasma urea in the elderly is 2 mmol l^{-1} higher than adults in middle age,

creatinine being up to 30 μmol l^{-1} higher. As in younger groups, levels are higher in men than women, owing to differences in muscle mass.

Water and Electrolytes

Potassium

Total body potassium appears to fall with age, even if allowance is made for the decrease in lean body mass. This appears to be due, at least in part, to reduced intake. The reduction in body potassium is probably unimportant unless additional losses occur. Thus, diuretic therapy may lead to hypokalaemia, this being seen only rarely with such treatment in younger subjects. Potassium supplements are often required in elderly patients, particularly if they are also receiving digoxin, since hypokalaemia is an important factor in digoxin toxicity. It is probably unnecessary to give potassium supplements prophylactically since adverse reactions to oral potassium can occur. Plasma potassium concentrations should be monitored and supplements given if hypokalaemia develops.

Sodium and Water

The ability of the kidney to conserve salt and water falls with increasing age. The renal response to vasopressin appears to be reduced and renal adaptation to sodium depletion is slower. Hyponatraemia is more common in the elderly, although the reference range for plasma sodium concentration appears no different in patients over 65 years of age compared with younger subjects, provided acutely ill patients or those receiving drug therapy are excluded. Causes of hyponatraemia include:

1. Postoperative fluid retention as a result of nonosmotic stimulation of vasopressin secretion. Stimuli of vasopressin secretion include preoperative fluid restriction, stress, perioperative pain and drugs.

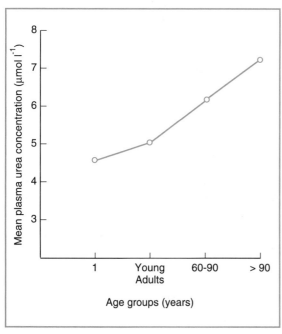

Figure 18.1 Mean plasma urea concentrations in different age groups. The urea concentration is slightly higher in adults compared with infants, significant increases occurring in fit elderly subjects owing to a decline in renal function.

2. Inappropriate antidiuretic hormone secretion owing ectopic secretion by
tumours. In addition to carcinoma of
the bronchus, malignancies of the bladder, prostate, pancreas and lymphoid
tissue are associated with this syndrome. Hypothyroidism is also an important cause of inappropriate antidiuretic hormone (ADH) secretion in
the elderly. This results possibly from
the central nervous system effects of
thyroid hormone deficiency. Other
drugs associated with inappropriate
ADH secretion include narcotic analgesics, carbamezapine, phenothiazines,
monoamine oxidase inhibitors and cytotoxic drugs, particularly vincristine.

3. Sulphonylurea drugs used in the treatment of non-insulin-dependent diabetes
mellitus (NIDDM) are also associated
with inappropriate vasopressin secretion in this age group, although hyponatraemia is less common with agents
used currently, such as glibenclamide,
than with chlorpropamide.

4. In the elderly, diuretic therapy is also an
important cause of hyponatraemia, this
being found more commonly than hypokalaemia in patients receiving thiazide
diuretics. Hyponatraemia may be severe
and can present as fits or coma. The
main cause appears to be volume
depletion leading to appropriate ADH
secretion, as a result of stimulation of
volume receptors overriding osmotic
control.

Hypernatraemia is almost always caused
by dehydration and occurs either because
dehydration is not accompanied by thirst or
if patients are unable to respond to
increased thirst. Hypernatraemia may be
found in many acute illnesses in the elderly
if these illnesses cause confusional states or
reduced mobility. Excessive water loss may
occur as a result of diabetes insipidus, this
being due most often to malignancy with
intracranial metastases.

KEY POINTS

**RENAL FUNCTION AND ELECTRO-
LYTES**

■ Kidney function declines progressively with age in the absence of
renal disease

■ Hyponatraemia is common, causes
including diuretic therapy and inappropriate secretion of ADH

■ Body potassium content falls with
age and diuretic therapy may cause
hypokalaemia

Endocrine Function

Sex Steroids and Gonadotrophins – Females
The most obvious change in endocrine
function occurring with age is the abrupt
decline in ovarian oestrogen production at
the menopause, with atrophic changes
occurring in target organs, including the
genital tract and breast. Progressive loss of
bone mass also occurs. Increased secretion
of pituitary gonadotrophins occurs as a
result of reduced negative feedback from
ovarian steroids, the increase in serum
follicle-stimulating hormone (FSH) concentration being greater than for luteinizing
hormone (LH). The ovary loses its ability to
convert androstenedione to oestrone (ar-
omatisation) and the postmenopausal ovary
produces mainly androgens.

Sex Steroids and Gonadotrophins – Males
Testosterone production and spermatogenesis decline with age in males, although
changes are gradual. Age-related vascular
changes are thought to impair Leydig cell
function. Pituitary gonadotrophin levels in
serum rise gradually after the age of 40 years
with more pronounced increases occurring
in patients over 70 years.

Thyroid Function
Thyroid hormone concentrations appear to
differ little between healthy elderly and
younger subjects, although levels are often

lower in elderly subjects admitted to hospital, as a consequence of disease. Both hypo- and hyper-thyroidism may develop for the first time in the elderly, the clinical presentation often being atypical. Thus, the features of hyperthyroidism include breathlessness, heart failure, disordered gastrointestinal function and weight loss. Hypothyroidism is relatively common among elderly inpatients and clinical features may be unusual, such as depression or resulting from hyponatraemia.

Glucose Tolerance and Diabetes Mellitus

Fasting blood glucose is affected little by age although glucose tolerance to a carbohydrate meal decreases from the third decade, even in the absence of type 2 diabetes mellitus. This is due to impaired peripheral glucose uptake rather than endogenous glucose production, and is a result of resistance to insulin action.

Metabolic Bone Disease

The prevalence of osteomalacia is increased in the elderly owing to lack of exposure to sunlight and poor nutrition. Hypocalcaemia often occurs although the serum calcium concentration may be normal. Typically, the serum alkaline phosphatase activity is raised, although such a finding is nonspecific and other causes must be considered. These include Paget's disease of the bone, the prevalence of which increases in the elderly, in liver disease, and in renal failure.

Hypocalcaemia is more commonly caused by low serum albumin concentrations than by osteomalacia. Other important causes of hypocalcaemia include drug therapy. Frusemide increases the urinary excretion of calcium and increased renal losses of calcium may also occur during treatment of malignant diseases with cytotoxic drugs.

Hypercalcaemia is caused by the same diseases affecting younger adult patients (see chapter 9). In addition, hypercalcaemia is seen occasionally in patients given large doses of diuretics over a relatively short time period, e.g. in the treatment of pulmonary oedema.

Nutritional Disorders

Nutritional disorders other than osteomalacia occur. Many elderly people live alone and have a reduced income – factors which increase the risk of nutritional disorders. The intake of vitamin C is sometimes inadequate and scurvy may occur. Low serum vitamin B_{12} concentrations have been found in up to 10% of otherwise healthy elderly subjects. Some of these, but by no means all, have early pernicious anaemia. Serum albumin concentrations are often reduced in the elderly and very low protein intake may be a contributory cause. However, albumin synthesis is reduced in a variety of disorders including liver disease, infections and inflammatory diseases. Protein loss also occurs through wounds, in protein-losing enteropathies and in nephrotic syndrome. Impaired hepatic function is a more common cause of hypoalbuminaemia than malnutrition.

Medication and Biochemical Investigations

Many elderly subjects receive medical treatment, perhaps as many as 75%. In addition, a high proportion of these receive multiple drug treatment. A number of effects of drugs on biochemical tests have been discussed

KEY POINTS

ENDOCRINE FUNCTION AND NUTRITIONAL DISORDERS

- Hyperthyroidism and hypothyroidism may present with atypical clinical features

- Glucose tolerance declines with age owing to resistance to insulin action

- Nutritional disorders are common in the elderly, particularly those who live alone and many others occur, e.g. impaired glucose tolerance and hyperuricaemia are seen in patients receiving thiazide diuretics.

CHILDREN

Introduction

With the exception of investigations for inherited metabolic diseases, most of the investigations performed on children are similar to those carried out on adults. The requirement for small volumes of blood for analysis can often be met by modern laboratory analysers used for adult work, although special attention must be paid to sample handling, particularly as the haematocrit is higher in neonates than in older subjects. The blood volume is 50 times lower in neonates than in adults.

Sample Collection

Blood

The requirement for very small blood samples in neonates can be met most conveniently by collecting capillary blood following a heel or finger prick. A good peripheral circulation is required for the satisfactory collection of capillary specimens and, if necessary, the area should be rubbed gently or immersed in warm water prior to sampling. The temperature should not exceed 40°C as temperatures above 43°C may cause tissue damage. It is important to sample the fleshy part of the finger or heel to reduce the risk of injury and possible infection to underlying bones. Occasionally, blood samples of 1 ml can be obtained by this technique but it is more realistic to anticipate volumes of up to 400–500 μl. Venepuncture is often used in older children although taking such samples can be difficult and may involve physical restraint.

Urine

Special techniques for urine collection are available for babies being managed in incubators and urine collection bags are used in more mature babies. Timed urine collections are difficult to collect accurately even in older children; therefore investigations using random urine specimens are preferable if possible.

Reference Ranges

Reference ranges for biochemical tests are often less well established in children than adults although considerable data are available (see references). Comprehensive surveys of reference ranges in normal children are more difficult than in adults for ethical reasons and such ranges change with rapid growth and development. Chronological age is not always satisfactory for establishing reference data as many tests are interpreted best by considering physical development. Thus, correcting test results for differences in height, weight or body surface area is often undertaken as an aid to interpretation.

Neonatal Jaundice

Neonates have a relative polycythaemia although this decreases rapidly in the first few days of life, with metabolism of excess haemoglobin to bilirubin. Since the major enzyme which conjugates bilirubin in the liver (UDP glucuronyl transferase, see chapter 11) is not fully mature at birth unconjugated hyperbilirubinaemia and jaundice are extremely common. This is usually physiological although there are many other causes of neonatal jaundice (**Table 18.1**). Physiological jaundice is maximal within 2–5 days of delivery; it is more severe in premature infants, in whom it may persist for 2 weeks, and also if bruising has occurred perinatally. Unconjugated bilirubin is toxic to the central nervous system, causing kernicterus if it is deposited in the basal ganglia of the brain. Kernicterus is characterized by choreo-athetoid movements and has a high mortality. However,

Table 18.1 Causes of neonatal jaundice

Predominantly unconjugated
Physiological jaundice
Haemolytic disease
Breast milk jaundice
Hypothyroidism
Inherited metabolic disorders
◆ Crigler–Najjar syndrome
◆ Lucey–Driscoll syndrome
Haemorrhage, sepsis

Conjugated
Infection
◆ Cytomegalovirus, rubella, hepatitis A, B,
  Escherichia coli etc
Inherited metabolic disorders
◆ Galactosaemia
◆ α_1-Antitrypsin deficiency
◆ Cystic fibrosis
◆ Hereditary fructose intolerance
◆ Tyrosinosis
Parenteral nutrition
Congenital hepatic fibrosis
Biliary atresia

finding of a large proportion of conjugated bilirubin requires detailed investigation (**Table 18.1**). Methods of treating physiological jaundice include phototherapy, exchange transfusion and enzyme induction using phenobarbitone or antipyrine.

KEY POINTS

PHYSIOLOGICAL HYPERBILIRUBINAEMIA

■ Physiological hyperbilrubinaemia is very common

■ Physiological jaundice is caused by catabolism of haemoglobin together with immature conjugating enzymes

■ Physiological hyperbilirubinaemia of the newborn is predominantly unconjugated

■ Physiological jaundice may lead to kernicterus

jaundice has no effect on the central nervous system in adults, even if severe, since bilirubin does not cross the blood brain barrier. The blood brain barrier is immature in neonates and unconjugated bilirubin can therefore enter brain tissue if the binding sites for bilirubin on albumin are saturated. This is likely to occur at serum bilirubin concentrations >400 μmol l^{-1} in healthy babies, but at lower concentrations in acidotic neonates, because H^+ ions compete for the same binding sites on albumin. Other substances also compete with bilirubin for albumin binding including salicylates, sulphonamides and nonesterified fatty acids (NEFAs). Physiological jaundice may be severe enough to cause kernicterus.

Neonatal jaundice should be investigated if it is severe, prolonged or if it is detected unusually early. Blood specimens for bilirubin analysis need to be protected from the light during transport to the laboratory, as bilirubin is photolabile. Physiological jaundice is predominantly unconjugated and the

Acid–Base Homeostasis and Respiration

Fetal Monitoring

Blood pH is often measured in the assessment of fetal distress by collecting capillary blood after making a nick in the scalp using a tube inserted through the cervix. Lactate production is increased by an anoxic fetus, a blood pH <7.2 often being accepted as an indication for immediate delivery. *In utero*, the lungs are filled with liquid, this being forced out during labour, or absorbed. Towards term, pneumocytes in the lungs secrete a surfactant, the main constituent of which is the phospholipid lecithin (phosphatidylcholine). Surfactant lowers the surface tension within the alveoli, facilitating lung expansion after delivery. Deficiency of surfactant, due to immaturity or asphyxia, leads to respiratory distress syndrome, the main indication for ventilation or oxygen therapy in preterm neonates. Amniotic fluid can be sampled before delivery to assess lung maturity by measuring the lecithin:sphingomyelin ratio. Sphingomyelin production is relatively constant during gestation while lecithin production increases as the fetal lung matures, synthesis starting at about 32 weeks gestation. Measurement of the lecithin:spingomyelin ratio is often undertaken if induction of labour is being considered.

In the Neonate

Acid–base homeostasis is important in perinatal life, causes of disordered function including respiratory and nonrespiratory conditions (**Table 18.2**). Hypoxia may occur during birth as a result of cord occlusion or compression. Lactic acidosis occurs commonly if hypoxia is prolonged owing to poor tissue perfusion and anaerobic metabolism. If prolonged, asphyxia leads to apnoea and circulatory failure, while acidosis increases the risk of intracranial haemorrhage and impaired myocardial function. Respiratory failure is more common in premature infants. Several factors contribute to this including asphyxia, immaturity of the lungs and muscle weakness. Adequate ventilatory support is important in minimizing these abnormalities. Metabolic acidosis in neonates may have a variety of causes in addition to poor tissue perfusion, including sepsis, blood loss, congenital abnormalities, renal disease and inherited metabolic disorders.

Measurement of Blood Gases in Neonates

Blood samples for gas analysis can be taken in capillary tubes, although prewarming of the skin to dilate arterioles and arterialize the blood is essential for blood gas samples Results of blood gas analysis may be required rapidly in critically ill patients and thus the investigation is often undertaken using analysers sited in the clinical unit. Transcutaneous monitoring of PO_2 using an oxygen electrode placed on the skin is used widely in neonatal units. These devices require that the blood is arterialized by warming the skin to 43°C, with the danger of causing burns. Therefore, the electrodes must be repositioned frequently, every 4 h or so, to prevent this. In addition, electrodes drift and therefore frequent recalibration is necessary. An alternative to continuous monitoring is pulse oximetry in which light-emitting probes are attached to a hand or foot. Light is absorbed by the blood flowing beneath the probe and the characteristics of the light absorption can be used to calculate oxygen saturation of the blood. Pulse oximetry monitors changes in oxygen saturation although knowledge of the PO_2 is also required, as small changes in oxygen saturation may occur with large changes in the PO_2 at the upper end of the oxygen dissociation curve (*see* **Figure 7.7**).

Table 18.2 Causes of acidosis in the neonate

Respiratory
- Asphyxia
- Prematurity
- Central nervous system (CNS) abnormalities
  Drugs administered to the mother (analgesics, sedatives, anaesthetic)
  Trauma
- Mechanical abnormality
  Respiratory distress syndrome
  Diaphragmatic hernia
  Pneumothorax
  Obstructed airways
  Muscle weakness
- Cardiovascular
  Pulmonary hypertension
  Congenital heart disease
Nonrespiratory
- Renal dysfunction
- Poor tissue perfusion leading to lactic acidosis
  Congenital heart abnormalities
  Sepsis
  Haemorrhage
- Inherited metabolic disorders
  Amino acid disorders
  Organic acidaemias

Hypoglycaemia

Hypoglycaemia is considered in chapter 1.

Hypocalcaemia

The clinical features of neonatal hypocalcaemia include irritability, twitching, convulsions, poor feeding and vomiting. Biochemically, hypocalcaemia is defined as a total serum calcium concentration <1.8 mmol l^{-1} or a serum ionized calcium concentration <0.7 mmol l^{-1}. Calcium is actively transported across the placenta and fetal total and ionized calcium concentrations are higher than those in adults. These fall in the first few hours after birth, levels of parathyroid hormone being transiently low. Calcium concentrations are at their lowest at 1–2 days, thereafter increasing.

The causes of neonatal hypocalcaemia are outlined in **Table 18.3**. The physiological fall in serum calcium is often more pronounced following birth asphyxia, in premature infants, and in infants born to diabetic mothers. Primary hypoparathyroidism is rare although inherited X-linked forms occur. T-cells are deficient in Di George's syndrome; other developmental abnormalities of organs derived from the embryonic neural crest also occur including thymic aplasia and hypoparathyroidism. Characteristic facies and cardiac abnormalities are

Table 18.3 Hypocalcaemia in infancy

Physiological
◆ Prematurity
◆ Birth asphyxia
◆ Infants of diabetic mothers
Hypoalbuminaemia
Hypoparathyroidism
◆ Primary
◆ Di George's syndrome
◆ Pseudohypoparathyroidism
Nutritional
◆ Low calcium intake
◆ High phosphate intake
◆ Vitamin D deficiency
Iatrogenic
◆ Exchange transfusion
◆ Parenteral nutrition

also seen. Cow's milk has a high phosphate content compared with human milk and infants fed unmodified cows milk may develop hypocalcaemia. Maternal vitamin D deficiency may lead to hypocalcaemia in neonates. Although it rarely occurs as an isolated defect, hypomagnesaemia may accompany hypocalcaemia. Hypocalcaemia is refractory to treatment if the hypomagnesaemia is not corrected. It is therefore important to investigate serum magnesium concentrations.

Renal Function and Electrolyte Balance

Urine is produced by the fetus from the ninth intrauterine week although the purpose of this is unclear, as toxic metabolites are eliminated via the placenta. Fetal urinary output approaching term is fairly large, up to 25 ml per hour, although this falls to 2–4 ml h^{-1} after birth. The GFR at birth is approximately 25% of that seen in older children. It increases rapidly in full-term infants during the first week of life and then more slowly, reaching adult values by 2 years of age. Plasma creatinine concentrations are similar to those seen in the mother at birth and fall to a mean value of 35 μmol l^{-1} after 1 week. Mean plasma values rise as muscle mass increases with growth, reaching adult values at puberty. Urea concentrations are more stable and do not increase at puberty.

Short Stature

The definition of short stature is determined by comparison of the patient's height compared with other children of the same age. The decision to investigate short stature is not always straightforward but in general this is not required in children less than -2 standard deviations below the mean height for their age. Evaluation should be undertaken in those who are more than -3 standard deviations below the mean for

Table 18.4   Causes of short stature

Constitutional growth delay
Endocrine
◆ Growth hormone deficiency
◆ Hypothyroidism
◆ Corticosteroid excess
◆ Precocious puberty
Nutritional
◆ Inadequate food supply
◆ Bowel disorders
    Coeliac disease
    Crohn's disease
Systemic disease
◆ Chronic renal failure
◆ Congenital heart disease
Chromosomal abnormalities
◆ Gonadal dysgenesis

their age and in those in whom a consistently low growth rate is observed.

Causes of short stature are outlined in **Table 18.4**. Several factors are important in control of growth. There is a relationship between parent's and children's height, although the height of children cannot be predicted accurately from that of the parents. Intrauterine growth is determined largely by maternal blood supply and appears to be little affected by hormonal factors. Body length at birth is a poor predictor of adult height. Nutritional deprivation after birth is caused either by inadequate intake (kwashiorkor, marasmus) or by malabsorption (coeliac disease, Crohn's disease). Linear growth occurs if growth hormone is deficient, although at less than half the normal rate. Growth is impaired more severely in the absence of

thyroid hormone. Gonadal steroids exert their major effect at the time of the pubertal growth spurt. Growth is impaired in severe systemic disease, such as chronic renal failure.

Investigation

An accurate history and examination, including an assessment of the parents' heights, are essential in addition to laboratory investigations. General investigations that may be helpful include renal and thyroid function tests.

FURTHER READING

Clayton BE, Jenkins P, Round JM. *Paediatric Chemical Pathology. Clinical Tests and Reference Ranges*. Oxford: Blackwell, 1980.

Green A, Morgan I. *Neonatology and Clinical Biochemistry*. London: ACB Venture Publications, 1993.

Faulkner WR, Meites S. *Geriatric Clinical Chemistry, Reference Values*. Washington: AACC Press, 1993.

Hodkinson M (ed). *Clinical Biochemistry of the Elderly*. Edinburgh: Churchill Livingstone, 1984.

Lipschitz DA. Nutrition and ageing. Chapter 6. In: Grimley Evans J, Franklin Williams T (eds). *Oxford Textbook of Geriatric Medicine*. Oxford: Oxford University Press. 1992, pp. 119–27

Tietz NW, Shue DF, Wekstein DR. Laboratory values in fit ageing individuals – sexagenarians through centenarians. *Clinical Chemistry* 1992; **38**: 1167–85

CASE 18.1

A 79-year-old man who lived alone was found in a confused state by neighbours. The history obtained by the general practitioner indicated that the patient had felt generally unwell and breathless for about 6 days. Ankle oedema was noted which the patient thought was of recent onset and there were crepitations in the base of both lungs. On admission to hospital an electrocardiogram (ECG) showed equivocal changes and some blood tests were undertaken. These showed:

sodium	141 mmol l^{-1}
potassium	3.9 mmol l^{-1}
urea	11.5 mmol l^{-1}
creatine kinase	140 U l^{-1}
lactate dehydrogenase	630 U l^{-1}

How would you interpret these results?

CASE 18.2

A 75-year-old man was admitted to a geriatric ward for investigation of weight loss and anaemia. He was noted to have atrial fibrillation and blood tests were undertaken to establish whether he had hyperthyroidism. These showed:

TSH	1.2 mU l^{-1}
free thyroxine (fT4)	12.4 pmol l^{-1}
free triiodothyronine (fT3)	3.9 pmol l^{-1}

Can these results be explained by thyroid disease?

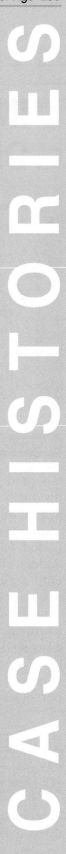

CASE HISTORIES

19

INHERITED METABOLIC DISEASES

INTRODUCTION

Inherited metabolic diseases, although individually rare, are important causes of ill-health in children. They may present as acute life-threatening illness in the neonatal period or become apparent later in childhood; rarely, clinical presentation is delayed until adult years. Inherited metabolic diseases occur because of abnormal gene expression leading to defective synthesis of a protein, usually an enzyme, which controls a key step in metabolism. Disease may result from an absence of the product of the enzyme action or be due to the accumulation of substrates (**Figure 19.1**).

INHERITED METABOLIC DISEASE IN NEONATES

Clinical Features

The clinical features of inherited metabolic disease are often nonspecific and include failure to thrive, feeding difficulties, vomiting, hypotonia and fits. There may be a symptom-free period after birth and it is important to establish whether there is a relationship between onset of disease and changes in feeding patterns, galactosaemia and hypolactasia presenting after the introduction of milk. An abnormal smell is characteristic of some disorders of amino acid and organic acid metabolism, while ambiguous genitalia suggest congenital adrenal hyperplasia. Neurological features occur in disorders of the urea cycle.

Laboratory Investigations

Laboratory investigations can be considered as several types. Basic investigations, such as determination of plasma glucose and blood gases, which are carried out as part of the normal care of a sick infant, may show results consistent with inherited metabolic disease (**Table 19.1**). However, such tests are nonspecific. Metabolic tests provide

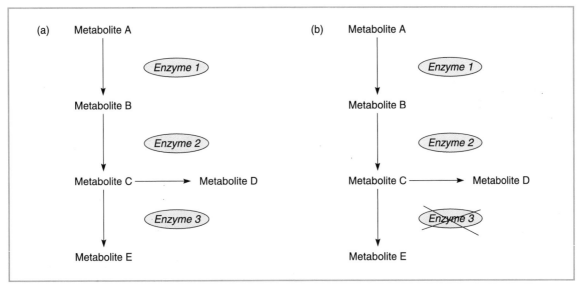

Figure 19.1   The effect of a defect in enzyme synthesis on a metabolic pathway. (a) In this hypothetical pathway metabolite A is converted to metabolite E via the intermediates B and C. Metabolite D is formed in small amounts by a minor reaction. (b) Metabolite E is not formed in significant amounts owing to a defect in the synthesis of enzyme 3. Metabolite C accumulates and more is converted to metabolite D. Clinical disease could result from a deficiency in metabolite E or because the larger amounts of metabolite C or D are toxic.

additional evidence and may suggest a particular group of conditions although diagnosis usually depends on a third level of investigation, the measurement of specific metabolites. It is possible to determine the activity of enzymes responsible for inherited metabolic disease although tissue culture of cells prepared from an appropriate biopsy may be necessary. Increasingly, the structural abnormality in deoxyribonucleic acid (DNA) causing inherited metabolic disease is being characterized (see below).

INHERITED METABOLIC DISEASE IN OLDER CHILDREN

Clinical presentation may occur as acute illnesses similar to those in neonates, particularly if precipitated by stress such as a severe infection or an operation. Other methods of presentation include mental retardation, dysmorphic features, or complications arising from disordered metabolism.

Disorders of Carbohydrate Metabolism

Disorders of carbohydrate metabolism are considered in chapter 1.

Disorders of Amino Acid Metabolism

Phenylketonuria

Phenylketonuria is due to an absence or deficiency of phenylalanine hydroxylase and is the commonest disorder of amino acid metabolism causing mental retardation. In the United Kingdom it occurs with an incidence of 1 in 10 000 births although it has been reported to occur in 1 in 5000 to 1 in 20 000 births in other countries.

Phenylalanine Metabolism   The metabolism of phenylalanine in outlined in **Figure 19.2**. Phenylalanine is dietary in origin and is catabolized mainly to tyrosine in the liver by phenylalanine hydroxylase, tetrahydrobiopterin being required as a cofactor. The

Table 19.1   Investigation of suspected inherited metabolic disease in a neonate

Test	Finding	Disorders
General Investigations		
Blood glucose	Hypoglycaemia	Defects of gluconeogenesis
		Organic acidaemias
		Galactosaemia
		Glycogen storage diseases
		Amino acid disorders
Blood gases	Metabolic acidosis	Organic acidaemias
		Lactic acidosis
		Renal tubular acidosis
Plasma electrolytes	Hyponatraemia	Congenital adrenal hyperplasia
Liver function tests	Hepatic dysfunction	Galactosaemia
		von Gierke's disease
		Hereditary fructose intolerance
		α_1-Antitrypsin deficiency
		Defects in gluconeogenesis
Urine analysis	Reducing substances	von Gierke's disease
		Hereditary fructose intolerance
	Ketones positive with hypoglycaemia	Defect in carbohydrate metabolism
	Ketones negative with hypoglycaemia	Defect in fatty acid oxidation
Metabolic Investigations		
Plasma lactate	Raised	von Gierke's disease
		Organic acidaemias
		Pyruvate dehydrogenase deficiency
		Defects of gluconeogenesis
Plasma ammonia	Hyperammonaemia	*See* **Table 19.2**
Plasma NEFA	Increased	Defect in fatty acid oxidation
Urinary sugars	Specific sugars are suggestive of particular defects in carbohydrate metabolism	
Urinary amino acids	Groups or specific amino acids are suggestive of particular disorders of carbohydrate metabolism	
Urinary organic acids	Specific acids are suggestive of particular organic acidaemias	

NEFA, nonesterified fatty acid.

enzyme is also present in leukocytes. If the enzyme is deficient, phenylalanine concentrations rise in blood and metabolism by alternative pathways occurs, producing phenyllactic acid, phenylacetic acid and many other metabolites, all of which are present in negligible amounts in normal subjects. These are excreted in the urine where phenyllactic acid causes a characteristic odour which may be detected in untreated patients. Persistent postnatal hyperphenylalaninaemia causes irreversible brain damage by complex mechanisms which include interference with brain amino acid metabolism and inhibition of neurotransmitter synthesis. Phenylalanine is a competitive inhibitor of tyrosinase, a key enzyme in the synthesis of melanin. Many different mutations producing phenylalanine hydroxylase deficiency have been described and hyperphenylalaninaemia also occurs owing to tetrahydrobiopterin deficiency, this also being caused by enzyme defects.

Clinical Features An infant with untreated phenylketonuria is normal at birth, since phenylalanine is transferred rapidly across the placenta. Thereafter phenylalanine accu-

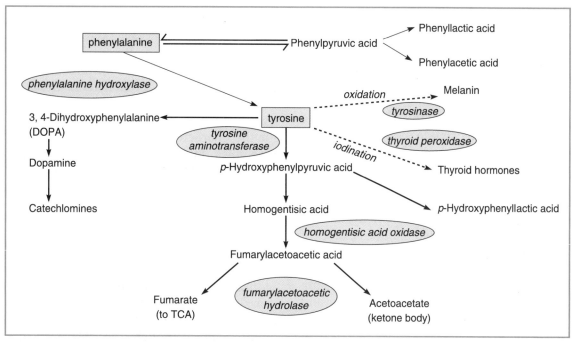

Figure 19.2 Outline of phenylalanine and tyrosine metabolism. Enzyme deficiencies causing inherited metabolic disorders are indicated in italics. TCA, tricarboxylic acid cycle.

mulates and mental development is obviously abnormal by 6 months in classical phenylketonuria. Some patients have fits and aggressive behaviour; microcephaly may occur. There is a tendency to hypopigmentation, blue eyes and fair hair being common.

Diagnosis Diagnosis must be made and treatment initiated within 1 month of birth if mental retardation is to be prevented. Thus, screening programmes have been introduced for neonates, using the Guthrie test. This is a microbiological assay in which a disk of filter paper containing blood from a heel prick is placed on plates impregnated with a microorganism, *Bacillus subtilis*, which requires phenylalanine for growth, the only source being the blood spot. Thus, growth of the organism is a positive test which must be confirmed by measuring blood phenylalanine concentrations.

Treatment Treatment is by a special diet in which protein is replaced by an amino acid mixture low in phenylalanine. Treatment should be continued for many years as excessive blood phenylalanine levels between 4 to 8 years leads to mental retardation. Even if treatment is instituted early some mental retardation may occur, although this is less severe than in untreated cases.

Other Causes of Hyperphenylalaninaemia In addition to phenylketonuria and tetrahydro-biopterin deficiency (which produces severe clinical features) partial deficiency of phenylalanine hydroxylase produces mild or atypical phenylketonuria.

KEY POINTS

PHENYLKETONURIA

- Phenylketonuria is the commonest inherited cause of mental retardation

- Phenylketonuria is caused by defective phenylalanine hydroxylase activity

- Screening programmes for phenylketonuria have been established based on the Guthrie test

Disorders of Tyrosine Metabolism

Tyrosine is a precursor of DOPA (3,4-dihydroxyphenylalanine), which in turn is converted to dopamine and catecholamines (**Figure 19.2**). Dopamine is a neurotransmitter in nuclei of the brain stem and changes in these together with a decrease of dopamine in the caudate nucleus and putamen occur in Parkinson's disease. Tyrosine is a precursor of melanin which is synthesized by a complex series of reactions initiated by tyrosinase, the activity of which is inhibited competitively by phenylalanine. Deficiency of tyrosinase is one cause of albinism.

Alkaptonuria is caused by a deficiency of homogentisic acid oxidase and homogentisic acid, a metabolite of phenylalanine and tyrosine, cannot be metabolized further and therefore accumulates and is excreted in urine. Homogentisic acid is deposited in connective tissue and converted to a dark pigment which is deposited in the sclerae and ear cartilages, causing ochronosis. Degenerative changes in joints also occur, leading to arthritis. The urine turns dark on standing.

Thyroid hormones are synthesized from tyrosine through an initial stage catalysed by thyroid peroxidase in which inorganic iodine is oxidized in the presence of hydrogen peroxide, iodide then replacing a hydrogen atom in tyrosine. Deficiency of thyroid peroxidase is one cause of goitre and hypothyroidism.

Tyrosinaemias I and II are inherited metabolic disorders resulting from enzyme deficiencies in the catabolic pathway by which tyrosine is converted to fumarate and acetoacetate. Tyrosinaemia II (tyrosine aminotransferase deficiency) is associated with corneal and skin abnormalities, with mental retardation occurring in some; the features appear to result from tyrosine accumulation. Tyrosinaemia I (fumarylacetoacetate hydroxylase deficiency) is associated with liver failure and renal tubular disorders owing to the accumulation of toxic metabolites.

Maple Syrup Urine Disease

Maple syrup urine disease (MSUD) is caused by a deficiency of the enzyme which decarboxylates oxoacids produced from the metabolism of branched-chain amino acids, leucine, isoleucine and valine. These oxoacids which accumulate are responsible for the characteristic odour in urine which resembles maple syrup. Clinical features include failure to thrive, feeding difficulties, lethargy and neurological dysfunction. Progressive deterioration occurs if the disease is untreated, with death in early childhood. Investigations often show the presence of metabolic acidosis and hypoglycaemia, the diagnostic test being plasma concentrations of branched-chain amino acids which are grossly elevated. Treatment is to introduce a diet that is deficient in branched-chain amino acids although the this may not produce a normal outlook, recurrent episodes of illness sometimes occurring.

Organic Acidaemias

The organic acidaemias are a group of inherited metabolic diseases in which carboxylic acids of low molecular weight accumulate. Organic acids are synthesized during the metabolism of amino acids, carbohydrates and fats. Many different disorders of organic acid metabolism have been described, the most prevalent forms being defects in branched-chain amino acids, proprionyl CoA, and fatty acid metabolism. Although individually they are rare, collectively the prevalence of organic acidaemias is similar to defects in amino acid metabolism. They may present as failure to thrive, vomiting, severe metabolic disturbances, and the sudden infant death syndrome. Metabolic abnormalities include hypoglycaemia, ketosis, lactic acidosis and hyperammonaemia. Diagnosis is by determination of specific organic acid concentrations in urine and analysis of enzyme activities.

Table 19.2 Important causes of hyperammonaemia

Transient hyperammonaemia
Severe illness in the newborn, e.g. sepsis, shock
Inherited metabolic disease
◆ Urea cycle disorders
◆ Organic acidaemias
Liver disease
◆ Reye's syndrome
◆ Other causes
High protein intake, particularly parenteral nutrition
Drugs, e.g. sodium valproate

gut and is also a product of the catabolism of amino acids in the liver. Ammonia is detoxified by conversion to urea in the liver by the urea cycle (**Figure 19.3**). Hyperammonaemia is associated with neurological dysfunction and may occur because of a deficiency of one of the enzymes involved in this cycle. In addition, hyperammonaemia is seen in organic acidaemias, due to severe illness in the neonatal period such as sepsis, and in Reye's syndrome. Raised blood ammonia concentrations may also be seen with parenteral nutrition, treatment with sodium valproate, and can occur transiently in neonates.

Hyperammonaemia

Hyperammonaemia may occur as a result of inherited metabolic diseases and also from acquired disorders (**Table 19.2**). Ammonia is produced by bacterial metabolism in the

Reye's Syndrome

Reye's syndrome is an acute illness seen in children below 15 years of age and is characterized by vomiting, signs of hepatic injury, central nervous system involvement and hypoglycaemia. The cause is unknown

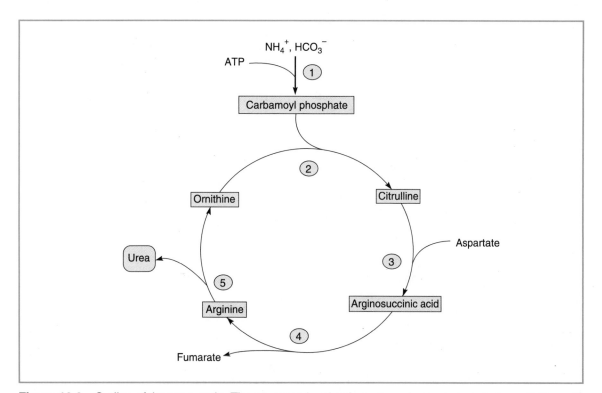

Figure 19.3 Outline of the urea cycle. The enzymes involved are: 1, carbamoyl phosphate synthetase; 2, ornithine carbamoyltransferase; 3, arginosuccinate synthetase; 4, arginosuccinate lyase; 5, arginase.

although salicylate use and viral causes have been implicated. The condition usually follows an upper respiratory tract infection which progresses to vomiting, convulsions and coma. Fatty vacuolization of the liver occurs although jaundice is rare. Elevations in serum transferases and ammonia are the major laboratory findings, together with a metabolic acidosis, prolonged prothrombin time and hypoglycaemia.

Cystic Fibrosis

Cystic fibrosis is a multisystem inherited metabolic disease which affects 1 in 2500 Caucasians; it is the commonest inherited metabolic disease affecting children. Cystic fibrosis is due to defective cystic fibrosis transmembrane conductance regulator (CFTR).

Molecular Basis

CFTR functions as a chloride channel in cell membranes. In most inherited metabolic diseases the defective protein is known before the gene is characterized but in this case, although the function of the protein was known, the gene responsible was identified before the protein product. The gene was cloned, sequenced and the protein structure predicted from the base sequence of the gene. Although over 200 mutations of the gene have been identified, over 70% of cases are caused by the deletion of a single amino acid, phenylalanine, which results in a functional change in the protein, impairing chloride transport. Defective ion transport at epithelial surfaces occurs due to impermeability to chloride resulting in abnormalities in the electrolyte contents of secretions. Secretions have a decreased water content and are therefore more viscous than normal. A correct ion and water content of secretions is essential for the normal function of proteins secreted at epithelial surfaces, these having digestive, lubricant and protective properties. In addition, viscous secretions may become inspissated in ducts, causing obstruction.

Clinical Features

The majority of patients present in infancy although some are not detected until adult years. Many organs are affected (**Table 19.3**), but the major clinical features result from abnormal function of the respiratory tract and pancreas. Nearly all patients develop progressive pulmonary disease, this being the commonest cause of death. Obstruction to small airways and infection are the major pathological changes, with progression leading to bronchiectasis. Pancreatic disease is often present from birth. Obstruction of ducts by inspissated secretions is followed by destruction of glandular tissue, the islets of Langerhans being spared until the disease is advanced, diabetes mellitus being, therefore, a late feature. Deficiencies of pancreatic enzymes leads to maldigestion of food, particularly fat and protein. Steatorrhoea is common, together with deficiencies of fat-soluble vitamins, and protein deficiency may occur. Failure of pancreatic enzyme secretion and digestion of intestinal contents leads to meconium ileus in the neonatal period and small bowel obstruction may also occur in older patients. Changes in the genitourinary tract are found in over 95% of male patients, obstruction of ducts leading to atrophy of Wolffian

Table 19.3 Clinical features of cystic fibrosis

Respiratory
◆ Recurrent bronchopneumonia, bronchiectasis
Intestinal
◆ Meconium ileus
Pancreatic
◆ Pancreatic insufficiency, steatorrhoea
◆ Diabetes mellitus
Genitourinary
◆ Infertility
Metabolic
◆ Sodium depletion
◆ Heat stroke

duct structures. Infertility is common in female patients.

Diagnosis

The diagnosis of cystic fibrosis is suggested by characteristic clinical features, accompanied by sweat chloride concentrations >60 mmol l^{-1}. This test involves collection of sweat, the flow of which is stimulated by pilocarpine iontophoresis, and subsequent determination of its chemical composition. Many other tests have been used for screening including measuring the albumin content of meconium and immunoreactive trypsin in blood, these both being raised soon after birth. DNA analysis is now available and can be used for prenatal diagnosis and detection of heterozygotes.

Treatment

Cystic fibrosis runs a variable course and survival has been increasing steadily in recent years. Over half the patients now survive into their late 20s and some beyond 50 years. Present treatment aims are to control infection, promote mucus clearance and improve nutrition. Postural drainage of the chest is important and symptoms suggestive of chest infection should have early treatment with antibiotics. Pancreatic enzyme supplements are often required and caloric requirements may be increased because of the extra work of respiration. Replacement of the defective gene by incorporating it in liposomes (lipid vesicles) and administering it by inhalation is being investigated.

KEY POINTS

CYSTIC FIBROSIS

- Cystic fibrosis is caused by a defect in chloride transport at epithelial surfaces

- Clinical features include recurrent lung infections and pancreatic insufficiency

- Sweat chloride concentrations exceed 60 mmol l^{-1} in cystic fibrosis

---

MOLECULAR DEFECTS IN INHERITED METABOLIC DISEASE
Gene Expression

The human genome contains between 50 000 and 100 000 genes which are assembled with proteins in chromosomes, forming chromatin. The genetic code in genes is determined by the sequence of purine (adenine, guanine) and pyrimidine (cytosine, thymine) bases which DNA contains, these being attached to a backbone of deoxyribose molecules that are linked by phosphate groups. Phosphate linkages are between $3'$ and $5'$ hydroxyl groups on adjacent deoxyribose molecules, one end of the DNA molecule having a free $5'$ hydroxyl group on deoxyribose, the other a free $3'$ group. The two chains of DNA are coiled around each other with opposite polarity, one in the direction $5' \rightarrow 3'$, the other $3' \rightarrow 5'$.

A triplet of bases (or codon) codes for a single amino acid. A gene is the section of DNA which contains the code for the amino acid sequence of a single polypeptide chain. The base sequence of most genes is greater than required for encoding a polypeptide chain, as coding regions (exons) are separated by intervening noncoding sequences (introns). Protein synthesis involves the copying or transcription of the gene sequence of DNA, including both exons and introns. An RNA polymerase enzyme copies the base sequence of one of the DNA strands (antisense) which acts as a template for the synthesis of a ribonucleic acid (RNA) transcript which is built up in the direction $5' \rightarrow 3'$. This has the same sequence as the DNA sense strand and it is edited by removing the introns and splicing the exons to produce a continuous coding sequence (**Figure 19.4**). This process occurs in the nucleus, the product, messenger RNA (mRNA), passing to the cytoplasm of the cell. In the cytoplasm mRNA associates with ribosomes, forming a template for protein synthesis. Amino acids in the cell are

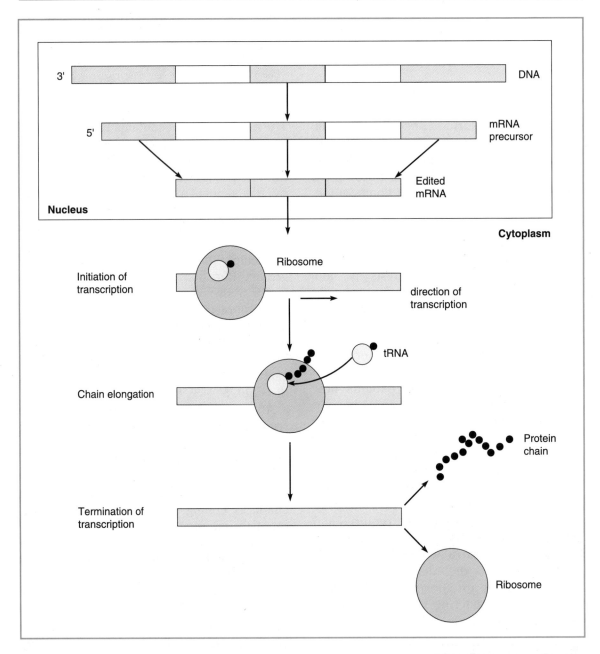

Figure 19.4 A schematic representation of the genetic control of protein synthesis. One of the double strands of DNA acts as a template for RNA synthesis.

attached to specific transfer RNAs, each of which contains a sequence of three bases that are complementary in mRNA. Thus, amino acids are incorporated into the polypeptide chain in an order determined by the base sequence of DNA.

Regulation of Gene Expression

The complete complement of genes is present in all nucleated cells, despite their widely differing functions. Only a small proportion of DNA is expressed at any one time, activity being reflected by changes in chromatin structure and the degree of methylation of genes, actively expressed genes being hypomethylated. Little is known about how changes in configuration are involved in gene transcription.

Parts of the DNA strands have regulatory functions. Promoter sequences are foun in the 5′ region of DNA which provide binding sites for regulatory signals for RNA polymerase, and enhancer sequences have also been identified. Specific transcription proteins bind to regulatory regions of the gene initiating transcription, the combination of particular binding sites in a gene and the presence or absence of transcription factors determining in which cell types the gene is transcribed. Genes are activated and repressed by external signals which act in at least three ways.

1. Endocrine signalling. In endocrine signalling a hormone or growth factor acts on distant target cells. There are two main mechanisms, lipid soluble hormones diffusing across cell membranes and interacting with proteins in the cytosol or nucleus, while peptides and growth factors bind to cell membrane receptors and act through the transduction of intracellular messengers.
2. Paracrine signalling in which the signalling cell affects target cells which are located close to it.
3. Autocrine signalling in which cells respond to substances they release themselves.

Genetic Diseases

There are three main categories of genetic disease:

1. Chromosomal abnormalities. Chromosomal abnormalities are caused by a lack, excess or abnormal arrangement of chromosomes. Down's syndrome (tris- omy 21) is an example of an autosomal chromosomal disorder and Kleinfelter's syndrome (47,XXY) is an example of a disorder affecting the sex chromosomes. Chromosomal abnormalities are beyond the scope of this book.
2. Polygenic disorders. Polygenic disorders are caused by the interaction of multiple genes and environmental factors. Genetic factors are important in many common diseases, including coronary heart disease, hypertension and diabetes mellitus. The aetiology of coronary heart disease is heterogeneous. While a small proportion of cases are caused by a single gene defect (e.g. familial hypercholesterolaemia) multiple factors contribute to the aetiology in the majority of patients. These interact, often also with environmental factors, each factor individually having a small effect but cumulatively producing clinical disease. An example of a multifactorial condition is polygenic hypercholesterolaemia (chapter 2), in which variations in proteins regulating lipoprotein metabolism, including apolipoproteins apoB and apoE, enzymes and receptors interact to produce high blood-cholesterol levels, particularly if combined with the environmental factor of high fat intake.
3. Monogenic disorders. Monogenic disorders are caused by single gene defects and follow a simple (Mendelian) pattern of inheritance. Many inherited metabolic diseases which occur as a result of single gene defects have a metabolic basis and up to 8% of children in hospital have one of these disorders. Some of these diseases are considered above while others are discussed elsewhere in this book (**Table 19.4**).

Single Gene Defects

Single gene defects are caused by mutations – changes in the structure of DNA which are

Table 19.4 Inherited metabolic diseases considered in this book

Autosomal dominant
- Acute intermittent porphyria
- Familial defective apolipoprotein B-100
- Familial hypercholesterolaemia
- Variegate porphyria

Autosomal recessive
- α_1-Antitrypsin deficiency
- Congenital adrenal hyperplasia
- Congenital erythropoietic porphyria
- Cystinuria
- Cystic fibrosis
- Galactosaemia
- Glycogen storage diseases
- Haemochromatosis
- Hereditary fructose intolerance
- Hypolactasia (neonatal)
- Phenylketonuria
- Wilson's disease

X-linked
- Glucose-6-phosphate dehydrogenase deficiency
- Lesch–Nyhan syndrome
- Testicular feminization

stable and heritable. These mutations may result in the substitution of one amino acid for another, with the possibility of altering the function of the resulting protein (missense mutations). Examples of such mutations are isoforms of apolipoprotein E, E2 and E4, the amino acid substitutions of which alter the receptor-binding function of apoE (see chapter 2). A mutation causing the deletion of a single base may produce a frameshift abnormality, every triplet following the mutation being altered. This can lead to gross changes in protein structure. In addition to coding for amino acids, base triplets (stop codons) also signal that the translation of the protein chain is complete. If a base change produces a stop codon premature termination of the protein will occur, resulting in a short protein with reduced function.

The cause of most mutations is unknown although they can arise from exposure to radiation, chemicals and viruses. In general, single gene defects are rare although heterozygous familial hypercholesterolaemia affects 1 in 500 of Northern European populations. More than one change in DNA sequence may affect the synthesis of a particular protein (genetic heterogeneity). Over 100 different mutations causing familial hypercholesterolaemia have been described.

Techniques of Gene Analysis

The characterization of inherited metabolic disease has been made possible by advances in technology which allow detailed analysis of gene disorders. Some understanding of the techniques is necessary to appreciate their application.

Gene Probes

The two strands of DNA may be dissociated by heating, reassociation (annealing) occurring on cooling. This process occurs specifically between nucleic acid strands that have identical or nearly identical base sequences. Gene probes consist of short lengths of DNA with a base sequence complementary to the gene. These probes can be synthesized from mRNA isolated from cells using reverse transcriptase enzymes (complementary or cDNA). If cDNA is radioactively labelled then it may be used to identify complementary sequences in genomic DNA. These DNA probes are relatively large and cannot recognize single base changes, although shorter synthetic DNA sequences can be prepared (oligonucleotide probes) which are able to differentiate a single base change, allowing abnormal DNA to be identified.

DNA Fractionation

It is possible to cleave DNA using bacterial enzymes, restriction endonucleases. These enzymes have specificity for particular combinations of bases and therefore the number of fragments of DNA produced by a particular enzyme depends on the base sequence. The fragments, or restriction length polymorphisms (RFLPs), are of different sizes and can therefore be characterized after separation by electrophoresis. Some occur within coding regions of DNA and hence can cause amino acid substitutions in gene products, while others occur in introns and thus have no effect. This technique demonstrates that considerable genetic diversity exists between individuals. RFLPs are inherited in a Mendelian fashion. Even if an RFLP does not involve a gene it may still be useful in investigating disease since if it occurs close to a particular gene it may be used as a marker to follow the pattern of inheritance of the gene. This type of analysis has been used in prenatal diagnosis although it is less specific than identifying mutations with oligonucleotide probes.

Gene Cloning

Genes must be isolated if their detailed structure is to be determined. This can be achieved by the process of gene cloning in which a fragment of DNA containing the gene is prepared using restriction enzymes and inserted into the DNA of a plasmid or bacteriophage. These simple organisms replicate in bacteria and through these organisms, genes that confer resistance to antibiotics may also be incorporated. Thus, bacteria containing the vector with the gene being studied may be selected by growing in a culture which contains the relevant antibiotic. Colonies containing the cloned DNA can be identified using a DNA probe, isolated and grown in large quantities. If genes can be isolated in large quantities the base sequence can be determined.

DNA Amplification

Small segments of DNA can be amplified using the polymerase chain reaction (PCR), which allows rapid identification of single base changes (**Figure 19.5**). For this two oligonucleotides are required which match the DNA sequence that flanks the area of interest. DNA strands are separated by heating and the oligonucleotides are added together with a heat-stable DNA polymerase and substrates for DNA synthesis. If present in excess, the oligonucleotides bind to the complementary sequences in DNA rather than the DNA strands reassociating, these acting as primers for DNA synthesis which occurs from the 3′ end of the oligonucleotides. Annealing occurs with cooling. The process can be repeated many times, the amount of DNA doubling with each cycle: 20 cycles produce a million-fold amplification of DNA. As the primers are flanking the area of interest in DNA on both strands the process, in effect, produces DNA between the two primers. By combining PCR with oligonucleotide probes, mutations can be identified more rapidly than with the previous techniques and therefore the technique can be used diagnostically to identify gene defects.

Detection of Mutations Using ARMS

An alternative approach for known mutations is to use oligonucleotide primers with a mismatched base at the 3′ end; thus this will not initiate PCR, the technique being the amplification refractory mutation system (ARMS). Two primers are used, one of which matches normal DNA, the other mutant DNA. Both will amplify DNA in heterozygotes but only one will in homozygotes. Because the results depend on the presence or absence of amplified DNA the products can be visualized with an appropriate probe rather than having to separate them by electrophoresis; hence diagnosis is more rapid than with other techniques.

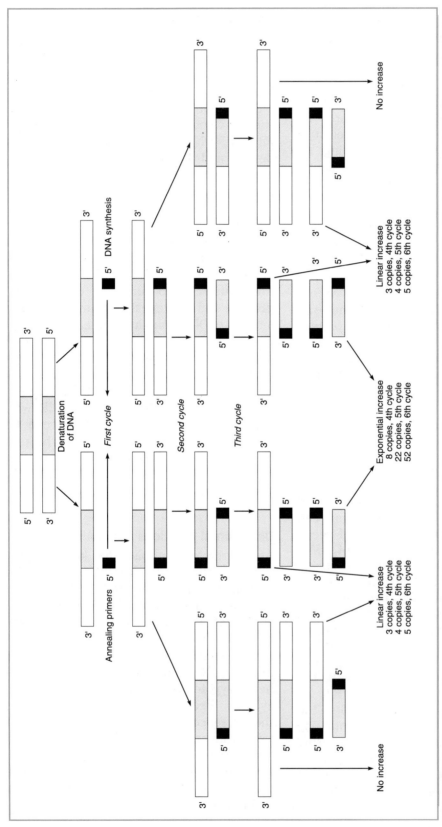

Figure 19.5 A schematic representation of the polymerase chain reaction. The section of DNA for amplification is designated by the green shaded areas. After dissociation of DNA primers with nucleotide sequences complementary to the flanking sequences are added. DNA is synthesized from the 3′ ends of the primers, the product having one chain truncated. In the second cycle short segments of DNA including only the section of interest are prepared, giving rise to double-stranded DNA which includes only this section in the third cycle. With further cycles, this increases exponentially while there is only linear increase of the truncated DNA species.

FURTHER READING

Markham AF. The polymerase chain reaction: a tool for molecular medicine. *British Medical Journal* 1993; **306**: 441–6

Meites S (ed.). *Paediatric Clinical Chemistry. Reference (Normal) Values.* Washington: AACC Press, 1989

Pollitt RJ. Amino acid disorders. Chapter 3. In: Houlton JB (ed.). *The Inherited Metabolic Disorders* (2nd edn). Edinburgh: Churchill-Livingstone, 1994, pp. 67–113

Rosenthal N. Regulation of gene expression. *New England Journal of Medicine* 1994; **331**: 931–3

Scriver CR, Beaudet AL, Sly WS, Valle D (eds). *The Metabolic Basis of Inherited Disorders* (7th edn). New York: McGraw-Hill, 1995

Warner JO (ed.). Cystic fibrosis. *British Medical Bulletin* 1992; **48**: 717–978

Weatherall DJ. *The New Genetics and Clinical Practice* (3rd edn). Oxford: Oxford University Press, 1992

CASE 19.1

A 3-months-old male infant was admitted because of failure to thrive and convulsions. Delivery was normal and at full term. He had an elder brother and sister who were normal. On examination he was hypotonic. Initial blood tests showed the following:

plasma sodium	137 mmol l^{-1}
plasma potassium	3.9 mmol l^{-1}
total CO_2	12 mmol l^{-1}
urea	3.5 mmol l^{-1}
blood glucose	3.7 mmol l^{-1}
ammonia	450 μmol l^{-1}

What are the possible diagnoses and what further investigations need to be carried out?

CASE 19.2

A male infant was normal at birth but developed jaundice by the fourth day after delivery. On examination hepatomegaly was detected. The following results of investigations were received:

serum total bilirubin	174 μmol l^{-1}
conjugated bilirubin	38 μmol l^{-1}
alanine aminotransferase	140 U l^{-1}
alkaline phosphatase	240 U l^{-1}
urine analysis	Positive for reducing substances

What is the most probable diagnosis?

PURINE AND URIC ACID METABOLISM

INTRODUCTION

Purines are constituents of nucleotides, including adenosine triphosphate (ATP), and thus they have a vital role in energy metabolism. In addition, they are constituents of nucleic acids, second messengers of hormone action, coenzymes, and carriers of activated intermediates in a variety of biochemical reactions. Almost all uric acid in man is produced from the catabolism of purine bases which are derived from endogenous nucleotides and from the diet. Uric acid is a metabolic end-product in man although some mammals possess an enzyme, uricase, which further metabolizes uric acid to the more soluble product allantoin. Many conditions lead to increases in serum urate concentrations and hyperuricaemia also results from inherited metabolic disease, due either to a defect in purine metabolism or because of enzyme deficiencies which affect urate metabolism secondarily. Because of its limited solubility, excess uric acid crystallizes and aggregates, leading to clinical disorders which include gout, nephrolithiasis and nephropathy. Other disorders of purine metabolism include immunodeficiency syndromes and orotic aciduria.

PURINE AND URIC ACID METABOLISM

Purine Synthesis

Purines are synthesized from amino acids, formate and carbon dioxide, the pathway being outlined in a simplified form in **Figure 20.1**. The first step of the sequence involves the addition of an amino group from glutamine to the ribose ring in 5-phospho-

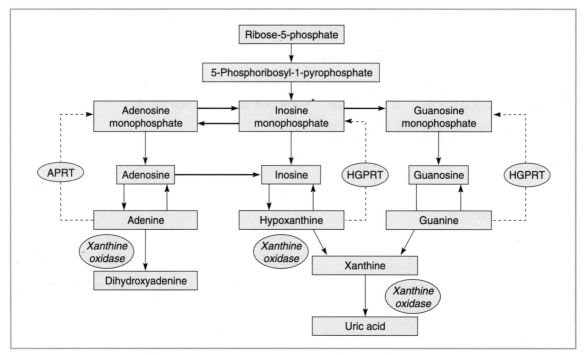

Figure 20.1 Outline of uric acid biosynthesis. Salvage pathways are shown by the dashed lines. HGPRT, hypoxanthine-guanine phosphoribosyl transferase; APRT, adenine phosphoribosyl transferase.

ribosyl-1-pyrophosphate (PRPP), this first committed step being the major site of regulation of synthesis, catalysed by PRPP amidotransferase. Purine monophosphates regulate the activity of this enzyme through negative feedback. Inosine monophosphate is a precursor of the major purines, adenine and guanine, with smaller amounts of xanthine and hypoxanthine also being found in man. Overproduction of purines by *de novo* synthesis leads to excessive urate production and gout. One cause of this is mutant forms of PRPP synthase which are not regulated by feedback inhibition. As a result, increased enzyme activity occurs leading to increased purine and thus increased urate synthesis.

Purine Salvage

Considerable amounts of energy are required for *de novo* purine synthesis in the form of ATP, and thus there is significant advantage in reutilizing purines for the synthesis purine monophosphates. Two mechanisms exist for this, hypoxanthine–guanine phosphoribosyl transferase (HGPRT) reconverting guanine and hypoxanthine to guanine and inosine monophosphates respectively. The Lesch–Nyan syndrome is caused by a deficiency of this enzyme. A separate enzyme, adenine phosphoribosyltransferase (APRT), salvages adenine by reconverting it to the corresponding monophosphate.

Purine Degradation and Urate Formation

Catabolism of purines occurs through a common pathway leading to uric acid formation. Nucleases cleave nucleotides from nucleic acids, these being further metabolized by nucleotidases. The metabolism of adenine nucleotides involves conversion to inosine via inosine monophosphate and also via adenosine. Deamination of the latter to inosine is controlled by adenosine deaminase, deficiency of which is associated with severe combined immunodeficiency syndrome. The conversion of both hypoxanthine to xanthine and xanthine to uric acid are controlled by the enzyme xanthine oxidase. The drug allopurinol is an inhibitor of xanthine oxidase and is used in the treatment of hyperuricaemia.

Urate Metabolism

The amount of uric acid in a normal man is approximately 7 mmol, about 2 mmol being produced each day. Approximately 80% of this is excreted in the urine, the remainder being excreted in the bile with partial degradation in the gastrointestinal tract by bacteria, forming carbon dioxide and ammonia. Uric acid, in the form of sodium urate, is filtered freely by the glomerulus, most being reabsorbed – mainly in the proximal tubule. Tubular secretion of urate also occurs, this being the most important mechanism leading to urinary urate excretion. Tubular secretion of urate appears to be inhibited by excess excretion of other organic acids, including ketones and lactate.

KEY POINTS

URATE METABOLISM

- Uric acid is the end-product of purine metabolism

- 80% of uric acid is excreted by the kidney

- The solubility of urate in both serum and urine is limited

HYPERURICAEMIA

Serum urate levels are higher in men than women and tend to rise with age. Reference ranges are 0.12–0.42 mmol l^{-1} in men and 0.12–0.36 mmol l^{-1} in women, these being similar to concentrations seen in children. The increase in males takes place at puberty. The prevalence of gout is very low if serum urate levels are within the reference ranges, this increasing as serum urate rises and approaches 20% when serum urate levels have exceeded 0.54 mmol l^{-1} for more than 4 years.

The clinical consequences of hyperuricaemia include gout and renal disease, these resulting from the physical properties of uric acid. Uric acid has an acidic dissociation constant (pK_a) of 5.75 and therefore is largely ionized at pH 7.4. Most urate in serum appears in the form of a sodium salt. This is more soluble than uric acid although precipitation of sodium urate in soft tissues occurs if serum levels above the normal reference range are maintained. The pH of urine is generally lower than serum and at a pH of 5.75, 50% of urate is in the form of uric acid, this being less soluble than the sodium salt.

Mechanisms of Hyperuricaemia

The causes of hyperuricaemia are outlined in **Table 20.1**. Mechanisms of hyperuricaemia are increased production, decreased excretion, or both.

Increased Production

Idiopathic (Primary) Hyperuricaemia In many subjects with hyperuricaemia in whom urate production has been measured the rate of synthesis is increased, although the mechanisms are unclear (idiopathic hyperuricaemia). Increased availability of substrates leading to urate synthesis, PPRP and glutamine, have been implicated. Intracellular levels of PRPP may be high because of increased PRPP synthase activity. In addition to PRPP, glutamine is a substrate for the rate-limiting step in purine biosynthesis and therefore excess of this could lead to increased purine production. However, the importance of this mechanism has not been established.

Inherited Metabolic Disease Both partial and severe defects in HGPRT activity have been

Table 20.1 Causes of hyperuricaemia

Increased urate production
Idiopathic
Inherited metabolic disorders
◆ Altered activity of enzymes of purine metabolism
  PRPP synthase
  HGPRT
◆ Secondary to other enzyme defects
  Type 1 glycogen storage disease (glucose-6-phosphatase deficiency)
Increased cell turnover
◆ Malignant disease
  Myeloproliferative and lymphoproliferative disorders, multiple myeloma, polycythaemia rubra vera
◆ Disorders of erythrocyte production
  Haemoglobinopathies, thalassaemia, pernicious anaemia
Increased urate synthesis
◆ Ethanol

Decreased renal excretion of urate
Reduced glomerular filtration rate
Inhibition of tubular secretion by organic acids
◆ Starvation, diabetic ketoacidosis, lactic acidosis
Drug therapy
◆ Aspirin, thiazide diuretics

---

described; these lead to increased intracellular levels by decreasing utilization, since the salvage pathways of purine metabolism are less active. In these conditions the increase in urate production is primary. Inherited metabolic diseases can also cause secondary increases in urate concentrations. Increased turnover of ATP occurs in glucose-6-phosphatase deficiency (type I glycogen storage disease), limited release of glucose trapping phosphate and depleting of ATP. Hyperuricaemia occurs in other glycogen storage diseases owing to reduced ATP resynthesis following consumption of glucose by muscular activity, as the enzyme deficiencies limit substrate availability.

Ethanol-Induced Hyperuricaemia Ethanol ingestion leads to increased serum urate concentrations by two mechanisms, increased production and decreased renal excretion. Increased production is due to accelerated ATP degradation, this resulting from acetate synthesis from ethanol. Acetate is metabolized to acetyl coenzyme A; synthesis of this utilizes ATP and some of the resulting AMP is degraded. Increased lactate production also occurs as a result of ethanol ingestion, hyperlactataemia increasing serum urate levels by competing for the same renal tubular excretory mechanism and inhibiting urate excretion.

Severely Ill Patients In severely ill patients increased urate production may occur, the basis being tissue hypoxia leading to increased ATP degradation. Impaired supplies of nutrients in addition to tissue hypoxia in such patients causes reduced resynthesis of ATP, leading to accelerated degradation.

Malignancy Hyperuricaemia often occurs in myeloproliferative and lymphoproliferative disorders. Increased cell turnover occurs, leading to increased urate synthesis.

Disorders of Erythrocyte Production A similar mechanism is responsible for hyperuricaemia in disorders of erythrocyte production, increased turnover of bone marrow cells occurring in haemolytic anaemia, thalassaemia and pernicious anaemia.

Decreased Urate Excretion

Decreased excretion of urate is a more common cause of hyperuricaemia than increased production and is due to both primary and secondary causes.

Primary (Idiopathic) The majority of patients with gout have decreased urate excretion, the cause of which is unknown, although decreased tubular secretion is thought to be responsible.

Secondary Decreased urate excretion is found in renal failure as a result of a fall in the glomerular filtration rate. Increased tubular reabsorption occurs in states of extracellular fluid volume depletion, such as dehydration and diuretic therapy. Decreased tubular secretion results from the accumulation of organic acids which share tubular secretion mechanisms with urate, these including ketoacids, lactic acid and salicylates at low concentrations. Several other drugs impair urate excretion by mechanisms that have not been fully clarified and include indomethacin, theophylline and β-adrenoreceptor blockers.

Hyperuricaemia in Pregnancy

Serum urate levels fall normally in pregnancy owing to water retention. However, levels rise in pre-eclampsia and eclampsia, due to reduced renal clearance. Increased maternal serum urate concentrations are associated with increased perinatal mortality.

KEY POINTS

HYPERURICAEMIA

- Hyperuricaemia is caused by over-production or decreased urinary excretion of urate

- Hyperuricaemia may lead to gout, renal disease and nephrolithiasis

- Hyperuricaemia in pre-eclampsia is associated with increased perinatal mortality

---

GOUT

Gout is characterized by recurrent attacks of acute arthritis in which crystals of monosodium urate are found in leukocytes in the synovial fluid of affected joints. Although only a minority of patients with hyperuricaemia develop gout, serum urate concentrations are or have been elevated in all patients. Deposits of sodium urate (tophi) may be found in soft tissues, particularly around the joints of the extremities and the ears. Renal disease and urinary tract stones also occur.

Causes

Arthritis and fever appear to result from interaction of urate crystals with polymorphonuclear leukocytes, leading to the release of cytokines such as interleukin 1 and leukotriene B4.

Clinical Features

Gout predominantly affects males, the peak incidence being between the fourth and sixth decades. It often presents as an acute monoarticular arthritis although gout commonly progresses to affect many joints. The big toe is the site of the first attack in around 50% of cases and is involved in 90% of patients. Other joints in the legs and also those in the arms are affected commonly. Affected joints are inflamed; fever and leukocytosis often develop. Attacks last from a few hours to weeks and usually resolve completely. If untreated, attacks recur with increasing frequency and progression to chronic gout may occur. This is characterized by deposits of sodium urate around joints, leading to joint swelling, bone erosion and joint destruction. Tophi occur in the ears and around joints.

Diagnosis

Several other arthritic conditions have clinical features which resemble gout, these being differentiated by finding the characteristic urate crystals in leukocytes from synovial fluid from affected joints. The finding of a high serum urate concentration is highly suggestive of gout in patients with characteristic clinical features, although gout is not inevitable in patients with hyperuricaemia and other forms of arthritis may occur coincidentally. In addition, finding a normal serum urate concentration does not exclude gout, as hyperuricaemia may have occurred in the past.

Management

Acute attacks are treated with anti-inflammatory drugs, colchicine or indomethacin often being used. Although they have no role in the treatment of acute attacks, drugs that reduce serum urate concentrations are important in long-term management. Allopurinol inhibits xanthine oxidase and thus uric acid synthesis, serum urate levels may also be reduced by drugs that promote urate excretion, uricosuric agents (e.g. probenecid).

Complications

Renal Disease

Deposition of sodium urate crystals in renal interstitial tissue may occur in chronic hyperuricaemia while deposition of crystals in the collecting ducts or renal pelvis may occur in patients with increased urinary urate excretion. Rarely, this may lead to acute renal failure, the cause usually being rapid lysis of malignant cells during chemotherapy.

Nephrolithiasis

Reduction of serum urate concentrations with uricosuric therapy leads to mobilization of urate deposits, causing transient increases in urinary urate concentrations and a risk of crystaluria and nephrolithiasis.

KEY POINTS

GOUT

- Acute gout results from the crystals of monosodium urate in synovial fluid causing an inflammatory response

- Deposits of sodium urate around joints and other soft tissues occur in chronic gout

- Complications of gout include renal disease and nephrolithiasis

---

DEFECTIVE HYPOXANTHINE-GUANINEPHOSPHORIBOSYL TRANSFERASE ACTIVITY

Low HGPRT activity reduces the salvage of purines and therefore less PRPP is utilized (**Figure 20.1**). This leads to increased *de novo* purine synthesis and hence urate production.

Lesch–Nyhan Syndrome

The Lesch–Nyhan syndrome is a rare X-linked disorder caused by a profound deficiency of HGPRT activity. Excessive urate production occurs although the main clinical features are neurological. These include self-mutilation, choreoathetosis, spasticity and mental retardation.

Partial HGPRT Deficiency

Partial HGPRT deficiency is found in around 1% of adults with gout. The onset of gout is earlier than for most patients and the prevalence of nephrolithiasis is high (75%). Mild neurological dysfunction occurs occasionally.

FURTHER READING

Fox IH, Palella TD, Kelley WN. Hyperuricemia: a marker for cell energy crisis. *New England Journal of Medicine* 1987; **317**: 111–2

Scott JT. Asymptomatic hyperuricaemia. *British Medical Journal* 1987; **294**: 987–8

Simmonds HA. Purine and pyrimidine disorders. Chapter 8. In: Holton JB (ed.). *The Inherited Metabolic Diseases* (2nd edn). Edinburgh: Churchill Livingstone, 1994, pp. 297–349

Wilson JM, Young AB, Kelley WM. Hypoxanthine–guanine phosphoribosyltransferase deficiency. The molecular basis of the syndrome. *New England Journal of Medicine* 1983; **309**: 900–10

CASE 20.1

A 52-year-old man presented with acute pain in his left ankle three days after twisting it while walking. On examination the point was acutely inflamed and tender.

serum urate concentration   0.68 mmol l^{-1}

Does this patient have gout?

21

IRON AND PORPHYRIN METABOLISM

INTRODUCTION

Iron and porphyrins are both required for the synthesis of haem which, since it has the property of binding oxygen reversibly, is an essential constituent of proteins involved in oxygen transport. In addition to haemoglobin these proteins include myoglobin, which binds oxygen in muscle, and cytochromes which are respiratory chain enzymes and oxidases. As iron and porphyrins are both haem precursors they are considered together, although disorders affecting their metabolism are quite distinct.

IRON METABOLISM

The normal adult contains approximately 70 mmol (4 g) iron, 70% of this being found in haemoglobin, and 5–10% in other haem-containing proteins. Iron has two major roles in the body; first, as a constituent of haemoglobin it is involved in oxygen transport and second, in cytochromes and other proteins ferrous and ferric ions are inter-converted with the loss or gain of an electron. Iron is lost from the body by desquamation and bleeding, very little appearing in urine. The daily losses by desquamation amount to around 1 mg per day and the average menstrual loss is 28 mg per cycle. Thus, in the absence of an additional source of bleeding, losses are 1 mg per day in men and 2 mg per day in women during reproductive life, these being the daily requirements to maintain balance. Additional amounts are required in pregnancy, as iron is needed by the fetus.

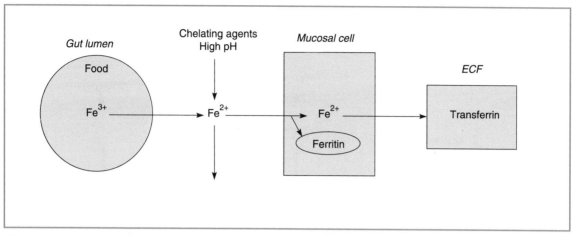

Figure 21.1   Factors affecting absorption of iron. Ferric (Fe^{3+}) ions in food are converted to ferrous (Fe^{2+}) ions, these being absorbed by enterocytes. Chelating agents and a high intraluminal pH interfere with absorption. There is control of iron assimilation from the enterocyte by sequestration within the cell. ECF, extracellular fluid.

Iron Absorption

Iron is present in meat, unrefined cereals, vegetables and fruit although amounts vary widely. The diet of most people contains 10–14 mg per day although not all of this is readily available. In animal-based foods iron is present mainly as haem in which iron is present in the ferrous (Fe^{2+}) form, which is readily absorbed. Iron is mainly in the ferric (Fe^{3+}) form in vegetables, complexed to phytates, phosphates and other ions. This is absorbed less readily. Gastric acid converts some Fe^{3+} to Fe^{2+}, facilitating its absorption.

There appears to be a mechanism for regulating the entry of iron into the body operating within enterocytes (**Figure 21.1**). Iron crosses the brush border by active transport, most absorption occurring within the duodenum. However, some of the iron which enters the enterocyte is not transferred to the submucosa but becomes sequestered within the cell; the amount depends on the body stores of iron. Enterocytes are formed within the crypts of Lieberkuhn and migrate to the villi, eventually being extruded from the tips of these approximately 5 days after they were formed. Thus, sequestered iron contained within the enterocytes will be lost. Less iron is sequestered by this mechanism when the body stores are low, and if excess iron is present, as with oral supplements, the mechanism can be saturated.

Iron Transport

Iron which escapes mucosal sequestration is bound to transferrin and transported to sites of utilization, mainly the bone marrow. As 1/120 of the haemoglobin in the body is broken down daily, around 350 μmol is transported from the reticuloendothelial system, where effete erythrocytes are broken down, to the bone marrow for the synthesis of new cells (**Figure 21.2**).

Iron Stores

Iron is stored in cells as ferritin and haemosiderin. Ferritin forms soluble complexes with an outer protein shell and an inner core of Fe^{3+}. Small amounts of ferritin appear in the circulation, there being a close correlation between serum ferritin levels

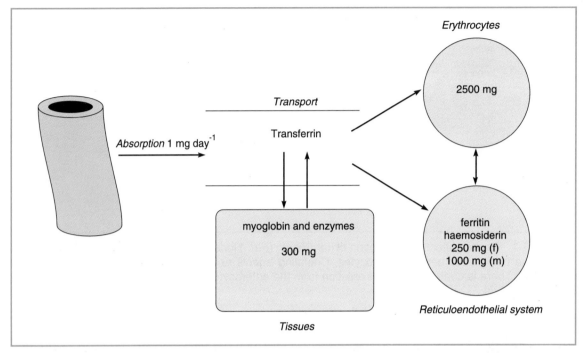

Figure 21.2 Outline of iron metabolism.

and iron stores. Haemosiderin is an insoluble complex which is probably formed from ferritin. If body stores of iron are increased the amount of haemosiderin formed also increases, excess giving rise to siderosis.

Assessment of Iron Metabolism

Serum Iron

Serum iron concentration varies from 13 to 32 μmol l^{-1} in men while levels are lower in women, 11–29 μmol l^{-1}, these falling during pregnancy. Values are low in iron deficiency although this finding is nonspecific as low levels also occur in several other conditions which are not necessarily associated with depleted iron stores, including chronic inflammatory diseases, infections, trauma, neoplasia and renal disease. High levels are found in iron poisoning, in conditions of iron overload (haemosiderosis and haemochromatosis), hepatitis and haemolytic anaemia.

Serum Transferrin and Iron-Binding Capacity

Most iron is transported in serum bound to transferrin (chapter 3), one molecule of which is able to bind two molecules of iron. However, transferrin is only 30–40% saturated with iron under normal circumstances. In iron deficiency the synthesis of transferrin is increased while the amount of iron bound or the degree of saturation of transferrin with iron is decreased, often to less than 10%. As a result, the amount of iron that serum can bind, the total iron binding capacity (TIBC), increases. Such findings are not specific for iron deficiency, and may occur in pregnancy. The serum TIBC decreases in haemochromatosis.

Serum Ferritin

Ferritin in serum differs chemically from the storage form found in tissues, and normally contains little iron. The range in healthy subjects is 15–350 μg l^{-1} in men and 8–300 μg l^{-1} in women, these falling with depleted tissue iron stores. Levels are increased if tissue iron stores are very high, and in chronic inflammatory disorders, infections, neoplasia and liver disease. Serum ferritin concentrations are more closely related to body iron status than serum iron, TIBC or transferrin.

Tissue Iron Stores

Iron stores in the reticuloendothelial system and may be assessed directly by biopsy of bone marrow or liver.

DISORDERS OF IRON METABOLISM

Iron Deficiency

Iron deficiency occurs when the rate of loss or utilization of iron exceeds the rate of absorption; the causes are outlined in **Table 21.1**. Gastrointestinal blood loss is a common cause of iron deficiency in men and postmenopausal women. Such a finding should raise the possibility of an occult gastrointestinal malignancy being present and, in the absence of other positive findings, the faeces should be tested for occult blood.

Clinical features result from impaired cellular growth. Although all cells require iron for growth the effect on erythrocytes is most obvious because of their high turnover and requirements for iron. Anaemia is the main clinical feature of iron deficiency although the gastrointestinal tract and other tissues may also be affected. The onset is usually insidious with nonspecific features which include tiredness, weakness, palpitations and dyspnoea on exertion. Angular stomatitis and glossitis also occur and thinning and flattening of the nails with koilonychia sometimes develops. There is an increased susceptibility to infection due to impaired T-lymphocyte function and reduced neutrophil bactericidal activity.

Laboratory findings include reduced serum ferritin and iron, and increased transferrin concentrations. In iron deficiency, the

Table 21.1 Causes of iron deficiency

Decreased iron intake
- Dietary deficiency
- Impaired absorption

Increased utilization
- Growth spurts

Increased physiological iron loss
- Repeated pregnancies

Pathological iron loss
- Menorrhagia
- Gastrointestinal bleeding
- Bleeding from the genitourinary tract
- Pulmonary haemosiderosis
- Repeated blood donations

serum ferritin concentration falls and transferrin rises (or TIBC increases) before decreases are seen in serum iron concentration, although this also occurs before anaemia develops. The anaemia is hypochromic with reduced mean corpuscular volume and mean corpuscular haemoglobin. Iron deficiency is treated by oral supplements, ferrous sulphate or gluconate usually being given. Excess free iron in the gastrointestinal tract can cause nausea, abdominal pain and constipation, although this is usually due to excess amounts being given.

Iron Overload

Iron overload can arise from excessive absorption or from parenteral administration in the form of blood transfusions. Iron accumulation in patients receiving regular blood transfusions is predictable and excessive iron absorption can also arise from high intake. Primary haemochromatosis is an autosomal recessive condition which appears to be caused by excessive iron absorption resulting from both increased cellular uptake and increased transfer of iron from the enterocytes to the extracellular fluid (ECF). As there is no route for excess to be lost from the body, iron accumulates causing siderosis when excess iron stores are present, and haemochromatosis if tissue damage results.

Primary haemochromatosis usually presents in middle age with clinical features which result from organ damage caused by excess tissue iron. These include cardiomyopathy, cirrhosis, diabetes mellitus, hypogonadism and pituitary failure. Additional factors, such as chronic ethanol abuse and hepatitis, may contribute to organ damage. The mechanism of tissue damage probably relates to the toxicity of excess iron, which inhibits cellular enzymes. It is possible that excess iron also promotes the formation of highly reactive products of oxidative reactions, free radicals, which damage both lipids and proteins. Iron overload is treated by regular infusions of desferrioxamine, a chelating agent which binds iron and is excreted in urine.

KEY POINTS

IRON METABOLISM

- Iron assimilation into the body is regulated by enterocytes

- Transferrin is the major iron-transporting protein in serum

- Iron is stored in cells in ferritin and haemosiderin

- Serum iron concentration is a poor indicator of tissue iron stores

PORPHYRIN METABOLISM

Haem consists of a porphyrin ring which is complexed with iron (Fe^{2+}). Porphyrins are synthesized from glycine and succinate by a series of enzyme-dependent reactions partly located in mitochondria and partly in cell cytoplasm (**Figure 21.3**). Although all cells synthesize haem, requirements are particularly high in the bone marrow because of erythropoiesis, and in the liver, where there is a high turnover of haem-containing enzymes which are required for hormone and drug metabolism. The major control point for haem biosynthesis is the step in which 5-aminolaevulinic acid (ALA) is formed, the regulatory enzyme being ALA synthase. The activity of ALA synthase is in turn controlled by the end-product of the biosynthetic sequence, haem. Thus, if the intracellular content of haem is high ALA synthase is inhibited and little fresh haem is synthesized. Increased utilization of haem-containing enzymes leads to increased synthesis of enzymes and depletion of intracellular haem content, ALA synthase will be derepressed and more haem will be synthesized. A partial deficiency of a haem-synthesizing enzyme will produce a second rate-limiting step in haem biosynthesis, although this may be normal unless demands for haem are unusually high. However, a consequence of a deficiency will be increased synthesis of intermediates higher in the biosynthetic sequence than the partial block (**Figure 21.4**). The majority of the ALA produced is converted to haem, although small amounts of intermediates are lost from the pathway. These porphyrinogens are unstable and are oxidized to porphyrins, either within the body or following excretion.

DISORDERS OF PORPHYRIN METABOLISM

The Porphyrias

The porphyrias are a group of disorders resulting from partial deficiencies of enzymes required for the biosynthesis of haem (**Table 21.2**), which lead to overproduction of haem precursors, and are associated with characteristic clinical features. Complete deficiencies are incompatible with life, as haem-containing proteins play a key role in respiration. The porphyrias are not common; porphyria cutanea tarda has the highest incidence in Europe and North America as 1:25 000. Despite this,

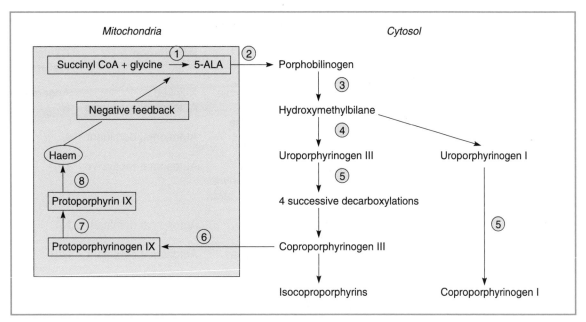

Figure 21.3   The biosynthesis of haem. Enzymes controlling the stages of this pathway are numbered. Uroporphyrin and coproporphyrin, which are not intermediates of haem synthesis, are produced by nonenzymatic oxidation of the corresponding porphyrinogens. (1) 5-aminolaevulinic acid (ALA) synthase; (2) porphobilinogen synthase; (3) porphobilinogen deaminase; (4) uroporphyrinogen synthase; (5) uroporphyrinogen decarboxylase; (6) coproporphyrinogen oxidase; (7) protoporphyrinogen oxidase; (8) ferrochelatase.

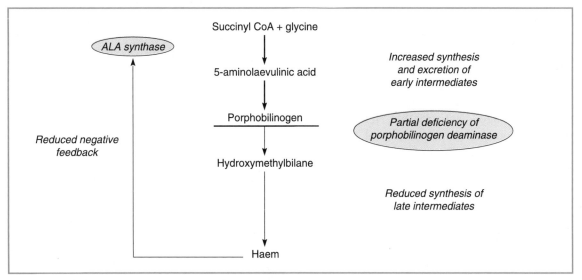

Figure 21.4   Site and consequences of the enzyme deficiency in acute intermittent porphyria. ALA, 5-aminolaevulinic acid; CoA, coenzyme A.

they are an important group of disorders as the clinical features are varied and can result in presentation to a number of different clinical specialties.

Pathophysiology of the Porphyrias

The clinical features of the porphyrins fall into two major groups, photosensitivity and those arising from neurotoxicity. Skin

Table 21.2 Disorders caused by haem-synthesizing enzyme deficiencies

Enzyme location (see Figure 21.2)	Enzyme	Disease	Inheritance	Clinical features
1	ALA synthase	Sideroblastic anaemia	X-linked	Anaemia
2	Porphobilinogen synthase	Porphobilinogen deficiency porphyria	Autosomal recessive	N
3	Porphobilinogen deaminase	Acute intermittent porphyria	Autosomal dominant	N
4	Uroporphyrinogen synthase	Congenital erythropoietic porphyria	Autosomal recessive	D
5	Uroporphyrinogen decarboxylase	Porphyria cutanea tarda		D
6	Coproporphyrinogen oxidase	Hereditary coproporphyria	Autosomal dominant	N/P
7	Protoporphyrinogen oxidase	Variegate porphyria	Autosomal dominant	N/P
8	Ferrochelatase	Erythropoietic protoporphyria	Autosomal dominant	N/P

ALA, 5-aminolaevulinic acid; N, neuropathic; P, psychiatric features; D, dermatopathic features.

changes include erythema, itching, oedema, bullae formation, atrophy and scarring on exposure to light. Photosensitivity occurs when porphyrins are produced in excess, this being found in all disorders of porphyrin synthesis except acute intermittent porphyria and sideroblastic anaemia. Because of their structure, porphyrins in the skin absorb light and become excited and re-emit the absorbed energy, causing local tissue damage. Neuropathic features include abdominal pain, peripheral neuropathy and psychiatric symptoms. These occur in all porphyrias in which the synthesis of ALA is increased, this being neurotoxic.

The porphyrias are conditions with acute attacks and remissions. In acute attacks the characteristic clinical features occur with increased production and excretion of metabolites, the pattern of which is determined by the enzyme deficiency. However, in remission clinical features may be absent and a less abnormal metabolite pattern is seen. The mechanism of acute attacks precipitated by drug administration results from acute changes in haem utilization. Drugs precipitating porphyrias are metabolized by cytochrome enzymes in hepatic microsomes (**Table 21.3**). Enzyme synthesis increases if active drug metabolism is occurring and therefore the utilization of haem increases, leading to increased haem synthesis. Rapid accumulation of metabolites distal to ALA synthase but proximal to the defective enzyme occurs, precipitating an acute attack.

Porphyrias are sometimes subclassified according to the organ which is the major site of porphyrin accumulation – hepatic, erythropoietic or both (erythrohepatic).

KEY POINTS

PATHOPHYSIOLOGY OF PORPHYRIAS

- Cutaneous features are caused by excess porphyrins

- Neuropathic features are caused by excess 5-aminolaevulinic acid

- Metabolites which accumulate are produced between ALA synthase and the defective enzyme

- Drugs metabolized by haem-containing enzymes precipitate acute attacks

Table 21.3 Drugs and acute attacks of porphyria

Known to precipitate attacks	Safe
Barbiturates	Amitriptylene
Carbamazapine	Aspirin
Oestrogens	Glucocorticoids
Progestagens	Insulin
Sulphonamides	Penicillins
Tolbutamide	Phenothiazines
Valproate	Tetracycline

Congenital Porphyrias

Acute Intermittent Porphyria

Acute intermittent porphyria is caused by porphobilinogen deaminase deficiency. The abnormal metabolites that accumulate are ALA and porphobilinogen (not porphyrinogens), therefore photosensitivity is not a clinical feature but psychiatric changes and neurological attacks occur, often including acute abdominal pain. Peripheral neuropathy is a common feature, this being predominantly motor. The condition is rarely apparent before puberty and following this is episodic, attacks lasting for a few days to several months. These attacks are often precipitated by alcohol or drugs which are metabolized by haem-containing enzymes. The condition may remain latent throughout life.

Investigation Urinary excretion of ALA and porphobilinogen increases during acute attacks, although this also occurs in some other porphyrias. Metabolite levels fall after attacks and may be normal in patients with latent disease. In such cases the enzyme deficiency can be demonstrated in erythrocytes or cultured skin fibroblasts. Asymptomatic carriers can also be identified by DNA analysis.

Variegate Porphyria and Hereditary Coproporphyria

These conditions have some clinical features in common with acute intermittent porphyria, variegate porphyria being caused by a deficiency in protoporphyrinogen oxidase (enzyme 7, **Figure 21.3**) and hereditary coproporphyria by a coproporphyrinogen oxidase deficiency (enzyme 6, **Figure 21.3**). Increased production of ALA and porphobilinogen occur in both conditions and therefore, as in acute intermittent porphyria, neuropathic features are found. However, in contrast to acute intermittent porphyria, cutaneous manifestations may also be seen as porphyrinogens are also produced in excess. In hereditary coproporphyria, the defective enzyme converts coproporphyrinogen III to protoporphyrinogen IX and therefore coproporphyrinogen III accumulates, this being oxidized to coproporphyrin III. Both protoporphyrin and coproporphyrin accumulate in variegate porphyria because the conversion of protoporphyrinogen to protoporphyrin is defective. Coproporphyrin is partly excreted in the urine, but mainly in stools, faecal excretion being the route of elimination of protoporphyrin. Therefore, in contrast to acute intermittent porphyria, in both conditions, even if latent, there is a marked increase in faecal porphyrins.

Congenital Erythropoietic Porphyria

Congenital erythropoietic porphyria is caused by defective uroporphyrinogen synthase (enzyme 4, **Figure 21.3**). The pattern of inheritance, autosomal recessive, differs from most other porphyrias which, with the exception of porphyria cutanea tarda, are autosomal dominant. Most cases of congenital erythropoietic porphyria present in infancy although a late-onset form with milder clinical features has been described. The condition is characterized by extreme photosensitivity which may lead to mutilation of exposed areas, particularly the face and hands. Brown discoloration of the teeth, erythrodontia, is common and is caused by deposition of porphyrins. The enzyme deficiency leads to overproduction of the type I isomer of uroporphyrinogen, presumably as a result of nonenzymatic condensation of hydroxymethylbilane. Uroporphyrinogen I is not an intermediate of haem biosynthesis, and further metabolism to uroporphyrinogen I and the corresponding porphyrins occurs. Formation of haem from uroporphyrinogen III is not impaired and ALA and porphobilinogen do not accumulate; neuropathic features do not therefore occur. Investigations include the measurement of porphyrins in erythrocytes where they accumulate and determination of the isomer type of urinary porphyrin excretion.

Porphyria Cutanea Tarda

Porphyria cutanea tarda is not the result of a single pattern of inheritance but rather represents a group of disorders which cause a defect in a single enzyme, uroporphyrinogen decarboxylase (enzyme 5, **Figure 21.3**). This results in the overproduction of intermediates of the uroporphyrinogen decarboxylase reaction and uroporphyrin, which result in skin lesions similar to those seen in other cutaneous porphyrias although the onset is often later (between the fifth and seventh decades). Increased ALA and porphobilinogen production do not occur and therefore there are no neuropathic clinical features. Familial porphyria cutanea tarda has a similar pattern of inheritance to most other porphyrias – autosomal dominant. It is frequently latent unless some other condition is present, usually liver disease caused by alcohol abuse. Sporadic and toxic forms of the disease also occur, the latter resulting from exposure to polyhalogenated aromatic hydrocarbons, particularly hexachlorobenzene. Porphyria cutanea tarda is characterized by increased urinary excretion of uroporphyrin and faecal isocoproporphyrins.

Protoporphyria

A defect in ferrochelatase (enzyme 8, **Figure 21.3**) causes protoporphyria, although the condition is often latent. The dominant clinical feature is photosensitivity and neuropathic features do not occur. The characteristic biochemical feature is accumulation of protoporphyrin in erythrocytes.

Porphyrin Metabolism in Other Diseases

Increased excretion of haem precursors occurs in many diseases unassociated with inherited abnormalities of haem synthesis. These include lead poisoning, as lead inhibits several stages of haem synthesis. Coproporphyrin is normally excreted in the bile, although a small proportion is excreted by the urine. Biliary excretion may be impaired in hepatobiliary dysfunction leading to increased urinary excretion of coproporphyrin. Faecal excretion of porphyrins increases following gastrointestinal haemorrhage.

Sideroblastic Anaemia

Sideroblastic anaemia is a diverse group of disorders in which characteristic erythroid precursors, ringed sideroblasts, are seen in bone marrow. Acquired causes are more common than inherited, as various drugs inhibit haem biosynthesis. A rare X-linked disorder also occurs resulting from a deficiency in ALA synthase (enzyme 1, **Figure 21.3**). Defective haem synthesis occurs without porphyria, as the stage of impaired synthesis is proximal to porphyrinogen synthesis.

ABNORMAL HAEMOGLOBIN DERIVATIVES

Abnormal derivatives of haemoglobin sometimes occur which inhibit the oxygen-carrying capacity of blood. They may be detected by finding characteristic haemoglobin absorption spectra in red cell lysates.

Methaemoglobinaemia

When the iron in haemoglobin is oxidized from the ferrous (Fe^{2+}) to ferric (Fe^{3+}) state methaemoglobinaemia results. A small amount of circulating haemoglobin is continuously oxidized, although this is normally reduced by a cytochrome enzyme which is continuously regenerated by methaemoglobin reductase. The amount of circulating methaemoglobin is usually less than 1% of circulating haemoglobin levels, the proportion increasing if a deficiency of one of the reducing enzymes occurs or if some abnormal haemoglobins are present (M haemoglobinopathies). In addition, methaemoglobinaemia may be caused by toxins or drugs, including nitrites and sulphonamides. If the amount of methaemoglobin is greater than 10% of haemoglobin, cyanosis usually results while symptoms, including breathlessness, may occur if the amount exceeds 35%. Methaemoglobinaemia resulting from toxic causes or enzyme deficiency may be treated by giving a reducing agent such as methylene blue.

Sulphaemoglobin

Sulphaemoglobin is not a normal constituent of blood but is produced as a result of abnormalities similar to those which cause methaemoglobinaemia if sulphur-containing products of enteric bacterial metabolism are also present.

Carboxyhaemoglobin

Carbon monoxide has a much higher affinity for the oxygen-carrying site than oxygen and thus impairs the oxygen-carrying capacity of the blood (Chapter 22).

FURTHER READING

Cavill I, Jacobs A, Wormwood M. Diagnostic methods for serum iron status. *Annals of Clinical Biochemistry* 1986; **23**: 168–71

Elder GH. The porphyrias. Chapter 9. In: Holton JB (ed.). *The Inherited Metabolic Diseases* (2nd edn). Edinburgh: Churchill Livingstone, 1994, pp. 351–78

Elder GH. Molecular genetics of disorders of haem synthesis. *Journal of Clinical Pathology* 1993; **46**: 977–81

Elder GH, Smith SG, Smyth SJ. Laboratory investigation of the porphyrias. *Annals of Clinical Biochemistry* 1990; **27**: 395–412

Peters TJ, Pippard MJ. Disorders of iron metabolism. Chapter 79. In: Cohen RD, Lewis B, Alberti KGMM, Denman AM (eds). *The Metabolic and Molecular Basis of Acquired Disease.* London: Baillière Tindall, 1990, pp. 1870–84

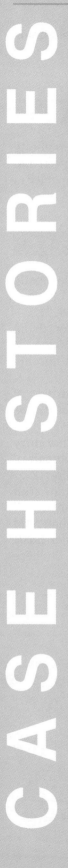

CASE 21.1

A 19-year-old woman was seen by a number of doctors. She had vague complaints which included abdominal pain and psychiatric symptoms. When referred to an endocrinologist the physical sign of wrist drop was elicited; there were no skin signs. Urine was analysed for porphobilinogen and a gross excess was present. Quantification of urinary porphyrin metabolites showed:

aminolaevulinic acid (ALA)	250 μmol 24 h^{-1}
porphobilinogen	48 μmol 24 h^{-1}
uroporphyrin	140 nmol 24 h^{-1}

What disorders could she be suffering from?

CASE 21.2

A 52-year-old man who was known to drink excessive amounts of alcohol developed blisters on his hands and face. The following were the results of investigations undertaken:

serum bilirubin	15 μmol l^{-1}
serum alanine aminotransferase (ALT)	230 U l^{-1}
serum alkaline phosphatase	80 U l^{-1}
serum γ-glutamyl transferase (GGT)	240 U l^{-1}
urinary porphobilinogen	12 μmol l^{-1}
urinary uroporphyrin	2500 nmol l^{-1}
urinary coproporphyrin	550 nmol l^{-1}

Explain these results.

TOXICOLOGY AND THERAPEUTIC DRUG MONITORING

INTRODUCTION

Toxicology is concerned with the diagnosis and treatment of acute and chronic poisoning by external agents. There are millions of chemicals and drugs and a systematic approach to disease resulting from these is obviously beyond the scope of the present text. However, a relatively limited number of different types of poisoning present commonly to District hospitals and these require analytical facilities to be available for their detection and quantification. The estimation of drugs levels is often required for diagnosis but they are most useful when an antidote or specific therapy is available to lessen the effects of the drug or toxin. Drugs commonly taken in overdose, either accidentally or with suicidal intent, are considered in the present chapter, together with monitoring drug levels to manage therapy.

SPECIFIC DRUGS AND TOXINS

The diagnosis of drug overdose can usually be established from the history and examination and confirmed by laboratory investigation, although no history may be available in unconscious or confused patients. In addition, the history may be unreliable in patients who have taken intentional overdoses due to psychiatric factors. Measurement of drug levels is essential under such circumstances, particularly if no characteristic clinical signs are detected.

Paracetamol

Paracetamol is metabolized mainly in the liver, in therapeutic doses by glucuronidation and sulphation with small amounts being metabolized by cytochrome enzymes to N-acetyl-p-benzoquinone imine. This is a toxic metabolite but the small amounts produced normally are inactivated by glutathione which is present in relatively small amounts. Larger amounts of the toxic metabolite are produced if overdoses of paracetamol are ingested and, if hepatic glutathione is overwhelmed, liver damage may result. This damage results from binding of the metabolite to thiol groups on cysteine residues of intracellular proteins, thiol oxidation, lipid peroxidation and activation of hepatic macrophages. Renal failure occurs usually, but not always, in patients with hepatic necrosis. There is variation in the susceptibility of individuals to the toxic effects of paracetamol, this increasing with the chronic ingestion of enzyme-inducing agents such as alcohol and anticonvulsant drugs. A single dose of 10 g can cause toxic effects.

Early signs and symptoms of paracetamol poisoning are nonspecific and include anorexia, nausea and vomiting: unconsciousness is not a feature. In severe overdoses, signs of hepatoxicity develop between 24 and 48 h with right hypochondrial tenderness, hyperbilirubinaemia, clotting abnormalities and elevated serum transaminase activities. Encephalopathy may follow. Antidotes to the toxic effects of paracetamol are available, including N-acetyl cysteine and methionine, both precursors of glutathione. Serum paracetamol levels are predictive of the probability of liver damage occurring and a nomogram is available indicating this risk (**Figure 22.1**). Patients presenting within 4 h should have gastric lavage. Serum levels are best determined between 4 and 12 h and maximum benefit of treatment is achieved if instituted within 10 h of ingestion, although treatment may be beneficial up to 24–30 h. N-acetyl cysteine is given intravenously while methionine can be given orally. Intravenous therapy is preferable in pa-

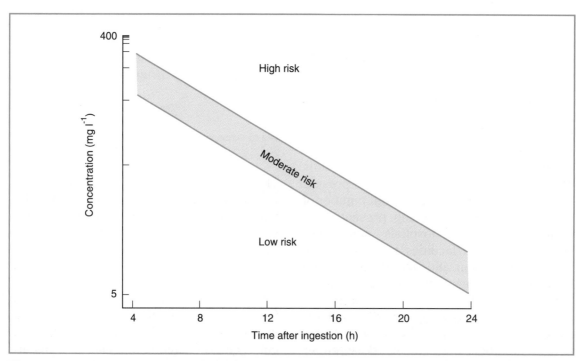

Figure 22.1 Nomogram of the relationship between prognosis and serum levels of paracetamol.

tients who have vomited and this also avoids the variability inherent in treatment with oral agents.

KEY POINTS

PARACETAMOL OVERDOSE

■ Unconsciousness is not a feature of paracetamol overdose

■ A single dose of 10 g can cause toxic effects

■ Overdose is best treated within 12 h by intravenous *N*-acetyl cysteine or oral methionine

---

Salicylates

The upper limit of the therapeutic range for salicylate levels is 350 mg l^{-1}. The clinical picture of moderate overdose occurs with serum levels of 500–750 mg l^{-1} while severe toxicity typically occurs with levels >750 mg l^{-1}. The clinical features of a moderate overdose include nausea, vomiting, tinnitus, hyperpnoea, pyrexia, sweating and hypokalaemia although loss of consciousness is unusual. This can occur in severe overdose, together with ketosis, severe dehydration and convulsions.

The metabolic effects of salicylate are responsible for many of the clinical features. It uncouples oxidative phosphorylation, leading to increased CO_2 production and O_2 consumption. This, together with a direct stimulatory effect of salicylate on the respiratory centre, leads to increased respiration and a metabolic alkalosis. As a compensatory response urinary bicarbonate excretion increases, limiting the change in pH. In some patients, particularly children and severely poisoned adults, the blood pH may fall below normal due to a metabolic acidosis. There are several contributory factors to the development of metabolic acidosis, including increased lactate production as a result of uncoupling of oxidative phosphorylation, increased lipoly-

sis leading to increased ketone body formation, and inhibition of carbohydrate metabolism, causing the accumulation of organic acids derived from the Krebs cycle. Volume depletion can also occur for several reasons. These include vomiting, leading to loss of gastrointestinal secretions, increased renal excretion of water and electrolytes as a result of metabolic alkalosis and a central effect sometimes seen is hyperpyrexia. This can lead to excessive sweating.

Treatment includes gastric lavage up to 24 h after ingestion, as salicylate may remain unabsorbed in the gastrointestinal tract for long periods. Salicylate is partly conjugated in the liver but is also excreted unchanged by the kidney. Salicylic acid is a weak acid and thus has no net charge at a pH of around 6. In its uncharged form salicylate is filtered by the glomerulus but also partly reabsorbed in the renal tubules, while ionized salicylate is much less readily reabsorbed. The excretion of salicylate is increased fourfold at a pH of 8 compared with a pH of 7: this is the rationale for increasing the pH of the urine of patients with overdose. This can be achieved by infusing sodium bicarbonate intravenously, supplementation with additional fluids being necessary in dehydrated patients to ensure adequate renal perfusion. Potassium losses should be corrected. In severely affected

---

KEY POINTS

SALICYLATE OVERDOSE

■ Unconsciousness is seen only rarely in salicylate overdose

■ Symptoms can occur with serum levels >500 mg l^{-1}

■ Salicylate overdose may cause respiratory alkalosis or metabolic acidosis

■ Salicylate overdose is treated by gastric lavage and by increasing urinary excretion through increasing the pH of urine

patients haemodialysis or haemoperfusion may be required.

Ethanol

Acute Ethanol Toxicity

The effects of acute alcohol toxicity are very well known. However, features such as abnormal behaviour or loss of conscious-ness may be due to other conditions such as hypoglycaemia or head injury, even when alcohol is detected in the breath. Alcohol ingestion can cause severe hypoglycaemia and also interacts with a number of other drugs, particularly cerebral depressants. Severe overdoses of alcohol cause cerebral depression. There are no specific antidotes. Measurement of blood levels is unnecessary in the majority of intoxicated patients but are useful in two circumstances. First, in the differential diagnosis of coma, or where an additional cause of abnormal behaviour is suspected, e.g. head injury. Second, where cerebral depression is present and treat-ment such as dialysis is being considered to reduce the blood ethanol levels.

Ethanol has diverse metabolic effects (**Table 22.1**). It is oxidized mainly in the liver with the production of large amounts of reducing equivalents which are transported into mitochondria by the malate–aspartate shuttle for further metabolism. However, within the cytosol reduced nicotinamide adenine diphosphate (NADH) forces the equilibrium of the lactate dehydrogenase reaction towards formation of lactate and

Table 22.1   Metabolic effects of alcohol

Hypoglycaemia
Lactic acidosis
Hepatic enzyme induction
Hepatic toxicity
Dyslipidaemia
Hyperuricaemia
Hypogonadism
Cushing's-like syndrome
Porphyria cutanea tarda
Thiamine deficiency

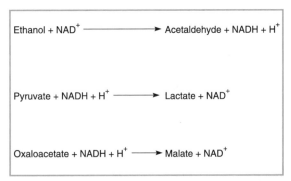

Figure 22.2 The effect of ethanol on carbohy-drate metabolism. The production of excess reduced nicotinamide adenine diphosphate (NADH) favours the formation of lactate from pyruvate and malate from oxaloacetate, reducing the amount of carbohydrate being oxidized by the tricarboxylic acid (TCA) cycle.

oxaloacetate is also converted to malate (**Figure 22.2**). Thus, less pyruvate and oxaloacetate are available for conversion to glucose and gluconeogenesis is inhibited. Hypoglycaemia and mild metabolic acidosis can occur.

Chronic Alcohol Abuse

Chronic alcohol abuse can lead to multiple abnormalities. In addition to the acute metabolic effects outlined above chronic alcohol excess produces changes in the liver, which include the accumulation of fat owing to reduced lipid oxidation and the induction of increased activity of some enzymes. One of these, γ-glutamyl transfer-ase (GGT), is monitored in serum as an indicator of alcohol abuse, although it is important to bear in mind that increased activities also occur in other conditions (see chapter 12). Further histological changes are seen including alcoholic hepatitis and portal cirrhosis. Gastritis and oesophagitis are common and the prevalence of carcino-mas of the head and neck, oesophagus and stomach is increased. Acute pancreatitis is a recognized complication. Nutritional disor-ders such as thiamine deficiency occur and haemopoiesis is affected, the commonest abnormality being an increase in erythro-cyte size (mean corpuscular volume). Like

GGT, this is often measured as an index of chronic alcohol abuse. Nervous system features include behavioural changes, loss of memory, peripheral neuropathy, Wernicke's encephalopathy and Korsakov's psychosis, these being linked to thiamine deficiency. Effects on the cardiovascular system include hypertension and cardiomyopathy. Moderate alcohol ingestion appears to be protective against cardiovascular death, possibly by raising high-density lipoprotein (HDL)-cholesterol levels. There is some evidence that red wine has a greater cardioprotective effect than other forms of alcohol, some hypothesizing that this is due to the presence of additional antioxidants. Further metabolic effects of alcohol include hyperuricaemia and hypercortisolism.

The safe limit of ethanol ingestion is usually considered to be 21 units per week for men and 14 units per week for women, one unit being a half pint of beer, a glass of wine or a single measure of spirits. A survey of medical students has shown that many drink more than the recommended maximum – to an extent that may well compromise their academic performance.

KEY POINTS

ETHANOL TOXICITY

- Ethanol interacts with other drugs to cause cerebral depression

- Metabolic effects of acute toxicity include hypoglycaemia and metabolic acidosis

- Laboratory tests often abnormal in chronic alcohol abuse include GGT and mean corpuscular volume

---

Methanol

Methanol is used extensively as a solvent, particularly as a windscreen wash solution, and it is sometimes used as a substitute for ethanol. The intoxicating effect of methanol is less than that of ethanol although acute toxicity associated with its use is greater because it is metabolized to formaldehyde and formic acid. Clinical features include severe malaise, vomiting, abdominal pain, coma and visual impairment, which may be permanent. Severe metabolic acidosis with a large anion gap occurs, partly owing to the direct effect of formic acid but also because formate increases the hepatic production of lactate, and ketosis also occurs. Treatment is directed at correcting the metabolic acidosis by administering bicarbonate, thereby inhibiting the metabolism of methanol to toxic metabolites and increasing the removal of methanol by dialysis, haemodialysis being more effective than peritoneal dialysis. The metabolism of methanol can be slowed because it is oxidized by the same enzymes that metabolize ethanol – the affinity of these for ethanol is much greater than for methanol. Thus ethanol can be considered as an antidote to methanol, this being administered orally or intravenously.

Ethylene Glycol

Ethylene glycol is a sweet-tasting alcohol which is widely used as an antifreeze in cars. It is not particularly toxic directly although it can produce nervous system depression in large doses. Toxicity is mainly due to its metabolites, glycoaldehyde, oxalic acid and other organic acids being formed by the action of alcohol dehydrogenases. Glycoaldehyde produces nervous system depression and severe metabolic acidosis with a large anion gap may occur owing to the formation of oxalate and other acids. Tissue deposition of oxalate as its calcium salt causes damage to several organs, including the heart and kidney. Symptoms include nausea, vomiting, slurred speech, ataxia, fits and coma. Respiratory depression and cardiovascular failure can also occur.

For reasons similar to those in methanol poisoning ethanol infusion is used to prevent the formation of toxic metabolites. Gastric lavage is undertaken and serum levels and acid–base status monitored. General supportive measures include correcting the acidosis with bicarbonate and ensuring that hydration is adequate. Haemodialysis may be used to increase the elimination of ethylene glycol.

Barbiturates

Although the use of intermediate-acting barbiturates as hypnotics has declined, long-acting barbiturates are still used as anticonvulsant drugs and overdoses occasionally occur. Features of severe overdose include cerebral depression leading to coma, respiratory depression and circulatory failure. General measures are very important in management; respiratory support and careful nursing care are required. Barbiturates are well absorbed by activated charcoal. Haemoperfusion or haemodialysis is used to remove barbiturates in severely affected patients.

Antidepressants

Overdoses of tricyclic antidepressants block the synaptic uptake of noradrenaline and serotonin; they have anticholinergic actions and cause cardiac arrhythmias. Symptoms generally develop within 2 h of ingestion but may be delayed up to 6 h; these include restlessness, confusion and hallucinations, with fits and coma occurring in severe overdoses. Other features include urinary retention, constipation, fever, hypotension and metabolic acidosis; pulmonary oedema may develop. The severity of overdose correlates with serum levels. Therapy includes respiratory support and control of arrhythmias and seizures.

Carbon Monoxide

Since the conversion of domestic gas supplies from coal gas to natural gas the main sources of carbon monoxide are car exhaust fumes and domestic appliances from which the fumes are incorrectly vented. Carbon monoxide is absorbed rapidly through the lungs and binds avidly to haemoglobin, blocking oxygen binding – its affinity for haemoglobin is over 200 times greater than oxygen. Thus, carbon monoxide poisoning causes tissue anoxia. Clinical features include shortness of breath, rapid respiration, headache, confusion, nausea, vomiting and diarrhoea, with respiratory depression occurring if poisoning is severe. Although the characteristic cherry-red colour of the skin and mucous membranes sometimes occurs this is rare. Cyanosis is also seen. In severe toxicity cardiac arrhythmias, hypotension and heart failure occur.

Some elevation in blood carbon monoxide levels is seen in smokers, although these are less than those seen in toxicity. It has been suggested that the elevated carbon monoxide levels in smokers damage the vascular endothelium, predisposing to atherosclerotic changes and possibly explaining, at least in part, the excess vascular risk of smoking. Blood levels of 20–30% are associated with mild toxic symptoms, 50-60% with moderate features and higher levels with severe clinical features.

Binding to haemoglobin is reversed when exposure ceases, the half-life being reduced in patients breathing 100% oxygen. Treatment involves removal from the source of poisoning and administration of 100% oxygen. Hyperbaric oxygen is even more effective in reducing the half-life of carbon monoxide.

Iron

Iron overdoses are not infrequent in small children who mistake tablets for sweets. High oral doses cause gastrointestinal irritation and ulceration. The absorption of large amounts leads to cardiovascular, hepatic and central nervous system toxicity. Vascular toxicity results from the release of vasoactive substances, such as histamine and serotonin, which lead to fluid loss from the vasculature. Clinical features include vomiting and diarrhoea, hypotension, metabolic acidosis, leukocytosis, fits and coma. Jaundice, elevation of liver enzymes and clotting abnormalities are seen if liver damage occurs. Overdose is confirmed by serum iron measurement, levels greater than 50 μmol l^{-1} being associated with serious effects and severe poisoning occurring with levels >90 μmol l^{-1}. Treatment includes desferrioxamine, a chelating agent, given intravenously or intramuscularly. This can also be included in lavage solutions. Electrolyte and H$^+$ abnormalities may need correction.

Heavy Metal Poisoning

Poisoning with heavy metals occurs mainly as a result of industrial or environmental exposure. The clinical features associated with three forms of heavy metal poisoning are outlined in **Table 22.2**.

THERAPEUTIC DRUG MONITORING

Therapeutic drug monitoring (TDM) is the measurement of drugs in body fluids as an aid to controlling dosage. The pharmacological response to some drugs can be established relatively easily by the clinical effect (e.g. antihypertensives or analgesics) while laboratory tests may indicate the response to others (e.g. hypolipidaemic or anticoagulant drugs). However, measurement of serum levels of some drugs is a valuable adjunct to clinical features in assessing the therapeutic response or possible toxic side-effects. Several factors lead to a different therapeutic effect of a particular drug between individuals, including body mass and clinical state. In addition, there is considerable heterogeneity with regard to drug metabolism owing to differ-

ences in the bioavailability of drugs, volume of distribution, protein binding, and rate of metabolism and excretion.

Therapeutic drug monitoring is potentially of benefit where there is a clear difference between the therapeutic and toxic effects and where serum levels correlate well with therapeutic and toxic effects Therapeutic drug monitoring is of little benefit when the desired effect can be assessed by clinical or laboratory measurement.

Digoxin

Digoxin is used in the treatment of cardiac failure and atrial fibrillation, and is often given to elderly subjects who may be vague about taking drugs. Side-effects include anorexia, nausea, vomiting, confusion, arrhythmias and heart block. The bioavailability from different formulations varies. The therapeutic range for digoxin is commonly held to be 1.0–2.6 nmol l^{-1} for serum levels measured at least 6 h after the last dose. Clinical toxicity is almost invariably present with levels >3.0 nmol l^{-1}. However, the correlation between serum levels and therapeutic effect is not particularly good. Reasons for this include:

1. Altered sensitivity of digoxin receptors. Receptor sensitivity is enhanced by electrolyte disturbances, such as hypokalaemia, hypercalcaemia and hypomagnesaemia, and by concomitant illnesses such as hypothyroidism.
2. Nonspecificity of the assay used to estimate digoxin. Inactive metabolites of the drug are often quantified and substances occur in the serum of some patients which react like digoxin in radioimmunoassays (digoxin-like immunoreactive substances). Examples of such substances are other steroids, particularly bile acids which accumulate in liver disease.

Table 22.2 Heavy metal poisoning

Metal	Sources	Clinical features	Pathophysiology	Laboratory findings
Lead	Petrol fumes, paint, water pipes, occupational	Anaemia	Inhibition of haem synthesis	Blood lead >1.2 μmol l^{-1} Increased erythrocyte protoporphyrin Increased urinary porphyrin precursors
		Encephalopathy (children), peripheral neuropathy Renal dysfunction	Neurotoxicity Nephrotoxicity	Aminoaciduria, Fanconi syndrome, uraemia
Cadmium	Occupational	Renal dysfunction	Nephrotoxicity	Proteinuria, increased β_2-microglobulin, urinary excretion >0.1 μmol day^{-1}
		Emphysema (following inhalation) Testicular damage Osteomalacia	Alveolar macrophage necrosis, enzyme release Vasoconstriction Impaired calcification	
Mercury	Occupational, paints, fungicides	Pneumonitis (inhalation) Gastrointestinal symptoms (ingestion of salts) Encepalopathy Nephropathy	Airway damage Epithelial damage Neuronal degeneration Nephrotoxic	Glycosuria, aminoaciduria, proteinuria, uraemia

Serum levels of digoxin are measured for three main reasons:

1. To assess patient compliance, particularly when there has been a poor response to treatment.
2. To investigate the possibility of toxicity. Plasma potassium should also be measured if digoxin toxicity is being investigated, as symptoms of toxicity occur at lower levels in the presence of hypokalaemia. Serum levels should not be taken as the sole guide to toxicity as there is considerable overlap between therapeutic and toxic levels.
3. To assess the therapeutic effect.

Theophylline

Theophylline relaxes bronchial smooth muscle and is used in the treatment of asthma and occasionally in left-ventricular failure. Theophylline is sometimes prescribed as aminophylline, a combination that includes ethylenediamine, which increases the solubility of theophylline twentyfold. Side-effects include nausea, diarrhoea, arrhythmias and fits. There is a well-defined therapeutic range, 55–110 μmol l^{-1}. The half-life of the drug is increased in heart failure, cirrhosis and by some drugs, including oral contraceptives. A decreased half-life is seen in smokers, heavy drinkers and with drugs that induce hepatic enzymes. Toxic symptoms occur with increasing frequency at serum concentrations >110 μmol l^{-1} and are sometimes seen at levels within the therapeutic range. Monitoring of serum levels is valuable when investigating toxicity and when optimizing dosage.

Anticonvulsant Drugs

Anticonvulsant (antiepileptic) drugs are usually administered initially in low doses, these being increased gradually until sei-

zures are controlled. Sometimes a combination of drugs is necessary when fitting continues with a single agent, despite adequate serum concentrations. Interactions between anticonvulsants occur.

Phenytoin is widely used – successful prescription depending on a knowledge of its pharmacokinetics. Approximately 90% is bound to serum albumin, the therapeutic effect being due to the free fraction. Phenytoin is metabolized in the liver by hydroxylation, this process showing saturation kinetics. Thus, the half-life of the drug increases with high doses. Phenytoin induces the activity of some hepatic enzymes, including those metabolizing vitamin D, bilirubin and folic acid. Thus, serum bilirubin levels are often lower in patients receiving phenytoin, and osteomalacia may occur. Adverse effects on the central nervous system include nystagmus, ataxia, tremor, lethargy, dysarthria, vomiting and coma. Convulsions may also occur together with hepatotoxicity, rashes and gum hyperplasia. The therapeutic range is 40–80 μmol l^{-1} and while higher levels are required to control seizures in some patients, clinical signs of toxicity become apparent in many subjects with levels >80 μmol l^{-1}. Conversely, effective control may be achieved in many patients with lower levels. Monitoring of plasma levels is useful when initiating therapy, when there is deterioration in previously adequate control, in the investigation of toxicity or if additional drugs are prescribed, particularly if these alter phenytoin metabolism, e.g. by displacing phenytoin from protein-binding sites. Phenytoin clearance is increased in pregnancy.

Sodium valproate is approximately 90% protein bound, although the proportion of the free drug increases with high doses. Valproate inhibits the metabolism of other anticonvulsants and displaces phenytoin from protein. However, this effect is usually masked by increased metabolism and phenytoin levels usually fall. Side-effects are usually minor and include anorexia, nausea, vomiting, drowsiness, weight gain, alopecia and thrombocytopaenia. No generally accepted therapeutic range has been established and toxic effects show no clear relationship with serum levels. Thus TDM is not recommended.

Phenobarbitone is a second-line drug for epilepsy, as is primadone which is converted to phenobarbitone and another active metabolite after absorption. Approximately 50% of phenobarbitone is protein bound. Most is metabolized by hepatic microsomal enzymes, although up to 30% is excreted unchanged in the urine. The half-life is very long, up to 100 h. Adverse effects include sedation, nystagmus and ataxia. The therapeutic range is wide, 40–170 μmol l^{-1}. Although some patients are well controlled with higher levels, tolerance to the therapeutic effect develops in long-term therapy. There is a poor correlation between serum levels and toxic effects. Monitoring of levels is of limited value under most circumstances although TDM may be useful in combination therapy, levels rising if valproate is added. Serum levels are also be useful in suspected toxicity.

Carbamazepine is metabolized in the liver and its metabolites also have anticonvulsant actions. It induces its own metabolism and thus serum levels fall when treatment is established; metabolism is also induced by phenytoin and phenobarbitone, although inhibited by valproate. Adverse effects include central nervous system symptoms (blurring of vision, diplopia and dizziness), depression of cardiac conduction, skin rashes, leukopaenia and water retention. There is considerable individual variability in the metabolism of carbamazepine and the therapeutic effect depends on both the drug and a metabolite. Thus, the therapeutic range is relatively wide, 17–42 μmol l^{-1}. Some patients require levels >42 μmol l^{-1} to show a therapeutic response, although side-effects become increasingly frequent at higher levels. Monitoring serum levels is useful in patients in whom seizures are difficult to control.

Lithium

Lithium is used widely in the treatment of acute mania and in the prophylaxis of manic-depressive illness. Lithium is not protein bound in serum and is excreted unchanged in the urine, although significant tubular reabsorption occurs. The half-life is determined by the volume of distribution and clearance, steady-state levels occurring within 5 days of starting treatment. Adverse effects are common if the serum level is >1.5 mmol l^{-1} and serious with concentrations >2.0 mmol l^{-1}. These include central nervous system effects, tremor, drowsiness, ataxia, tinnitus, blurred vision and dysarthria. Polyuria may occur owing to reduced sensitivity of the renal tubule to vasopressin. Thyroid enlargement is sometimes seen. The therapeutic range of lithium is 0.5–0.8 mmol l^{-1} in the prophylaxis of manic-depressive illness and up to 1.3 mmol l^{-1} in the treatment of acute mania. Monitoring serum levels is essential when treatment is introduced and it is advisable to measure concentrations periodically in patients on maintenance therapy.

Aminoglycoside Antibiotics

Aminoglycoside antibiotics have a wide spectrum of activity against Gram-negative organisms. They have limited solubility in water and must therefore be given parenterally. There is little protein binding and aminoglycosides are excreted in urine without metabolism. Adverse effects include nephrotoxicity and ototoxicity. They have a bacteriostatic effect and in addition are bactericidal at higher concentrations. Peak levels of gentamicin of 5–10 mg l^{-1} are recommended although trough levels of >2.5 mg l^{-1} with an 8-hourly dosage regime are associated with toxicity. Monitoring is important in seriously ill patients to ensure that adequate serum levels are attained, in patients with impaired renal function and in patients on prolonged treatment.

Cyclosporin

Cyclosporin is an immunosuppressive drug that is used widely following organ grafting to prevent transplant rejection. Gastrointestinal absorption is variable and metabolism occurs mainly in the liver. The drug is bound to erythrocytes and monitoring is undertaken by measuring whole-blood levels. Adverse effects include nephrotoxicity, hepatoxicity, hypertension and hyperkalaemia. Nephrotoxicity is dose-related, the risk increasing at blood levels >170–330

nmol l^{-1}. There is, however, considerable overlap between the levels seen in rejection and toxicity.

FURTHER READING

Bray GP. Liver failure induced by paracetamol. *British Medical Journal* 1993; **306**: 157–8.

Collier DJ, Beales ILP. Drinking among medical students – a questionnaire survey. *British Medical Journal* 1989; **299**: 19–22.

Hallworth M, Capps N. *Therapeutic Drug Monitoring and Clinical Biochemistry*. London: ACB Venture Publications, 1993.

CASES HISTORIES

CASE 22.1

A 72-year-old man who lived alone was admitted after neighbours noticed that he was very confused. An empty tablet bottle was found in his flat although it was unlabelled. No abnormal findings were elicited on examination although he was breathing deeply. The following investigations were performed:

plasma sodium	142 mmol l^{-1}
plasma potassium	4.9 mmol l^{-1}
total CO_2	11 mmol l^{-1}
urea	7.4 mmol l^{-1}
creatinine	134 μmol l^{-1}
blood glucose	6.4 mmol l^{-1}
urinary ketones	negative

What diagnoses should be considered?

CASE 22.2

A 38-year-old woman was admitted to the accident room having been found unconscious in a bus shelter. No other history was available. The following were the results of the initial investigations:

plasma sodium	139 mmol l^{-1}
plasma potassium	4.9 mmol l^{-1}
total CO_2	4 mmol l^{-1}
urea	4.2 mmol l^{-1}
creatinine	138 μmol l^{-1}
blood pH	6.95
P_{CO_2}	2.1 kPa
P_{O_2}	13.7 kPa
blood ethanol	900 mg l^{-1}

How can these results be explained?

NEAR-PATIENT TESTING

INTRODUCTION

Most diagnostic investigations are carried out in a central laboratory, some distance from the wards or clinics. This is essential when investigations require sophisticated, expensive equipment and highly skilled dedicated staff to operate it. Such centralization of expertise provides economies of scale and is satisfactory for most clinical requirements. However, investigations are sometimes required urgently and while laboratories offer special services for emergencies it is often more convenient, particularly in critical care units, to have certain key tests available locally. Testing on site is speedier, circumventing the time taken to arrange urgent investigations with the laboratory and for transport of specimens. There are also obvious advantages in having certain key monitoring tests available in

Outpatients at the time of clinical consultation, as management decisions can be taken immediately.

Near-patient testing in the form of urine analysis has been available for many years, although these tests are only semiquantitative. Recently, there have been major technical developments in which more tests have been adapted to test strips (dry chemistries). Increasing clinical applications, coupled with rapid developments in microprocessors and data processing, have lead to the development of small desktop analysers suitable for use in the home, ward side-rooms, outpatient clinics and general practitioners' surgeries.

Near-patient testing can be considered under three groupings: urine tests, blood tests, and self-monitoring by patients in their own homes. A further type of near-patient testing is breath analysis, the most obvious example being the measurement of breath alcohol at the roadside for medico-legal purposes. Breath analysis will not be considered further in this chapter.

URINE TESTS

Testing for abnormal constituents in urine was one of the first types of diagnostic investigations carried out; the original method to detect glucose in urine, tasting, was rapidly replaced by chemical methods, for obvious reasons. The traditional type of chemical procedures using test tubes and liquid reagents has largely been replaced by dry chemistry technology. The tests are available individually although many of them are also incorporated into multi-test strips. The most widely used urine tests are for glucose, reducing substances, ketones, protein, pH, bilirubin and urobilinogen.

Glucose

Semiquantitative tests for detection of glucose are based on strips impregnated with glucose oxidase. This enzyme reacts specifically with glucose to form hydrogen peroxide which is then detected by forming a colour. The enzyme is specific for glucose although positive reactions can occur if the urine container is contaminated with hypochlorite, which then produces hydrogen peroxide. False-negative reactions can also occur, particularly if ascorbic acid is present in large amounts. Ascorbic acid reacts with hydrogen peroxide, preventing the latter forming a colour.

Glycosuria occurs if blood glucose concentrations exceed 10 mmol l^{-1}, as the capacity of the renal tubules to reabsorb filtered glucose is exceeded above this level. Glycosuria occurs in diabetes mellitus, but also if the renal threshold for glucose reabsorption is reduced. This often occurs in late pregnancy, even if diabetes does not develop. Glycosuria also occurs if renal tubular dysfunction is present, e.g. Fanconi

syndrome (see chapter 8). Testing urine for glucose should be undertaken as part of a full medical examination. It is sometimes used for home-monitoring of diabetes although there is wide variation in the renal threshold for glucose reabsorption and this rises with age.

> **KEY POINTS**
>
> **GLYCOSURIA**
> - Glucose excretion depends on the renal threshold, which is variable
> - The renal threshold for glucose excretion decreases in pregnancy
> - Other causes of glycosuria include diabetes mellitus and renal tubular disorders

Reducing Substances

Reducing substances, including glucose and other sugars (**Table 23.1**), may be detected by using a wet chemistry reaction in which the reagents are available in a tablet (Clinitest). Tests for reducing substances are used to screen neonates for inherited metabolic disorders. If found, more specific investigations are required to identify the reducing substance, e.g. sugar chromatography.

Ketone Bodies

Tests for ketone bodies are available in tablet and stick forms; these react with acetoacetate and acetone but not β-hydroxybutyrate. Testing for ketonuria is important in patients with newly diagnosed diabetes mellitus and can be used to differentiate poorly controlled non-insulin dependent from insulin-dependent diabetes. Monitoring is also useful in ketosis-prone patients, particularly during intercurrent illnesses, as an indicator of ketoacidosis.

Table 23.1   Reducing substances found in urine

Reducing substance	Causes
Glucose	Diabetes mellitus
	Late pregnancy
	Renal tubular disorders
Galactose	Galactosaemia
	Severe liver disease
Fructose	Excessive ingestion of some fruits
	Essential fructosuria
	Hereditary fructose intolerance
Pentoses	Excessive ingestion of some fruits
	Essential pentosuria
Lactose	Lactation
	Neonates
	Coeliac disease
Salicylates	Salicylate therapy
Drugs	Some penicillins
	Some cephalosporins
Creatinine	Concentrated urine
Homogentisic acid	Alcaptonuria

However, it is important to be aware that levels may be elevated during starvation, prolonged exercise and pregnancy. Some inherited metabolic disorders cause keto-naemia and hence ketonuria. Stick tests for blood ketones are also available, the applications being similar to those of urinary ketones.

Proteinuria

The principle of the stick tests for proteinuria is that of a colour change with an impregnated dye, albumin giving a stronger reaction than other proteins. The dye used is an indicator and highly alkaline urine specimens will give a false-positive reaction. This sometimes occurs in urinary tract infection. This is likely if infection is due to an organism which can split urea to form ammonia; *Proteus* species have this property. False-negative reactions occur if the urine is acidified. The interpretation and further investigation of proteinuria is discussed in chapter 8.

Bilirubin

The qualitative detection of bilirubin in urine is useful in the differential diagnosis of jaundice although it is important to use a fresh specimen of urine, as bilirubin degrades rapidly on exposure to light. Bilirubinuria results from the excretion of conjugated bilirubin and occurs in hepatic and cholestatic causes of jaundice but not in haemolysis (see chapter 10).

Urobilinogen

Urinary urobilinogen excretion is increased in haemolytic and hepatocellular disease. It is detected in laboratory tests by reaction with Ehrlich's aldehyde reagent; porphobilinogen, which is excreted in excess in some porphyrias, also reacts. These are differentiated by solubility, urobilinogen being soluble and porphobilinogen insoluble in organic solvents. A strip test for urobilinogen is available which is less sensitive to porphobilinogen.

BLOOD TESTS IN CLINICAL UNITS

Analysers used in clinical units vary in complexity from being equipment dedicated to a single or small number of related tests to compact, sophisticated analysers capable of a wide range of tests. Examples of such equipment in widespread use are blood glucose, gas, electrolyte, and bilirubin analysers.

Near-patient testing in critical care units offers physicians the advantages of very rapid results and convenience. However, the development of near-patient testing should not occur in isolation from the laboratory services of the hospital. The local laboratory should be involved in the selection and maintenance of analytical equipment in the clinical environment for several reasons:

1. While such equipment is generally reliable regular maintenance is required. This will usually involve fairly simple day-to-day maintenance with more extensive checking being undertaken from time to time.

2. Checking the performance of the instruments by quality assurance procedures is essential to ensure that accurate results are obtained. Although quality assurance has been used for many years the concept may be new to clinical staff who have not worked in laboratories.

3. Clinical staff must be trained in the use of the equipment, calibration procedures, simple quality assurance and proper record keeping. Cooperation from a lead clinician is very important to help ensure that use of equipment is limited to clinical staff who have received agreed training.

4. The results from extralaboratory equipment must be consistent with those from the laboratory as these will be required as back-up in the event of machine failure. Compatibility between near-patient testing equipment and the laboratory service should be considered at the time of purchase of equipment.

5. Spillage of blood may occur in the areas around desktop analysers and machines will, potentially at least, be contaminated with blood. Procedures must be introduced to minimize the risk from blood infected with agents such as hepatitis B and human immunodeficiency virus (HIV). Careful cleaning of desktop analysers must be adopted.

Blood Glucose Analysis

Blood glucose concentrations can be estimated in clinical areas using strips which have a similar chemical basis to that described for urinary glucose estimation. Results can be determined either by comparing visually the colour developed against a chart, or by using a simple meter. Both methods of assessment can give accurate results from finger-prick specimens although it is important to follow the instructions for use of the test strips, particularly with regard to the volume of blood and the time of incubation before washing the blood off.

Blood glucose measurement in critical care areas can be used to diagnose hyperglycaemia and hypoglycaemia, the latter condition often being too acute to wait for the results of laboratory analysis before starting treatment. Blood glucose monitoring is also used by diabetic patients for home monitoring (see chapter 1), and also in diabetic clinics.

KEY POINTS

NEAR-PATIENT TESTING

- Near-patient testing is undertaken in wards, clinics and patients' homes

- Advantages include immediacy of results, which are often necessary for clinical management

- Near-patient testing requires the active collaboration of clinical and laboratory staff

Blood Gas Analysis

Blood gas analysis has found applications in intensive care wards, operating theatres and neonatal wards where the rapid availability of results is essential for clinical care. The instruments used are similar to those in clinical laboratories and therefore there is usually comparability between results. Blood gas partial pressures (Po_2, Pco_2) and pH are estimated.

Blood Electrolyte Analysis

Analysers for the measurement of sodium and potassium have been developed which use ion-selective electrodes. Direct-reading ion-selective electrodes are usually used in clinical practice. These determine electrolyte concentrations without prior dilution of blood and results may differ from those obtained in laboratories using indirect-reading ion-selective electrodes for patients with hyperproteinaemia or hypertriglyceridaemia. This is because samples are diluted before analysis with indirect-reading ion-selective electrodes and therefore less plasma is sampled due to a volume displacement effect (see chapter 5).

Bilirubin Analysis

Bilirubinometers are used in obstetric units to monitor hyperbilirubinaemia in neonates. These instruments are simple spectrophotometers which quantify bilirubin on the basis of absorbance of light in serum. Chemical methods are usually used in clinical laboratories and results may differ at high concentrations, bilirubinometers giving low values. Falsely low results may also occur with haemolysed specimens.

Blood Cholesterol

Blood cholesterol measurement is available using desktop analysers, although such measurements have no clinical application in critical care units. The possible application of near-patient cholesterol measurement is rather in outpatient clinics, general practices and pharmacies as part of coronary heart disease (CHD) prevention programmes. The advantage of such testing is the immediacy of results in terms of feedback to the patients and for planning management of hypercholesterolaemia. It is important that cholesterol testing is not undertaken in isolation from assessment and appropriate management of other risk factors for CHD. In addition to total serum cholesterol, HDL cholesterol and serum triglyceride measurements are available. Such analysers can give accurate results although values are not as precise as laboratory measurements. Kits are being marketed for home estimation of serum cholesterol although these appear more technically demanding than desktop analysis and the application of such tests is not clear.

Other Investigations

It is technically feasible to undertake several other clinical investigations including blood urea, creatinine, uric acid, lactate, amylase, alanine and aspartate aminotransferase, lactate dehydrogenase, creatine kinase and γ-glutamyl transferase. However, the clinical requirements for these in acute clinical care units has not been demonstrated.

CONTINUOUS PATIENT MONITORING

The logical extension of the principle of providing biochemical tests in critical clinical areas is continuous patient monitoring. One area in which this is being undertaken is in monitoring blood gases by the application of electrodes to the skin, particularly in neonatal units where it has the advantage of reducing the need for repeated blood samples in infants with respiratory conditions (see chapter 19). There is considerable potential for the continuous monitoring of electrolytes, glucose and intermediary metabolites by extracorporeal systems or intravascular electrodes, although some technical difficulties remain to be overcome before these find widespread clinical applications.

FURTHER READING

Annotation. Home cholesterol monitoring. *Lancet* 1992; **340**: 1386

Marks V. Essential considerations in the provision of near-patient testing facilities. *Annals of Clinical Biochemistry* 1988; **25**: 220–5

Marks V. Stick testing. *British Medical Journal* 1991; **302**; 482–3

Scott A, Tattersall R. Self-monitoring of diabetes. Urine testing revisited and self-monitoring of blood glucose updated. Chapter 9. In: Alberti KGMM, Krall LP (eds). *The Diabetes Annual/2*. Amsterdam: Elsevier, 1986, pp. 120–36

Steinhausen RL, Price CP. Principles and practice of dry chemistry systems. Chapter 12. In: Price CP, Alberti KGMM (eds). *Recent Advances in Clinical Biochemistry, Volume 3*. Edinburgh: Churchill Livingstone, 1985, pp. 273–96.

CASE 23.1

A 29-year-old insulin-dependent diabetic patient was admitted to the accident and emergency department at the request of his general practitioner who had been called to see the patient after his blood glucose control worsened following an episode of diarrhoea and vomiting. The blood glucose concentration had been determined by home monitoring and was found to be 17.9 mmol l^{-1}. The patient was fully conscious and physical examination was unremarkable. The results of his blood tests were as follows.

sodium	137 mmol l^{-1}
potassium	4.1 mmol l^{-1}
chloride	109 mmol l^{-1}
total CO_2	16 mmol l^{-1}
urea	7.2 mmol l^{-1}
creatinine	108 mmol l^{-1}
blood glucose	8.7 mmol l^{-1}

Comment on these results.

CHAPTER 24

BIOCHEMICAL INVESTIGATIONS IN CLINICAL PRACTICE

INTRODUCTION

An understanding of the pathophysiological basis of metabolic disease is essential for the effective use of biochemical tests in clinical practice. In addition, some appreciation of other factors related to biochemical investigations is also important, including their purpose, the processes involved in undertaking tests, and general factors which influence interpretation of results.

THE PURPOSE OF INVESTIGATIONS

There should always be a clear reason for undertaking investigations as unnecessary tests are uneconomic and involve some discomfort to the patient. There are many biochemical investigations, the purpose of which is to contribute to clinical care. The reasons for undertaking investigations include diagnosis, management, prognosis, and screening for disease.

Diagnosis

Diagnosis is based on clinical features, including history and examination, and investigations. Occasionally, biochemical tests are diagnostic of a particular disease, an example being the glucose tolerance test in diabetes mellitus. However, investigations more often confirm a diagnosis or indicate that a particular metabolic syndrome is present, such as hypercalcaemia, hyponatraemia or hypoglycaemia. Specific biochemical tests are often useful in the differential diagnosis of metabolic syndromes, such as parathyroid hormone (PTH) levels in hypercalcaemia.

Management

Biochemical abnormalities are important markers of metabolic disorders and thus monitored in management. Applications include:

1. Following the response to therapy in acute disorders. In diabetic ketoacidosis it is important to monitor the response of blood glucose concentrations after insulin administration to ensure that control is established without producing hypoglycaemia. In addition, accompanying metabolic disturbances such as hyperkalaemia require monitoring and treatment.
2. Assessing treatment in chronic disorders. Glycated haemoglobin concentrations are an important indicator of blood glucose levels over several weeks in diabetes mellitus and are used to assess whether treatment is adequate. The suppression of elevated serum thyroid-stimulating hormone (TSH) levels by thyroxine supplements are measured to assess the adequacy of hormone replacement in hypothyroidism.
3. Assessing drug therapy. Drug levels are monitored for three main reasons: to assess compliance, to check that therapeutic ranges are being achieved, and to investigate overdosage. The possibility of sensitivity to or toxicity from drug therapy must also be considered, abnormal liver function being a side-effect of many drugs. Efficacy is also monitored when appropriate, e.g. the response to lipid lowering drugs.

Urgent Tests

Requesting an investigation urgently implies that the result is required before the next routine delivery of test results to the ward. Urgent investigations involve considerably more organization than routine tests, and may require special venepuncture, portering services, and special liaison with the laboratory. Additional cost is involved compared with routine investigations and therefore justification of urgent investigations is required. This is true particularly at night and at weekends when the laboratory is closed and an analyst must be called in. However, an excessive number of urgent requests during a normal working day also causes problems by deflecting staff from other tasks. The key question in justifying an urgent request is whether receiving the result within the next half-hour rather than at the end of the day will influence the management of the patient during the intervening period. If not, the test is not urgent. Occasionally, a metabolic emergency may be too acute to wait the half-hour or so it may take to get a result back from the laboratory, an example being acute hypoglycaemia. If hypoglycaemia is suspected blood should be taken for a blood glucose estimation but the condition should be treated if a low blood glucose concentration is confirmed by a reagent strip test. The specimen for blood glucose should be analysed urgently if the patient fails to respond to glucose infusion.

It is sometimes important to take blood specimens at the time of an emergency admission although immediate results are not required for effective short-term management. Thus, if a patient presents with acute chest pain at 03.00 hours the immediate management is unlikely to be altered by a result of serum cardiac enzyme activities at that time, although the information may be useful for later management decisions. This requirement could be met by taking the blood but postponing analysis until the next day.

Prognosis

Tests are sometimes used to provide information about the course of a disease.

An example is the serial measurement of tumour markers in patients with malignant disease, falling levels being evidence for a response to treatment, while rising levels following an initial response indicating the possibility of recurrence. Measuring risk factors is a form of prognosis assessment. The treatment of hypercholesterolaemia in patients with established coronary heart disease (CHD) has been shown to improve prognosis and thus measuring serum cholesterol in patients with ischaemic heart disease allows assessment of the possible benefits of specific treatment.

Screening

Screening is undertaken to detect the presence of disease which is not apparent and for which there is no specific indication on clinical grounds. For screening to be effective certain criteria should be met.

1. The disease has a significant effect on the length or quality of life.
2. There is a period during the natural history of the disease in which irreversible damage does not occur and during which the condition may be detected.
3. Treatment is available which is acceptable and effective during the asymptomatic period.
4. An effective screening test should be available.
5. The prevalence of the disease and benefits of therapy should justify the cost of screening.
6. A population at risk can be defined.

Biochemical screening tests are undertaken to detect specific conditions such as inherited metabolic disorders or hypercholesterolaemia, or more general biochemical screening (profiling) in which a large number of tests are performed on a single sample to detect latent disease.

Inherited Metabolic Disease

Screening for some inherited metabolic diseases, particularly phenylketonuria and neonatal hypothyroidism, fulfils many of the criteria outlined above. Thus, untreated, phenylketonuria causes brain damage and the prognosis is improved if the condition is diagnosed and treated effectively early in infancy. Although the incidence of the condition varies it occurs, on average, in 1:10 000 births. The population at risk, the newborn, is easily defined and an effective screening procedure, the Guthrie test, is available.

Hypercholesterolaemia

The case for some other screening procedures is less clear, e.g. measuring cholesterol in the general adult population. Although hypercholesterolaemia is common and easily detected the benefits of treatment have not been clearly established in the absence of other risk factors for CHD, such as pre-existing CHD, hypertension and diabetes mellitus. However, in patients with multiple risk factors treatment of hypercholesterolaemia reduces the incidence of CHD, induces regression of atherosclerotic lesions and, in patients with existing CHD, improves mortality. Thus screening for hypercholesterolaemia is likely to be effective in high-risk patients but cannot, at present, be recommended for the general population.

Biochemical Profiling

Undertaking multiple biochemical tests simultaneously in fit subjects with the hope that something will turn up (well-population screening) cannot be recommended as such approaches have a low efficiency in detecting disease. Similarly, nonselective biochemical tests at the time of outpatient attendance or admission to hospital rarely provide useful information, even though the prevalence of disease will be higher than in the general population.

Functionally Related Test Groups

Performing several tests simultaneously that are related to the assessment of a particular organ function differs from screening. For example, the combination of a serum transaminase and alkaline phosphatase activity is helpful in the differential diagnosis of hyperbilirubinaemia and time is often saved if these are measured in parallel rather than sequentially. Other tests that are often grouped in this way include electrolytes, urea and creatinine (urea and electrolytes), and calcium, phosphate, albumin and alkaline phosphatase (bone chemistry).

THE MECHANICS OF INVESTIGATIONS

Blood Collection

Blood for biochemical analysis is collected from arteries, veins and capillaries, depending on the type of test and the age of the patient. The majority of samples from adults are obtained by venepuncture. Venepuncture requires careful attention to technique and consideration of factors that may cause spurious test results. Normally, blood should not be taken from an arm into which an intravenous infusion is being given because there is communication between veins. Thus, a blood sample may be contaminated unless the infusion is interrupted for several minutes. Fasting is required for some tests as a recent meal may cause changes, e.g. increased triglyceride and glucose concentrations. A tourniquet to obstruct venous return is usually required although this increases the filtration pressure across capillary walls, causing transfer of water and small molecular weight constituents, with resulting concentration of larger molecular weight substances. Increases of 10% in proteins and protein-bound constituents occur within a few minutes of venous stasis. The posture of the subject also affects fluid distribution,

haemodilution occurring with a change from standing to lying.

Blood is taken into syringes or evacuated tubes. If syringes are used the needle must be removed before expelling the blood into the tube as failure to do this often results in a severely haemolysed sample. Blood may also be haemolysed during a difficult venepuncture, haemolysis causing spurious elevations of substances such as potassium, which have high intracellular concentrations.

Anticoagulants and Specimen Preservation

Serum is satisfactory for most biochemical tests although clotting takes 15–30 min. Using plasma shortens the time for separation of cells and therefore is often used for emergency tests. In addition, the yield of plasma is greater than that of serum and is preferable for small samples. An anticoagulant is also required in collection tubes if whole blood is required for analysis, e.g. blood gases and lactate determinations. Heparin is widely used for this purpose, causing little interference in most tests although it is not suitable for blood counts. The anticoagulant action of the chelating agent ethylene diamine tetra-acetic acid (EDTA) results from its calcium-binding properties and it is widely used in haematology because it preserves the cellular elements of blood. It is unsuitable for the analysis of divalent metals because these are removed by chelation. In addition, EDTA is a sodium or potassium salt and therefore values for these would be elevated spuriously. It also inhibits enzymes that require divalent metals as cofactors. Sodium fluoride inhibits glycolytic enzymes and is used for glucose analysis, although it is not particularly effective as an anticoagulant and therefore is usually used in combination with an oxalate salt.

Urine Collection

Biochemical analyses in urine are carried out using either random specimens or timed collections, usually for 24 h although different periods are sometimes used. Timed 24-h collections have the advantage that they correct for diurnal variations in the excretion of the test substance although they are demanding to collect. Careful instruction of the patient is required. This should include a warning against washing the collection bottle as this may contain a preservative essential for the particular test. The patient should also be warned if the preservative is acid. Just before the start of the collection the bladder should be emptied and the urine discarded. All subsequent voids are placed in the collection container and it is important to empty the bladder at the end of the collection period to complete the save. If there is a suspicion that the collection is incomplete, measurement of urinary creatinine excretion may be helpful, as this is relatively constant in an individual.

Specimen Transport

Clear identification of specimens is mandatory and is the responsibility of the person taking the blood specimen. Information must also be provided on age and, if necessary, sex (see reference ranges). Specimens are usually transported to the laboratory in plastic bags to contain any spillages that may occur. Labelling of these with specific warning stickers is necessary if specimens are potentially hazardous, e.g. from patients with hepatitis or from a patient at high risk of human immunodeficiency virus (HIV) infection.

The conditions of transport may be vital. Specimens for bilirubin should be protected from the light to avoid photodegradation and some tests require specimens to be maintained at 4°C, e.g. lactate and some hormones.

KEY POINTS

BLOOD COLLECTION

- Always check that the correct anticoagulant is being used
- Blood should be taken with minimal venous stasis
- Specimens must be labelled correctly
- Possible biohazards must be indicated
- Special transport conditions must be followed

THE INTERPRETATION OF INVESTIGATIONS

Reference Ranges

The most obvious question to consider when interpreting a test result is whether it is normal. As a guide, results are compared with those obtained from a population who are thought to be disease free. These data are gathered in two ways: (i) by measuring the concentration of the test substance in a population which appears to be free of disease; and (ii) by assessing the values for health for a test which may be defined by associations between particular values and disease, these often being defined by epidemiological surveys.

Population-Based Reference Ranges

These are determined by the concentration of the test in a representative group of the general population who appear to be free of disease. The group should be large enough to allow sex differences and age-related changes to be assessed. The values for many tests have a Gaussian distribution and in such cases the reference data, by convention, are taken as ±2 standard deviations of the mean (**Figure 24.1**, serum sodium). This definition includes 95% of the population tested.

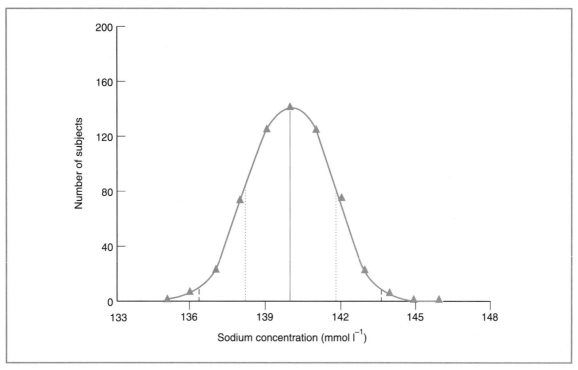

Figure 24.1 The values of serum sodium obtained from a healthy population. These are distributed evenly around the mean (solid bar) and therefore the distribution is Gaussian or normal. The dotted lines represent ±1 standard deviations (SD) and the values for 66% of the population fall within these. The dashed lines (±2 SD) include 95% of the population. By convention the reference range is taken as ±2 SD.

Sometimes the distribution of the data is not Gaussian (**Figure 24.2**, serum total bilirubin) and therefore different statistical techniques must be used to determine the reference range. One method that is used is to transform the values of the test to logarithms and assess whether the distribution is converted to Gaussian. If it is Gaussian then the reference range can be determined in the way outlined above using the log-transformed data. Alternatively, the reference range can be defined as the values between the 2.5th and 97.5th percentiles, thus including 95% of the population. The example given in **Figure 24.2** is more complex than this for two reasons. First, there is a second peak of frequency of bilirubin concentrations. This occurs because two populations have been included in the sampling procedure, subjects with no

abnormality in bilirubin metabolism and a small group who have Gilbert's disease, this not being apparent clinically. The reference range in this case was defined as the point of intercept between the curves of the two populations. Second, the data are not transformed to Gaussian by log conversion; more than 50% of the values for the subjects without Gilberts disease lie to the right of the dotted line, this representing the mode.

The term reference range is preferable to normal range for several reasons.

1. The term normal has a particular statistical meaning, and refers to a Gaussian pattern of distribution. In this sense the use of the word normal does not relate to health.
2. The definition of a reference range which includes 95% of a healthy popula-

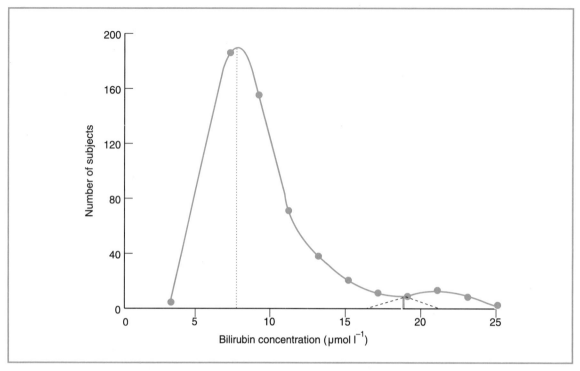

Figure 24.2 The distribution of total serum bilirubin from a population who were apparently healthy and gave no history of liver disease or jaundice. Two peaks are seen, the larger one including healthy subjects while the smaller peak includes subjects with Gilbert's disease. The concentrations from the two populations overlap and the probable distribution of each is interpolated by the dashed lines. The cut-off value for the upper limit of the reference range was taken at the point at which the two curves cross (solid line). Even if the subjects with Gilbert's disease are excluded bilirubin values are not Gaussian, as they are skewed to the right of the mode (dotted line).

tion excludes 2.5% at the lower end and 2.5% at the upper end. Thus, some people who appear to be healthy, i.e. normal, are excluded from the reference range.

3. Despite excluding subjects with obvious clinical conditions it is likely that not all subjects who provide specimens to establish a reference range are healthy. Some may well have latent disease, e.g. undiagnosed type 2 diabetes mellitus.

4. A test result within the reference range cannot be taken to imply normality in the sense of being nonpathological, as tests do not discriminate perfectly between healthy and diseased populations under all circumstances.

Reference Ranges Defined by Disease Risk

The concept that values of a particular test in a population who are free of disease imply normality in a clinical sense is not always correct. Thus, 25% of the population in many Northern European countries have serum total cholesterol concentrations 6.5 mmol l^{-1} without any clinically obvious evidence of disease. However, a cholesterol value of 6.6 mmol l^{-1} cannot be regarded as normal, since it carries an increased risk of developing coronary heart disease (*see* **Figure 2.10**). In the case of serum cholesterol concentrations, the 'reference values' on which the interpretation of a patient's results is based are defined by the association cholesterol concentrations with the subsequent risk of developing CHD. Thus, this is low if the cholesterol concentrations are <5.2 mmol l^{-1}, moderately increased for values 6.5 mmol l^{-1}, while the risk is high if values are 7.8 mmol l^{-1}.

Factors Affecting Reference Ranges

Tests may vary with various factors, two important ones being age and gender. An example of a test that varies with age is alkaline phosphatase – activity in serum is higher when active bone growth is occurring. Gonadal steroid secretion is higher in adults than children, differs in men and women, and falls at the menopause. Plasma creatinine concentrations are related to muscle mass and are therefore lower in children than adults, and values in men are higher than those in women. Renal function declines in the elderly in the absence of disease, and therefore plasma creatinine concentrations tend to be higher in this age group than in young adults. With computerization of laboratory data it is possible to assign age- and gender-specific

reference ranges to results, provided the appropriate information is supplied with the request.

The changing values of a test with age are not always caused by ageing *per se*. Thus, serum total cholesterol concentrations increase with age in Western populations but this is not inevitable in all societies. The increase seen represents the increasing prevalence of hypercholesterolaemia in the populations in which it occurs.

Variation in Test Results

If a patient has had a previous investigation it is important to consider whether any difference seen in a subsequent result is significant. Every test has some inherent variability due to two main factors, variation in the analysis and variation in the patient.

Analytical Variation

Analytical variation is the differences in test results which are due to the technical process of measurement. These may be occasional or random errors which occur owing to unforeseen circumstances, or systematic variations that are inherent in the particular procedure being used for measurement.

Random Error

The most obvious type of analytical variation is when a result is obtained which bears no relation to the clinical state of the patient, sometimes due to the wrong result being reported. This type of random error is very rare and results from a mismatch between the specimen and the patients details. The error may have occurred within the laboratory, but also in the ward through mislabelling of specimens at the time of venepuncture.

Systematic Variation

Systematic variation in analytical results can occur because the analysis is inaccurate or

---

KEY POINTS

REFERENCE RANGES

- Most reference ranges include 95% of a healthy population

- 5% of healthy subjects will have a result which falls outside the reference range

- Some reference ranges are defined by disease risk rather than the values seen in the general population who appear free of disease

- A result within the reference range does not exclude disease

- Reference ranges of some tests are affected by age and sex

imprecise. The accuracy of an analytical method is a measure of how closely results approach the true values and is affected by the type of method used and factors such as standardization procedures. Precision is the reproducibility of a method and is often expressed as a coefficient of variation. To calculate this, repeated analysis of a single sample is undertaken:

Coefficient of variation (CV, %) =

Standard deviation (SD)/mean × 100

Laboratories participate in quality assurance schemes and from these obtain data on inaccuracy (or bias) and imprecision. Thus, laboratories have data on the analytical variability of a particular test.

The effect of these factors on test results is illustrated for cholesterol in **Figure 24.3**. An internationally agreed standardization programme for cholesterol measurement has been agreed which allows inaccuracy to be assessed. If it is assumed that the standardization in a particular laboratory agrees with this, analytical variation will largely be due to imprecision, and the effect of this on test results for CVs of 3% and 5% are shown. The effect of a CV of 3% on a test result with a true value of 6.2 mmol l^{-1} is that values will vary between 5.9 and 6.5 mmol l^{-1}.

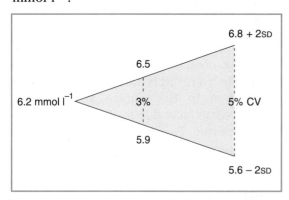

Figure 24.3 The effect of analytical imprecision on cholesterol results. An assay with a coefficient of variation (CV) of 3% will give results of 5.9–6.5 mmol l^{-1} at a true value of 6.2 mmol l^{-1} while a CV of 5% will give results of 5.6–6.8 mmol l^{-1}. (Reproduced with permission from *Clinical Chemistry*, 1988; **34**: 193–201.)

Biological Variation

Test results in an individual vary due to nonanalytical factors in addition to those affecting the analysis, some of which have been considered above.

1. Recumbency.
2. Age.
3. Sex.
4. The menstrual cycle. Variations in female sex hormones occur during the menstrual cycle but other tests also vary to a small extent, including serum proteins and cholesterol.
5. Exercise. Strenuous exercise increases the activity in serum of muscle enzymes such as creatine kinase owing to increased permeability of muscles.
6. Some tests show circadian variation, cortisol in blood being highest at 06.00–08.00 hours.
7. Drug therapy. Many drugs have metabolic side-effects; those for thiazide diuretics include impaired glucose tolerance, hypercalcaemia, hypokalaemia, hyperuricaemia and metabolic alkalosis.

The Diagnostic Utility of Laboratory Investigations

The diagnostic utility of laboratory investigations may be considered in terms of the criteria of sensitivity, specificity, predictive value, and efficiency.

The sensitivity of a test is the frequency with which it is positive in a particular condition while the specificity is a measure of the frequency of negative results. A perfect test would discriminate completely between healthy subjects and those with a particular disease and thus have 100% sensitivity and 100% specificity (**Figure 24.4**). However, in practice some patients with the disease will have a negative result and some without the disease will have a positive result. Thus in **Figure 24.2**, the values of total bilirubin from healthy sub-

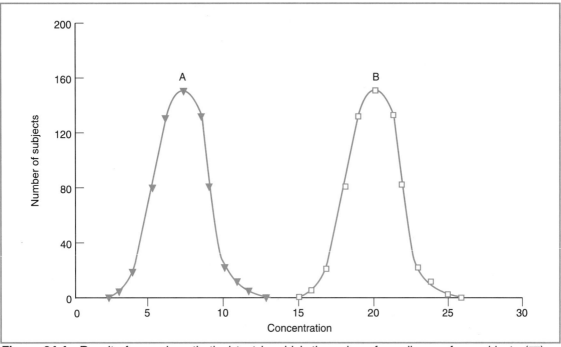

Figure 24.4   Results from a hypothetical test in which the values from disease free subjects (▼) are completely separated from those with a disease (□). The test has 100% specificity and sensitivity. However, this rarely occurs in practice and these data should be compared with Figure 24.2.

jects and patients with Gilbert's disease overlap.

The predictive value of a positive test result is the percentage of positive results that have the condition being considered while the predictive value of a negative result is the percentage of all results that are truly negative. The efficiency of a test is the percentage of patients who are correctly classified. These assessments of tests depend on the prevalence of the disease being considered and the cut-off value chosen to indicate the presence of the disease, this often being different from the limits of the reference range. In general, tests will perform less well if applied to a population with a low incidence of the disease. Thus, the predictive value of an elevated serum creatine kinase activity is greater in a coronary care unit where the incidence of myocardial infarction is high, compared with a general ward where the proportion of false-positive results will be higher.

It is important in screening procedures to avoid false-negative results, as harm will result from a missed diagnosis. Therefore high sensitivity is important and although false-positive results may occur these can be identified by further investigations. However, specificity is important if a test is being used to select patients for a form of treatment that has serious side effects, e.g. cytotoxic drug therapy. The diagnostic utility of a test must be considered when deciding cut-off values for clinical decision making.

FURTHER READING

Fraser CG. *Interpretation of Clinical Chemistry Laboratory Data*. Oxford: Blackwell, 1986
Galen RS, Gambino SR. *Beyond Normality: The Predictive Value and Efficiency of Medical Diagnosis*. New York: John Wiley, 1975

CASE 24.1

The following serum electrolyte values were obtained from a patient in intensive care who had suffered a road traffic accident. Two blood specimens were drawn simultaneously and analysed in the laboratory and also using an electrolyte analyser in intensive therapy unit.

Test	Laboratory result	Result from ITU analyser
Sodium (mmol l^{-1})	189	142
Potassium (mmol l^{-1})	1.9	3.4

Both results were checked and found to be 'correct'. What could be going on?

CASE 24.2

Blood was received in the laboratory from a patient being investigated following an episode of viral hepatitis. The condition had resolved clinically and he was free of any symptoms. The results were:

serum total calcium   0.2 mmol l^{-1}
serum albumin   37 g l^{-1}

Can you think of any explanation?

CHAPTER 1

Case 1.1

The glucose tolerance test was normal. Glycosuria is a common finding in pregnancy and may be due to diabetes mellitus which can present for the first time in pregnancy. This is important to establish as complications may occur in both the fetus and the mother. More commonly, glycosuria is caused by a reduced renal threshold for glucose, which returns to normal after delivery.

Case 1.2

The history is suggestive of diabetic ketoacidosis and the blood glucose concentration is very high. The plasma total CO_2 level may be reduced due to metabolic acidosis or respiratory alkalosis (see chapter 7). Metabolic acidosis occurs in DKA owing to increased ketone body formation – acetoacetate and 3-hydroxybutyrate being weak acids. The plasma urea is most likely elevated because excess glucose excretion causes an osmotic diuresis, leading to fluid loss and dehydration. Metabolic acidosis causes exchange of K^+ and H^+ across cell membranes. Elevation of plasma potassium levels is observed in some patients, despite increased urinary losses occurring as a result of the osmotic diuresis interfering with renal tubular reabsorption of potassium.

Case 1.3

The results show that the patient has hypoglycaemia – C-peptide levels being virtually undetectable. This suggests endogenous insulin secretion is suppressed and therefore an insulinoma is extremely unlikely. The most probable cause is factitious hypoglycaemia resulting from insulin injection and this proved to be the case.

CHAPTER 2

Case 2.1

This patient has a family history of premature coronary disease, tendon xanthomas and a very high total and LDL cholesterol level with near-normal triglycerides. The diagnosis is therefore familial hypercholesterolaemia. Other risk factors for coronary disease should be assessed and if found appropriate action should be taken. Dietary advice should be given, although it is extremely unlikely that this will produce a large enough fall in cholesterol concentration to reduce significantly the risk of coronary disease. He will almost certainly need drug therapy, an HMG-CoA reductase inhibitor being the agent of choice. The chances of a child of a patient with heterozygous FH inheriting the condition are 50%. The cholesterol should be tested in any brothers and sisters of the patient and also in his children.

Case 2.2

Gross hypertriglyceridaemia is found in chylomicronaemia syndrome, when the abnormality is either lipoprotein lipase or apoC-II deficiency. Secondary causes include uncontrolled type 1 diabetes mellitus and alcohol abuse. The patient admitted drinking 42 units of alcohol a week, the equivalent of 21 pints of beer. He was not hyperglycaemic but one test of liver function, serum γ-glutamyl transferase activity, showed a mildly raised level. Alcohol-induced hypertriglyceridaemia responds poorly to drug treatment – the only effective therapy is to strictly limit alcohol intake. Massive hypertriglyceridaemia predisposes to acute pancreatitis.

In patients with hypertriglyceridaemia it is usually important to ensure that the blood specimen was taken fasting. That was not the case here although the hypertriglyceridaemia was too gross for this to be important.

Case 2.3

In the absence of additional risk factors hypercholesterolaemia of this degree, if caused by elevated LDL, predisposes to coronary disease to only a small extent in premenopausal women. The patient did not smoke, was not obese or diabetic and was normotensive, although the family history was positive. A full lipid profile was investigated rather than just the total cholesterol level, which was measured for screening purposes. This showed that the HDL cholesterol was very high, 2.6 mmol l^{-1}. Therefore, her serum lipid profile was not atherogenic and does not require active treatment. However, the tests should be repeated after menopause as this causes the LDL cholesterol concentration to increase.

Case 2.4

The skin nodules were cutaneous xanthomas and the yellow streaks were palmar xanthomas – both features of familial dysbetalipoproteinaemia, in which raised cholesterol and triglyceride concentrations and a characteristic broad β-band on electrophoresis occur. Diabetes mellitus, hypothyroidism and obesity predispose to the condition. It is often responsive to diet and the hyperlipidaemia resolved in this patient when she lost 9 kg in weight. Some patients require drug treatment and an agent effective against both lipids, such as a fibric acid analogue, is used.

CHAPTER 3

Case 3.1

The concentration of total protein is increased while that of albumin is reduced, indicating an increase of another protein, such as immunoglobulin. Thus, the protein results are consistent with a paraproteinaemia due to multiple myeloma. Hypercalcaemia is present, a recognized complication of multiple myeloma, and the phosphate together with the alkaline phosphatase are normal which is usual in this condition. Anaemia and a high ESR are common in myeloma. Further investigations should include protein electrophoresis to establish if a paraprotein band is present. If found the paraprotein should be quantified and type of protein established. Other immunoglobulins should be measured and the urine should be tested for Bence–Jones protein.

Case 3.2

Protein, albumin and calcium concentrations are normal although the initial electrophoresis result suggested that a paraprotein band was present. The band was not present when the investigations were repeated suggesting that the initial result may have been an error. The sample was re-examined and it was found to be plasma, the blood having been initially taken into a tube that contained heparin as an anticoagulant and then transferred to a clotted (serum) tube. Thus, the original protein band was fibrinogen which is normally removed in the clotting process.

Case 3.3

Crohn's disease is an inflammatory bowel disease which is often associated with protein-losing enteropathy. The patient suffered a relapse and the albumin result is consistent with protein loss. The calcium is low because approximately 50% is normally bound to albumin although this is not the physiologically active fraction.

CHAPTER 4
Case 4.1

The most severe abnormality is the plasma phosphate level and the most common cause of hypophosphataemia in hospital populations is the intravenous infusion of glucose (see chapter 9). This is because glucose is phosphorylated prior to glycolysis. Hyperglycaemia occurred because the rate of glucose infusion was greater than the rate of metabolism. The albumin level is low, probably owing to protein losses into the gut. Hypocalcaemia is present because of the hypoalbuminaemia, albumin binding approximately 50% of the calcium in the blood.

Case 4.2

The findings of petechial haemorrhages are consistent with vitamin C deficiency (scurvy). This condition is sometimes seen in elderly patients who have a poor diet. If this is a possibility investigations should be undertaken early, as replenishment occurs when patients start a normal diet. Leukocyte ascorbate levels are a better index of tissue stores than plasma concentrations.

Case 4.3

The patient is moderately obese as his body mass index (BMI) is 33 kg m^{-2}. The health risks of obesity include CHD, hypertension and Type 2 diabetes mellitus (see **Table 4.6**). The total cholesterol concentration is not markedly elevated although the triglyceride concentration is slightly increased and the high-density lipoprotein cholesterol level is low, increasing the risk of CHD. His blood pressure is elevated, he takes little exercise and he has a positive family history of CHD in a first-degree relative. He would benefit from diet and increased exercise patterns.

CHAPTER 5

Case 5.1

The low total CO_2 and high blood glucose levels are consistent with diabetic ketoacidosis in which severe hypertriglyceridaemia is an uncommon complication. Two factors could contribute to the hyponatraemia: the elevated triglyceride levels by decreasing the fractional water content of plasma, and hyperglycaemia by causing an osmotic shift of water from the intracellular (ICF) to the extracellular fluid (ECF). The osmolality is elevated but if the contribution from glucose and urea are deducted, the osmolality is normal (285 mmol kg^{-1}).

Case 5.2

The patient has hyponatraemia with a low plasma osmolality, water excess or volume depletion with water replacement being possibilities. There was no obvious route of fluid loss and clinically the patient was not dehydrated; inappropriate antidiuretic hormone (ADH) secretion appears the most likely diagnosis. A mass was detected on chest X-ray which proved to be a carcinoma of the bronchus.

Case 5.3

The increase in sodium and urea concentrations with only minimal elevation of plasma creatinine suggests dehydration, which could be due to the loss of hypotonic fluids. The other main possibility is that the patient has hyperosmolar nonketotic diabetic coma and therefore it is very important to estimate the blood glucose level; this was marginally raised (8.9 mmol l^{-1}). The patient was febrile and was found to have a urinary tract infection. This was treated and she was rehydrated. After she recovered she gave a history of feeling unwell for several days and not eating or drinking during this period.

CHAPTER 6

Case 6.1

The potassium concentration is unbelievably high and a telephone call to the ward established that she was well and did not have a cardiac arrhythmia. It transpired that the blood specimen had been taken at 5.00 p.m. on the previous day but had not been delivered to the laboratory until the following morning. Repeat analysis using a fresh specimen showed a potassium concentration of 3.9 mmol l^{-1} and thus the apparent hyperkalaemia was due to a storage artefact occurring in unseparated blood. The possibility of artefactually raised plasma potassium concentrations should always be considered in the differential diagnosis of hyperkalaemia.

Case 6.2

Diabetic ketoacidosis is unlikely in view of the urine analysis and the low sodium and high potassium results, together with the clinical history, suggest mineralocorticoid deficiency. The low total CO_2 is consistent with a metabolic acidosis and the high urea concentration with volume depletion, both of which occur in Addison's disease.

Case 6.3

The abnormal results may be explained by diuretic therapy. Many patients receiving diuretic therapy do not develop hypokalaemia but this may develop, even if supplements are being given. Hyponatraemia also occurs, particularly in the elderly, possibly because volume depletion causes nonosmotic vasopressin secretion, leading to water retention. Volume depletion also causes secondary hyperaldosteronism which increases potassium and H^+ excretion in the distal tubule. The raised total CO_2 reflects a metabolic alkalosis. The glomerular filtration rate falls in the elderly and therefore urea and creatinine concentrations are often higher than in younger patients.

CHAPTER 7

Case 7.1

The T_{CO_2} is reduced, possibilities for this including metabolic acidosis and respiratory alkalosis. In view of the magnitude of the change metabolic acidosis is more likely and calculation of the anion gap shows that this is increased, 33 mmol l^{-1}. Possible causes include renal failure, diabetic ketoacidosis, poisoning and lactic acidosis. Although the patient has mild uraemia, the plasma creatinine concentration is normal and renal impairment will not explain the results. Blood glucose concentration was normal, alcohol was detected in blood in small amounts (90 mg l^{-1}), but the blood lactate was grossly elevated at 18 mmol l^{-1}.

Case 7.2

The major findings are an extremely high total CO_2 concentration with a low chloride value. A raised total CO_2 concentration can be caused by metabolic alkalosis or respiratory acidosis, although the degree of abnormality suggests a metabolic alkalosis. Such a marked abnormality is characteristic of pyloric stenosis, resulting from acid without bicarbonate loss from the gut. Chloride and potassium are also lost, explaining these abnormalities. The urea level is raised owing to dehydration.

Case 7.3

The pH is very low and therefore an acidosis is present. The P_{O_2} is low and the P_{CO_2} is high, suggesting that this is due to respiratory failure. The arterial bicarbonate concentration is slightly low and this should be raised by renal compensation in respiratory acidosis. This is likely to be due to a metabolic component, most probably lactic acidosis occurring as a result of muscular effort in breathing, combined with tissue hypoxia.

Case 7.4

The low total CO_2 suggests that a metabolic acidosis is present and the high chloride concentration indicates that this is a hyperchloraemic metabolic acidosis. The anion gap is normal. This can occur with acetazolamide (diamox) treatment which is often used to treat glaucoma. Acetazolamide is a carbonic anhydrase inhibitor

CHAPTER 8

Case 8.1

The total CO_2 concentration is reduced because a metabolic acidosis is present, this being due to reduced H^+ excretion and impaired bicarbonate absorption and generation in the renal tubules. Hyperkalaemia occurs due to reduced excretion. The anion gap (26 mmol l^{-1}) is increased as a result of retention of acidic anions, such as phosphate and sulphate.

Case 8.2

The patient has hypokalaemia with mild uraemia and the raised total CO_2 suggests either a metabolic alkalosis or respiratory acidosis. The most likely cause is diuretic therapy, the abnormality in total CO_2 being a metabolic alkalosis. The patient was receiving frusemide.

Case 8.3

In addition to ankle swelling the albumin concentration is low, suggesting that the patient may have developed the nephrotic syndrome. The raised urea and creatinine levels suggest that renal impairment is also present. Urinary protein excretion was estimated, this being 8.5 g 24 h^{-1}, confirming nephrotic syndrome. The creatinine clearance was reduced (28 ml min^{-1}) and diabetic nephropathy was confirmed by renal biopsy.

Case 8.4

Stones containing calcium are radio-opaque and also cystine stones, due to their sulphur content. Urine should be examined for cystine, arginine, ornithine and lysine content and the plasma calcium concentration should be measured. Further investigations include urinary oxalate and calcium excretion. This patient proved to have cystinuria.

CHAPTER 9

Case 9.1

Several features suggest hyperparathyroidism is the diagnosis. In addition to hypercalcaemia, the plasma phosphate concentration is low. The low total CO_2 and high chloride suggest that the patient has a hyperchloraemic metabolic acidosis; PTH inhibits renal tubular bicarbonate reabsorption. The ureteric colic was due to calcium-containing calculi, consistent with hypercalcaemia of long duration.

Case 9.2

Hypercalcaemia was caused by vitamin D and 1α-hydroxycholecalciferol treatment. The hypocalcaemia that developed postoperatively had been difficult to control and doses had gradually been increased. It is possible that the patient complied poorly with treatment initially, but developed hypercalcaemia when she took the medication regularly.

Case 9.3

The finding of hypocalcaemia together with a raised serum alkaline phosphatase activity in a patient of this age is suggestive of osteomalacia. This was confirmed by X-rays of the pelvis which revealed Looser's zones. The patient lived alone and rarely left his flat and therefore saw little sunlight. He responded well to vitamin D supplements.

Case 9.4

The two most probable causes of hypocalcaemia are malabsorption, causing vitamin D deficiency, and hypoparathyroidism. The latter proved to be the diagnosis in this case, confirmed by finding a very low level of PTH in serum.

CHAPTER 10

Case 10.1

The body mass index was 19 [weight (kg)/height^2 (m)]. The normal range is 20–25: The total serum calcium concentration is low and this is not corrected by adjusting for the reduced albumin level. The raised alkaline phosphatase activity is consistent with osteomalacia. Macrocytic anaemia may be due to folate or vitamin B_{12} deficiency and the erythrocyte folate levels were reduced in this patient while the vitamin B_{12} concentration in plasma was normal. Combined with the weight loss and diarrhoea these results suggest that the patient may be suffering from malabsorption. A jejunal biopsy was performed which showed marked villous atrophy. The patient started a gluten-free diet and 6 months later had gained weight, with almost complete recovery of jejunal morphology when the biopsy was repeated. She was suffering from coeliac disease.

Case 10.2

The hyperchylomicronaemia syndrome is characterized by very severe hypertriglyceridaemia (see chapter 1) and predisposition to acute pancreatitis. This patient has suffered repeated attacks and the onset of diarrhoea suggests that chronic pancreatitis may have supervened. The reduced absorption of fat in the fatty acid breath test is consistent with steatorrhoea. The characteristic radiological appearances of chronic pancreatitis were seen when endoscopic retrograde cholangio-pancreato-graphy (ERCP) was undertaken and pancreatic enzyme supplements were prescribed. This led to improvement in the diarrhoea.

CHAPTER 11

Case 11.1

Further analysis of the plasma bilirubin showed that is was predominantly unconjugated. Bilirubin was not found in the urine and urinary urobilinogen was not increased. The most likely cause of such findings in a young man in the absence of clinical features is Gilbert's disease, although mild viral hepatitis should be considered. Tests for hepatitis were negative.

Case 11.2

The liver function tests show an obstructive pattern with jaundice, a modest increase in ALT activity but a marked increase in alkaline phosphatase activity. The most probable cause is hepatic metastases resulting from the colonic tumour.

Case 11.3

The very slight increase in ALT could possibly be due to an excessive alcohol intake. Other laboratory investigations which may be abnormal in alcohol abuse include GGT, owing to induction of hepatic enzymes, and the MCV (mean corpuscular volume) of erythrocytes, which is increased. The plasma GGT activity in this patient was 375 U l^{-1}. Patients often do not admit their true alcohol consumption and the fact that this man indicated that his intake was the maximum safe daily intake did not rule out the possibility of a larger intake.

CHAPTER 12

Case 12.1

The increase in creatine kinase activity was very modest and fell quickly. The patient was given an intramuscular injection of an analgesic by his general practitioner before admission to hospital and this can cause some increase in muscle enzymes. There was no other evidence of myocardial infarction in this patient.

Case 12.2

There are many causes of increased serum amylase activity but values over 10 times the upper limit of normal are almost always due to acute pancreatitis, the clinical features in this case being consistent with this diagnosis. More modest elevations (>5 times the upper limit of normal) in amylase activity could be due to pancreatitis but also other causes of acute abdominal pain, such as a perforated peptic ulcer. Slight increases are seen in renal failure, since amylase is cleared by the kidney.

Case 12.3

The only abnormality here is an increase in serum alkaline phosphatase activity. This could be caused by cholestatic liver disease or bone disease. The serum γ-glutamyl transferase activity was normal and alkaline phosphatase isoenzyme determination showed an increase in the bone isoform. In this age group osteomalacia and Paget's disease of the bone are likely causes of the increased alkaline phosphatase activity. The patient proved to have Paget's disease.

CHAPTER 13

Case 13.1

The serum TSH is normal and the gonadotrophin levels are low – these should be increased in a postmenopausal subject. Therefore amenorrhoea appears to be secondary rather than a result of a premature menopause. Further investigation indicated that her serum prolactin concentrations were $>14\,000$ mU l^{-1} and a CT scan showed that she had a pituitary tumour.

Case 13.2

Although the growth hormone and prolactin levels are raised, the increases are fairly modest. Further investigations in a programmed investigation unit were undertaken with cannulation of a vein 30 min prior to blood sampling for repeat investigations. These demonstrated normal hormone concentrations. Both prolactin and growth hormone concentrations are raised by stress and a venepuncture is sufficient to cause this. Cannulation allows the stress of venepuncture to settle before blood sampling. No other abnormalities were found on detailed evaluation and the galactorrhoea settled after several more months.

Case 13.3

The blood glucose results during the glucose tolerance test indicate that the patient has impaired glucose tolerance (see chapter 1) and the growth hormone concentrations fail to suppress as they should. These findings are characteristic of acromegaly.

Case 13.4

The symptoms are suggestive of diabetes insipidus and this was supported by loss of weight and failure to concentrate urine during the water deprivation test. After the administration of vasopressin his urine osmolality increased to 670 mmol kg^{-1}. A CT scan of the base of the brain showed a small calcified lesion which proved to be a craniopharyngioma.

CHAPTER 14

Case 14.1

The serum TSH concentration is raised while the free T4 levels are normal, indicating subclinical hypothyroidism. Follow-up investigations showed positive for thyroid autoantibodies. This was treated by thyroxine replacement which reduced the TSH level but had no effect on serum cholesterol concentration. Thus, her hypercholesterolaemia did not appear to be secondary to the thyroid disorder. It responded to administration of a hydroxymethyl glutarate-coenzyme A (HMG-CoA) reductase inhibitor.

Case 14.2

Most patients with thyrotoxicosis have elevated T4 concentrations although these may occasionally be normal, T3 levels being raised. In this patient the free T3 concentration was 14 pmol l^{-1} and T3 toxicosis was diagnosed. In addition to the clinical features this diagnosis is also suggested by the low TSH level, this being suppressed by T3.

Case 14.3

The free T4 results are normal at all visits while the TSH concentrations are elevated on three but fall within the reference range on one occasion. The normal result at one visit suggests that the dose of thyroxine she is receiving is sufficient to correct her hypothyroidism. The most likely explanation was that she was taking her hormone treatment intermittently as free T4 concentrations are suppressed more rapidly than TSH levels. This proved to be the case as she admitted that she tended to forget to take her medication until the date for her next clinic visit approached and this reminded her.

CHAPTER 15

Case 15.1

Hyponatraemia with hyperkalaemia is suggestive of mineralocorticoid deficiency and the reduced total CO_2 may indicate that a metabolic acidosis, which is also found in this condition, is present. The clinical features are consistent with an Addisonian crisis and this was confirmed first by the response to steroid injections and second by the serum cortisol result, which was 50 nmol l^{-1}. The causes of this include autoimmune adrenalitis, tuberculosis and metastases to the adrenal glands. Auto-immune disease is the commonest cause and was responsible in this case.

Case 15.2

The results are almost identical to those in the previous case although in a baby a congenital abnormality of steroid biosynthesis is more likely than destruction of the adrenal glands. The infant has congenital adrenal hyperplasia.

Case 15.3

The blood gas and total CO_2 results indicate that the patient has a metabolic alkalosis and with hypokalaemia, suggesting mineralocorticoid excess. However, there were no somatic features of Cushing's disease present even though serum cortisol concentrations were 3200 nmol l^{-1} at 09.00 hours and 3700 at midnight; ACTH levels were very high. Further investigation revealed the presence of a small-cell carcinoma of the bronchus. Diabetes mellitus may be found as a complication of Cushing's syndrome.

CHAPTER 16

Case 16.1

The low testosterone result suggests primary testicular disease, the gonadotrophin levels being high owing to a lack of effective negative feedback inhibition. This was caused by cryptorchidism and at this age the prognosis for improved function is poor.

Case 16.2

The low levels of gonadotrophins suggest the presence of hypothalamic or pituitary disease (hypogonadotrophic hypogonadism). This was confirmed by a failure to respond to the injection of Gn-RH. This was an isolated lesion, thyroid and adrenal function being normal. The patient had no sense of smell and thus suffered from Kallman's syndrome.

Case 16.3

The prolactin concentration is normal. The serum testosterone concentration is slightly elevated for a woman and this, combined with the raised gonadotrophin levels affecting particularly LH, is suggestive of polycystic ovary syndrome. Ultrasound examination of the ovaries showed that multiple cysts were present.

CHAPTER 17
Case 17.1

Although a rare cause of hypertension, phaeochromocytoma should be considered as the condition is potentially curable by surgery. The clinical presentation of phaeochromocytoma is very variable and includes the features elicited in this patient. The determination of urinary 4-hydroxy-3-methoxymandelic acid (HMMA or VMA) was undertaken by the general practitioner, values being 52–79 μmol 24 h^{-1}, 2–3 times the upper limit of normal. The patient was referred to a specialist for further investigation and management. A benign tumour was removed successfully from the left adrenal gland.

Case 17.2

The symptom of flushing combined with diarrhoea is suggestive of carcinoid syndrome and this is investigated by measuring 5-hydroxyindole acetic acid (5-HIAA) excretion in urine, 5-HIAA being a metabolite of 5-hydroxytryptamine (5-HT). This patient proved to have carcinoid syndrome, the urinary 5-HIAA excretion being clearly elevated, 150 μmol 24 h^{-1}. The tumour was rectal in origin, with hepatic metastases. Excessive secretion of 5-HT produces diarrhoea and also bronchospasm, this being the origin of the breathlessness in this patient. The flushing is thought to be due indirectly to 5-HT secretion, as this causes the release of other mediators such as prostaglandins and histamine.

Case 17.3

Neuroblastoma is a common malignancy of childhood while phaeochromocytoma is extremely rare. Also in neuroblastoma the increase in homovanillic acid (HVA) excretion is more marked than increases in HMMA excretion, possibly because neuroblastomas are more primitive tumours and have a lower activity of dopamine β-hydroxylase, the enzyme which converts dopamine to noradrenaline (**Figure 17.1**).

CHAPTER 18

Case 18.1

Although the patient does not have a history of chest pain the clinical features suggest congestive cardiac failure of recent onset. The raised serum lactate dehydrogenase (LDH) activity and normal creatine kinase (CK) activity are consistent with myocardial infarction occurring at the time of the onset of symptoms, 6 days previously. The plasma urea concentration is raised. Although plasma urea concentrations increase with age owing to reduced renal function the level is higher than expected from this mechanism. Plasma urea levels also increase in congestive cardiac failure, due to decreased renal perfusion and this appeared to be the mechanism in this patient.

Case 18.2

The serum TSH level is within the reference range suggesting that thyroid disease is not the cause of the patients' symptoms. The fT4 is also normal although the fT3 is low. This is not necessarily caused by reduced thyroid function as reduced peripheral conversion of T4 to T3, with increased formation of reverse T3 occurs in nonthyroidal illness. The causes of this are poorly understood. The patient proved to have a carcinoma of the caecum.

CHAPTER 19

Case 19.1

The baby has severe hyperammonaemia and a low total CO_2 which suggests a metabolic acidosis. The causes of hyperammonaemia include disorders of the urea cycle and organic acidaemias, both inherited metabolic diseases. Hyperammonaemia may also occur through other causes including liver disease, Reye's syndrome and severe illness. However, in an infant inherited metabolic disease is a strong possibility. Metabolic acidosis is not a feature of urea cycle disorders but does occur in organic acidaemias. Analysis of urinary organic acids was undertaken, methylmalonic acid being found.

Case 19.2

In this age group important causes of hyperbilirubinaemia include physiological jaundice, biliary atresia and inherited metabolic diseases such as galactosaemia. In physiological jaundice hyperbilirubinaemia is unconjugated while conjugated bilirubin accumulates in biliary atresia and several inherited diseases. In this case a significant proportion is conjugated. The enlarged liver and reducing substances in the urine suggest galactosaemia and this was detected in urine using a specific test. The patient improved on a galactose-free diet, the diagnosis later being confirmed by demonstrating that galactose-1-phosphate uridyl transferase in erythrocytes was deficient.

CHAPTER 20

Case 20.1

The finding of a raised serum urate concentration in a subject with acute monoarticular arthritis is highly suggestive but not diagnostic of gout. Several other arthritic diseases have a pattern of onset similar to that seen in gout, including trauma, infection and pyrophosphate arthropathy. Although there was a history of trauma in this case aspiration of the joint showed typical urate crystals.

CHAPTER 21

Case 21.1

The finding of wrist drop suggests that a peripheral neuropathy is present, one group of causes of which are the neuropathic porphyrias. This was confirmed by the urinary ALA and porphobilinogen excretion values, both being significantly elevated. Uroporphyrin excretion was also slightly elevated although this occurs without increased synthesis of porphyrino-gens in acute intermittent porphyria by nonenzymatic condensation of porphobilinogen in urine if this is allowed to stand at room temperature. Porphobilinogen deaminase activity in the patient's erythrocytes was reduced.

Case 21.2

The skin lesions were on areas exposed to the light – such findings occur in the cutaneous porphyrias. The liver function test results are consistent with alcohol abuse, the GGT and ALT activities being elevated. The analysis of urine shows a large increase in uroporphyrin with a smaller increase in coproporphyrin excretion. These findings, together with the clinical features and normal porphobilinogen excretion, suggest porphyria cutanea tarda.

CHAPTER 22

Case 22.1

The findings are those of a metabolic acidosis with normal renal function and no evidence of diabetes mellitus. Possibilities include lactic acidosis, methanol or ethylene glycol poisoning, and salicylate overdose. Plasma salicylate was measured the result being 820 mg l^{-1}. An alkaline diuresis was induced and the patient made a full recovery.

Case 22.2

The alcohol level is too low to explain the unconscious state, 800 mg l^{-1} being the legal limit for driving. The pH and total CO_2 results show that the patient has an extremely profound metabolic acidosis. As with the previous case it is possible that other agents such as methanol had been ingested and lactic acidosis must also be considered. This diagnosis was confirmed by a plasma lactate result of 17.4 mmol l^{-1}. Lactic acidosis occurs occasionally in ethanol toxicity which was the precipitating cause in this patient, although most of the ethanol previously ingested had been metabolized by the time the patient was investigated.

CHAPTER 23

Case 23.1

The blood glucose concentration is only slightly elevated and considerably lower than the value found at home. However the total CO_2 is reduced, suggesting a metabolic acidosis which, when combined with the elevated blood glucose concentration, would suggest diabetic ketoacidosis. After finding the elevated blood glucose concentration the patient had given himself extra insulin, this having the effect of reducing the blood glucose concentration but not correcting the metabolic acidosis.

CHAPTER 24

Case 24.1

The confirmation of the results on repeat analysis shows that the concentration of the sodium in each of the samples is as reported although clearly there is something odd going on. It looks as though the specimen received in the laboratory is contaminated although this is extremely unlikely to have occurred in the laboratory. The explanation lay in the method of blood sampling which was through an indwelling cannula. This was kept patent by sodium citrate, this having a higher concentration than isotonic saline. The first specimen drawn was sent to the laboratory while the second was analysed in ITU. Although the cannula was flushed by aspirating, and the fluid was discarded before specimens were collected, this was insufficient to prevent contamination in the first specimen although the second was clear.

Gross effects of contamination such as seen in this case are obvious. However, if isotonic saline had been infused through the cannula contamination would not have been so apparent. Collection of blood for investigations through an indwelling cannula may be unavoidable in acutely ill patients: it is essential that cannulae are flushed adequately.

Case 24.2

The calcium result looks as though it is an artefact. Blood was collected for biochemical and haematological tests simultaneously by someone who was not very experienced at venepuncture. Too much was initially placed in the haematology tube, leaving insufficient for biochemical analysis. The phlebotomist therefore decanted excess blood from the haematology tube to correct the shortfall. However, the haematology tube contained EDTA as anticoagulant; the anticoagulation occurs as a result of chelation of calcium.

LIST OF ABBREVIATIONS

5-HIAA	5-hydroxyindoleacetic acid	CK-MB	creatine kinase muscle isoenzyme
5-HT	5-hydroxytryptamine (serotonin)	CoA	coenzyme A
ACE	angiotensin-converting enzyme	CRF	corticotrophin-releasing factor
acetyl CoA	acetyl coenzyme A	CRH	corticotrophin-releasing hormone
ACTH	adrenocorticotrophic hormone	CSF	cerebrospinal fluid
ADH	antidiuretic hormone	CT	computerized tomography
ADP	adenosine disphosphate	DHEA	dehydroepiandrosterone
AIDS	acquired immune deficiency syndrome	DHEA-S	androsendione
ALA	5-aminolaevulinic acid	DKA	diabetic ketoacidosis
ALP	alkaline phosphatase	DNA	deoxyribonucleic acid
ALT	alanine aminotransferase	DOPA	3,4-dihydroxyphenylalanine
ANP	atrial natriuretic peptide	ECF	extracellular fluid
API	α_1-protease inhibitor	ECG	electrocardiogram
apo	apolipoprotein	EDTA	ethylene diamine tetra-acetic acid
apoB	apolipoprotein B	ERCP	endoscopic retrograde cholangio-pancreatography
APRT	adenine phosphoribosyl-transferase	ESR	erythrocyte sedimentation rate
ARMS	amplification refractory mutation system	FH	familial hypercholesterolaemia
AST	aspartate aminotransferase	FSH	follicle-stimulating hormone
ATP	adenosine triphosphate	fT4	free thyroxine
ATPase	adenosine triphosphatase	FTI	free thyroxine index
AZT	zidovudine	G6PD	glucose-6-dehydrogenase
BMI	body mass index	GFR	glomerular filtration rate
BT-PABA	N-benzoyl-L-tyrosyl-p-aminobenzoic acid	GGT	γ-glutamyl transferase
CCK-PZ	cholecystokinin-pancreozymin	GH	growth hormone
CEA	carcinoembryonic antigen	GH-RH	growth hormone-releasing hormone
CETP	cholesterol ester transferase protein	GIP	gastric inhibitory protein/ glucose-dependent insulinotrophic peptide
CFTR	cystic fibrosis transmembrane conductance regulator	Gn-RH	gonadotrophin-releasing hormone
CHD	coronary heart disease		
CK	creatinine kinase		

Hb	haemoglobin	NIDDM	non-insulin-dependent diabetes mellitus
HBD	hydroxybutyrate dehydrogenase	NIDDY	non-insulin-dependent diabetes mellitus in the young
hCG	human chorionic gonadotrophin	OGTT	oral glucose tolerance test
HDL	high-density lipoprotein	PABA	p-aminobenzoic acid
HGPRT	hypoxanthine-guanine phospho-ribosyltransferase	P_{CO_2}	partial pressure of CO_2
		PCR	polymerase chain reaction
HIV	human immunodeficiency virus	PCV	packed cell volume
HLA	human leukocyte antigen	PEM	protein-energy malnutrition
HMG-CoA	hydroxymethyl glutaryl coenzyme A	Pi	protease inhibitor
		pK	dissociation constant (negative logarithm)
HMMA	4-hydroxy-3-methoxymandelic acid (see VMA)		
		pK_a	acidic dissociation constant
HONK	hyperosmolar nonketotic coma	P_{O_2}	partial pressure of O_2
hPL	human placental lactogen	PP	pyrophosphate
ICF	intracellular fluid	PRRP	5-phosphoribosyl-pyrophosphate
IDDM	insulin-dependent diabetes mellitus		
		PSA	prostate-specific antigen
IDL	intermediate-density lipoproteins	PTH	parathyroid hormone
		PUFA	polyunsaturated fatty acid
Ig	immunoglobulin (IgA, IgD, IgG, IgM)	RFLP	restriction fragment length polymorphism
		RNA	ribonucleic acid
IGF-1	insulin-like growth factor 1	RPB	retinol-binding protein
IGT	impaired glucose tolerance	rT3	reverse tri-iodothyronine
IL-1	interleukin 1	RTA	renal tubular acidosis
IL-6	interleukin 6	SCAD	short-chain acyl dehydrogenase
ITU	intensive therapy unit	SGOT	serum glutamate-oxaloacetate transaminase
K_m	affinity constant		
LCAD	long-chain acyl dehydrogenase	SGPT	serum glutamate-pyruvate transaminase
LCAT	lecithin:cholesterol acyl transferase		
		SHBG	sex-hormone-binding globulin
LDH	lactate dehydrogenase	SIADH	syndrome of inappropriate diuretic hormone secretion
LDL	low-density lipoproteins		
LH	luteinizing hormone	SLE	systemic lupus erythematosis
LH-RH	luteinizing hormone-releasing factor	T3	tri-iodothyronine
		T4	thyroxine
MCAD	medium-chain acyl dehydrogenase	TBG	thyroid-binding globulin
		TBPA	thyroid-binding prealbumin
MCV	mean corpuscular volume	T_{CO_2}	total CO_2
MEA-1	multiple endocrine adenomatosis syndrome	TDM	therapeutic drug monitoring
		TIBC	total iron-binding capacity
MEN	multiple endocrine neoplasias	TRH	thyrotropin-releasing hormone
MSUD	maple syrup urine disease	TSH	thyroid-stimulating hormone
NAD	nicotinamide adenine dinucleotide	UDP	uridyl diphosphate
		UTP	uridyl triphosphate
NADH	reduced nicotinamide adenine dinucleotide	VLDL	very-low-density lipoproteins
		VMA	vanillylmandelic acid (see HMMA)
NADP	nicotinamide adenine dinucleotide phosphate		
		WHO	World Health Organization
NAG	N-acetyl-β-D-glucosaminidase		
NEFA	nonesterified fatty acid		

REFERENCE RANGES

The following are reference ranges for results given in the case studies and also for other biochemical tests which are performed commonly. These should only be regarded as being a rough guide since differences may be seen in some laboratories.

PLASMA OR SERUM

Acid phosphatase (prostatic)	0–3.5 U l^{-1}
ACTH	<47 ng l^{-1}
Adrenaline	0.03–0.50 nmol l^{-1}
Alanine amino transferase:	
male	6–62 U l^{-1}
female	3–41 U l^{-1}
Albumin	38–48 g l^{-1}
Alkaline phosphatase:	
males	39–127 U l^{-1}
females	29–111 U l^{-1}
Ammonium	11–35 nmol l^{-1}
Amylase	70–300 U l^{-1}
α_1-Antitrypsin	1.4–4.0 g l^{-1}
Aspartate aminotransferase	<37 u l^{-1}
Bilirubin (total)	3–19 μmol l^{-1}
Caeruloplasmin	0.2–0.6 g l^{-1}
Calcium (total)	2.15–2.46 mmol l^{-1}
Calcium (ionized)	1.19–1.37 mmol l^{-1}
Cholesterol (total):	
desirable	<5.2 mmol l^{-1}
acceptable	<6.5 mmol l^{-1}
Cholesterol (HDL):	
males	1.0–1.5 mmol l^{-1}
females	1.2–1.8 mmol l^{-1}
Cholesterol (LDL)	<4.2 mmol l^{-1}
Cholinesterase (pseudo)	620–1400 u l^{-1}
Chloride	99–109 mmol l^{-1}
CO_2 (total):	
males	24–31 mmol l^{-1}
females	22–30 mmol l^{-1}
Copper	12–26 μmol l^{-1}
Cortisol:	
9 am	145–610 nmol l^{-1}
midnight	<170 nmol l^{-1}
C-peptide	0.18–0.52 nmol l^{-1}
Creatine kinase:	
males	<175 U l^{-1}
females	<140 U l^{-1}
Creatinine:	
males	68–108 μmol l^{-1}
females	57–94 μmol l^{-1}
Follicle-stimulating hormone:	
males	1.3–9.2 U l^{-1}
females,	
follicular phase	2–9 U l^{-1}
luteal phase	1–10 U l^{-1}
postmenopausal	>30 U l^{-1}
Glucose (fasting, plasma)	3.6–5.5 mmol l^{-1}
γ-Glutamyl transferase:	
males	<70 U l^{-1}
females	<40 U l^{-1}
Growth hormone (excludes deficiency)	>20 mU l^{-1}

Haemoglobin A_{1c}:

normal	<4.4%
acceptable control	<5.2%
IgG	8–16 g l^{-1}
IgA	1–4 g l^{-1}
IgM	0.6–2.6 g l^{-1}
Insulin-like growth factor 1	9–48 nmol l^{-1}
Insulin (fasting)	2.8–13.5 mU l^{-1}
Iron:	
males	13–32 μmol l^{-1}
females	11–29 μmol l^{-1}
Lactate	0.65–2.00 mmol l^{-1}
Lactate dehydrogenase	<430 U l^{-1}
Luteinizing hormone:	
males	3–12.6 mU l^{-1}
females,	
follicular phase	2–12 U l^{-1}
luteal phase	1–12 U l^{-1}
postmenopausal	>30 U l^{-1}
Magnesium	0.7–1.0 mmol l^{-1}
Noradrenaline	0.5–2.5 mmol l^{-1}
17-β Oestradiol:	
females,	
follicular phase	70–370 pmol l^{-1}
ovulatory peak	280–1720 pmol l^{-1}
luteal phase	90–870 pmol l^{-1}
males	<220 pmol l^{-1}
Osmolality	282–298 mmol kg^{-1}
Phosphate	0.80–1.44 mmol l^{-1}
pH	7.35–7.42
P_{CO_2}	4.5–6.1 kPa
P_{O_2}	12.0–14.0 kPa
Potassium (plasma)	3.4–4.4 mmol l^{-1}
Progesterone:	
females,	
pre-ovulation	<5 nmol l^{-1}
post-ovulation	>20 nmol l^{-1}
Prolactin	<450 mU l^{-1}
Protein (total)	59–72 g l^{-1}
Sex-hormone-binding globulin:	
males	10–40 nmol l^{-1}
females	20–95 nmol l^{-1}
Sodium	137–144 mmol l^{-1}
Testosterone:	
adult males	9–28 nmol l^{-1}

Thyroid-stimulating hormone (TSH)	0.15–3.0 mU l^{-1}
Thyroxine (free)	12–28 pmol l^{-1}
Thyroxine (total)	54–142 nmol l^{-1}
Transferrin	1.8–2.7 g l^{-1}
Triglycerides	0.45–1.80 mmol l^{-1}
Triiodothyronine (free)	3–9 pmol l^{-1}
Urate:	
males	0.15–0.42 mmol l^{-1}
females	0.12-0.39 mmol l^{-1}
Urea:	
males	3.1–7.9 mmol l^{-1}
females	2.5–6.4 mmol l^{-1}
Zinc	10.0–17.0 μmol l^{-1}

URINE

5-Amino laevulinic acid	0–40 μmol 24 h^{-1}
Calcium	2.5–7.5 mmol 24 h^{-1}
Copper	0.1–1.0 μmol 24 h^{-1}
Cortisol	35–255 nmol 24 h^{-1}
Creatinine	7.2–17.5 mmol 24 h^{-1}
Coproporphyrin	0–430 nmol 24 h^{-1}
Homovanillic acid	5.5–42.5 μmol 24 h^{-1}
5-Hydroxyindole acetic acid	<52 μmol 24 h^{-1}
4-Hydroxy-3-methoxymandelic acid (adults)	<34 μmol 24 h^{-1}
Magnesium	1–7 mmol 24 h^{-1}
Metadrenalines	1.5–4.5 μmol 24 h^{-1}
Microalbumin	<3.0 mg $mmol^{-1}$ creatinine
Oxalate:	
males	0.08–0.49 mmol 24 h^{-1}
females	<0.32 mmol 24 h^{-1}
Phosphate	15–50 mmol 24 h^{-1}
Porphobilinogen	0–16 μmol 24 h^{-1}
Protein	<0.1 g 24 h^{-1}
Urate	<6 mmol 24 h^{-1}
Urea	250–600 mmol 24 h^{-1}
Uroporphyrin	0–49 nmol 24 h^{-1}

INDEX

Numbers in *italics* refer to illustrations. Numbers in **bold** refer to tables.